Health Care: Assessment and Management

Health Care: Assessment and Management

Edited by Delilah Kinsley

hayle
medical

New York

Hayle Medical,
750 Third Avenue, 9th Floor,
New York, NY 10017, USA

Visit us on the World Wide Web at:
www.haylemedical.com

ISBN: 978-1-63241-627-8

Cataloging-in-Publication Data

Health care : assessment and management / edited by Delilah Kinsley.
    p. cm.
Includes bibliographical references and index.
ISBN 978-1-63241-627-8
1. Medical care. 2. Health services administration 3. Public health.
4. Public health--Evaluation. I. Kinsley, Delilah.
RA776 .H43 2019
613--dc23

Table of Contents

Preface

The main aim of this book is to educate learners and enhance their research focus by presenting diverse topics covering this vast field. This is an advanced book which compiles significant studies by distinguished experts in the area of analysis. This book addresses successive solutions to the challenges arising in the area of application, along with it; the book provides scope for future developments.

Healthcare involves the maintenance and improvement of health with the help of proper diagnosis, prevention and treatment of diseases, and other physical and mental impairments. Such care is usually provided by health professionals, including physicians, nurses, surgeons, midwives, nutritionists, etc. Several health care interventions are delivered outside of the health facilities. Some of these include the distribution of condoms, food safety surveillance and needle-exchange programs. The management and administration of health care is highly crucial in the delivery of health care services. Biomedical research, evidence-based practice and pharmaceutical research have contributed to the advancement of the health care sector. This book includes some of the vital pieces of work being conducted across the world, on various topics related to health care. It brings forth some of the most innovative concepts and elucidates the unexplored aspects of health care. The extensive content of this book provides the readers with a thorough understanding of the subject.

It was a great honour to edit this book, though there were challenges, as it involved a lot of communication and networking between me and the editorial team. However, the end result was this all-inclusive book covering diverse themes in the field.

Finally, it is important to acknowledge the efforts of the contributors for their excellent chapters, through which a wide variety of issues have been addressed. I would also like to thank my colleagues for their valuable feedback during the making of this book.

Editor

Persistent Borrelia Infection in Patients with Ongoing Symptoms of Lyme Disease

Marianne J. Middelveen [1], Eva Sapi [2] (iD), Jennie Burke [3], Katherine R. Filush [2], Agustin Franco [4], Melissa C. Fesler [5] and Raphael B. Stricker [5,*] (iD)

[1] Atkins Veterinary Services, Calgary, AB T3B 4C9, Canada; middel@telus.net
[2] Department of Biology and Environmental Science, University of New Haven, West Haven, CT 06516, USA; unh@evasapi.net (E.S.); katherine.r.filush@gmail.com (K.R.F.)
[3] Australian Biologics, Sydney, NSW 2000, Australia; Jennie.burke@australianbiologics.com.au
[4] School of Health Sciences, Universidad Catolica Santiago de Guayaquil, Guayaquil 090615, Ecuador; agustin.franco@optusnet.com.au
[5] Union Square Medical Associates, 450 Sutter Street, Suite 1504, San Francisco, CA 94108, USA; melissacfesler@gmail.com
* Correspondence: rstricker@usmamed.com

Abstract: Introduction: Lyme disease is a tickborne illness that generates controversy among medical providers and researchers. One of the key topics of debate is the existence of persistent infection with the Lyme spirochete, *Borrelia burgdorferi*, in patients who have been treated with recommended doses of antibiotics yet remain symptomatic. Persistent spirochetal infection despite antibiotic therapy has recently been demonstrated in non-human primates. We present evidence of persistent *Borrelia* infection despite antibiotic therapy in patients with ongoing Lyme disease symptoms. Methods: In this pilot study, culture of body fluids and tissues was performed in a randomly selected group of 12 patients with persistent Lyme disease symptoms who had been treated or who were being treated with antibiotics. Cultures were also performed on a group of ten control subjects without Lyme disease. The cultures were subjected to corroborative microscopic, histopathological and molecular testing for *Borrelia* organisms in four independent laboratories in a blinded manner. Results: Motile spirochetes identified histopathologically as *Borrelia* were detected in culture specimens, and these spirochetes were genetically identified as *Borrelia burgdorferi* by three distinct polymerase chain reaction (PCR)-based approaches. Spirochetes identified as *Borrelia burgdorferi* were cultured from the blood of seven subjects, from the genital secretions of ten subjects, and from a skin lesion of one subject. Cultures from control subjects without Lyme disease were negative for *Borrelia* using these methods. Conclusions: Using multiple corroborative detection methods, we showed that patients with persistent Lyme disease symptoms may have ongoing spirochetal infection despite antibiotic treatment, similar to findings in non-human primates. The optimal treatment for persistent *Borrelia* infection remains to be determined.

Keywords: Lyme disease; *Borrelia burgdorferi*; tickborne disease; chronic infection; spirochete culture

1. Introduction

Lyme disease (LD) and similar Lyme-like *Borrelia* infections are caused by members of the *Borrelia burgdorferi* (Bb) sensu lato complex or by members of the *Borrelia* relapsing fever complex such as *B. miyamotoi*, respectively [1–4]. Following initial infection, *Borrelia* spirochetes can evade host defenses, sequester in immune privileged sites such as joints or the central nervous system, and persist in pleomorphic forms [5–8]. Tickborne coinfections including *Babesia*, *Anaplasma*, *Ehrlichia*, *Bartonella* and *Rickettsia* may complicate the clinical picture [6,9,10]. If LD is not treated early in the course of infection, chronic illness may result and a variety of symptoms may develop. These symptoms include fatigue, musculoskeletal pain, arthritis, cardiac disease and neurological involvement with peripheral neuropathy, meningitis, encephalitis, cranial neuritis and cognitive dysfunction [6,8,11,12].

Although LD was first recognized in 1975, it remains a controversial illness and the topic of polemic debate [6,10,13–15]. One viewpoint claims that persistent Lyme disease symptoms are related to ongoing spirochetal infection despite antibiotic therapy. This scenario has been demonstrated in animal models including rodents, dogs and horses using various detection methods [16–36], and a recent study in non-human primates showing "persistent, intact, metabolically-active *B. burgdorferi* after antibiotic treatment of disseminated infection" offers the strongest support for this pathogenesis [37]. Furthermore, comparable studies have suggested persistent infection after antibiotic therapy as a cause of chronic symptoms in humans [38–60]. The opposing viewpoint claims that persistent Lyme disease symptoms may be due to spirochetal "debris" without active infection. While a number of studies from Europe and the USA have demonstrated persistence of Bb DNA or antigens in human bodily tissues or fluids, very few studies have demonstrated culture of live *Borrelia* spirochetes, the highest form of evidence for persistent infection in chronic Lyme disease patients [4,51,53,59].

In this pilot study, we present detailed evidence of persistent *Borrelia* infection despite antibiotic therapy in 12 randomly-selected North American patients with ongoing LD symptoms. Spirochetal infection was demonstrated by corroborative microscopic, histopathological and molecular detection of live *Borrelia* organisms in cultures of body fluids and tissues from these patients.

2. Methods

2.1. Subject Selection

Subjects included in the study were chosen at random from our North American patient population. All of the LD patients in the study were either clinically diagnosed with LD or had positive Bb serological testing prior to study participation. Serological testing for LD was performed by a Clinical Laboratory Improvement Amendments (CLIA)-certified laboratory (IGeneX Laboratory in Palo Alto, CA, USA), as described in detail elsewhere [60]. Subjects with Morgellons disease (MD) who were seropositive for LD were included in the study (see below) [61]. All subjects had been treated with antibiotics prior to the study, and symptomatic patients who remained on antibiotic treatment were included in the study.

2.2. Control Selection

Ten healthy subjects were recruited as controls after informed consent was obtained. These subjects were then tested serologically for LD and those who were negative were accepted as controls. Vaginal or seminal fluids were collected from negative controls and cultured for *Borrelia*, as described below. Culture pellets underwent PCR testing for *Borrelia* in a blinded manner at the University of New Haven and Australian Biologics, as described below.

2.3. Informed Consent

All subjects were adults who gave informed consent to participate in the study. Signed informed consent to collect specimens was obtained in accordance with the ethics approval requirements for sample collection of the Western Institutional Review Board, Puyallup, WA, USA (Study # 1148461). Approval for anonymous sample testing was also obtained from the Institutional Review Board of the University of New Haven, West Haven, CT, USA. Additional signed informed consent to publish the results was obtained from each subject.

2.4. Cultures

To avoid contamination, all cultures were performed under strict aseptic conditions in a laboratory that was free of *Borrelia* reference strains, and cultures of control and patient samples were processed in an identical manner. Inocula were placed in Barbour-Stoner-Kelly H (BSK) complete medium with 6% rabbit serum (Sigma-Aldrich, #B8291, St. Louis, MO, USA) containing the following antibiotics: phosphomycin (0.02 mg/mL) (Sigma-Aldrich), rifampicin (0.05 mg/mL) (Sigma-Aldrich), and amphotericin B (2.5 µg/mL) (Sigma-Aldrich), as described previously [62]. Inocula were prepared as follows:

A. Blood—whole blood (10 mL) was collected by venipuncture and left at room temperature to clot, then centrifuged at low speed to separate red blood cells from sera. The serum supernatants with a small amount of blood cells below the serum layer were collected and were inoculated into the BSK medium.

B. Skin—whole calluses or skin from lesions were removed from MD subjects by scraping with a scalpel blade.

C. Vaginal—vaginal secretions were collected by swabbing inside the vagina with sterile cotton-tipped swabs that were then introduced into the BSK medium.

D. Seminal—semen was self-collected into a sterile vial, then was pipetted into the BSK medium.

8 mL tubes of inoculated medium were filled to minimize the airspace present, thus providing a microaerobic environment, and incubated at 32 °C. Culture fluid was examined by darkfield microscopy for visible spirochetes weekly for up to 4 weeks. Cultures were concentrated by centrifuging the fluid at 15,000 g for 20 min, retaining the pellet and discarding the supernatant. For imaging, a small amount of culture pellet was resuspended in 50 µL 0.85% saline solution, washed and centrifuged again. The pellet was mixed with gelatin and then fixed with formalin for further staining.

2.5. Dieterle and Anti-Bb Immunostaining

Dermatological specimens and/or culture pellets from patients were fixed, sectioned and processed for specialized staining at either McClain Laboratories LLC, Smithtown, NY, USA, or the Department of Biology and Environmental Science, University of New Haven, West Haven, CT, USA, as previously described [59]. Dieterle silver-nitrate staining was performed at McClain Laboratories. Anti-Bb immunostaining was performed at McClain Laboratories or the University of New Haven. In brief, immunostaining was performed using an unconjugated rabbit anti-Bb polyclonal antibody (Abcam ab20950, Cambridge, MA, USA), incubated with an alkaline phosphatase probe (Biocare Medical #UP536L, Pacheco, CA, USA), followed by a chromogen substrate (Biocare Medical #FR805CHC), and counterstained with hematoxylin. Positive and negative controls were prepared for comparison purposes using liver sections from Bb-inoculated and uninfected C3H/HeJ mice followed by Dieterle and immunostaining. Culture pellets from mixed Gram-positive bacteria (*Streptococcus* and *Staphylococcus*) and Gram-negative bacteria (*Escherichia coli* and *Klebsiella*) were also prepared for comparison purposes as negative controls to exclude cross-reactivity with commonly encountered microorganisms.

2.6. Molecular Testing

Patient and negative control samples were submitted in a blinded manner to the laboratories performing polymerase chain reaction (PCR) amplification of DNA, as described below. PCR detection of *Borrelia* was performed for research purposes only. No data resulting from this study was used diagnostically.

2.7. PCR—University of New Haven

DNA was extracted from culture pellets as previously described [59]. Reactions of blinded samples were performed in triplicate.

Borrelia DNA in extracted samples was detected using a published TaqMan assay targeting a 139-bp fragment of the gene encoding the *Borrelia* 16S rRNA, as described previously [59,63,64]. Amplifications were conducted on a CFX96 Real-Time System (Bio-Rad, Hercules, CA, USA) with cycling of 50 °C for 2 min, 95 °C for 10 min, followed by 40 cycles of 95 °C for 15 s and 60 °C for 60 s, and fluorescent signals were recorded using CFX96 Real-Time software with the Cq threshold set automatically.

Nested PCR primers for the 16S rRNA, flagellin (Fla), OspC, uvrA and pyrG genes were used as previously described [59,64–66], with a final volume of 50 µL using 10 µL template DNA and final concentrations of 20 mM Tris-HCl (pH 8.4), 50 mM KCl (1 × Buffer B, Promega, Fitchburg, WI, USA), 2 mM $MgCl_2$, 0.4 mM dNTP mix, 2 µM of each primer, and 2.5 U Taq polymerase (Invitrogen, Carlsbad, CA, USA). The first reaction used "outer" primers and the second reaction used "inner" primers, and 1 µL of PCR product from the first reaction was used as template for the second. Cycling was programmed as follows: 94 °C for 5 min followed by 40 cycles of denaturation at 94 °C for 1 min, annealing for 1 min, and extension at 72 °C for 1 min, with a final extension step at 72 °C for 5 min. DNA products were visualized in 1–2% agarose gels.

PCR amplification was followed by Sanger sequencing. PCR products were extracted using the QIAquick Gel Extraction kit (Qiagen, Hilden, Germany) in accordance with the manufacturer's instructions. Eluates were sequenced in both directions, then were compared by BLAST analysis using the GenBank database (National Center for Biotechnology Information).

2.8. PCR—Australian Biologics

DNA was extracted from culture pellets using the DNeasy Blood and Tissue kit® (Qiagen) in accordance with the manufacturer's instructions. Samples were forwarded to Australian Biologics for *Borrelia* DNA and *Treponema denticola*/*Treponema pallidum* DNA testing. Blinded samples were run in duplicate with positive and negative controls using primers for the *Borrelia* 16S rRNA and rpoC gene targets, as previously described [59,67,68]. *Borrelia* DNA was detected by real-time PCR targeting the 16S rRNA gene and/or by endpoint PCR targeting the rpoC gene, as previously described [59,67,68], using the Eco™ Real-Time PCR system with software version 3.0.16.0. Thermal profiles were performed with incubation for 2 min at 50 °C, polymerase activation for 10 min at 95 °C then PCR cycling for 40 cycles of 10 s at 95 °C dropping to 60 °C sustained for 45 s. The PCR signal magnitude generated (ΔR) was interpreted as either positive or negative as compared to positive and negative controls.

For endpoint PCR, amplicons were visualized on 1–2% agarose gels and extracted from the gels using the QIAquick Gel Extraction kit (Qiagen) in accordance with the manufacturer's instructions. Sanger sequencing was used for gene analysis, as described previously [59,67,68].

2.9. PCR—University California Irvine

The presence of Bb sensu stricto DNA in a set of blinded samples was confirmed by the laboratory of Dr. Alan Barbour (University of California Irvine) by first quantitative PCR [69], and then by sequence of the PCR-amplified 16S-23S intergenic spacer [70]. The samples studied included specimens from two of the subjects in this paper, Case 2 and Case 10, as described below.

3. Results

3.1. Subject Histories

The clinical histories of the 12 study subjects with persistent Lyme disease symptoms (Cases 1–12) are provided below, and the clinical characteristics of the subjects are summarized in Table 1. All subjects had received treatment with 2–4 weeks of antibiotics as recommended by Lyme treatment guidelines endorsed by the Centers for Disease Control and Prevention (CDC) [14]. Six patients were taking antibiotics at the time of study sampling, as noted in Table 1. The type of Lyme IgM and IgG

Western blot reactivity detected in each patient is shown in Table 2. Persistent IgM reactivity was found in several patients, as described in other studies [37].

Table 1. Clinical Characteristics of Study Patients.

Case #	Age/Gender	EM Rash	Sx	MD Lesions	LD Seroreactivity	Co-Infections	Abx
Case 1	50F	No	MS, F	Yes	Negative	Unknown	Yes
Case 2	54F	Yes	MS, F	Yes	Negative	*Bab, Bart*	No
Case 3	63M	No	MS, F	No	Positive	*Bab, Ana*	Yes
Case 4	53F	Yes	MS, F	No	Negative, seroconverting to positive	*Bab, Ana*	Yes
Case 5	40F	No	MS, N	No	Positive	*Bab*	Yes
Case 6	42M	No	MS, N	No	Positive	None	Yes
Case 7	36F	No	MS, N	No	Positive	None	Yes
Case 8	39M	No	MS, N	No	Positive	Unknown	No
Case 9	71F	No	MS, F, N	No	Positive	None	No
Case 10	72M	No	MS, F, N	No	Positive	None	No
Case 11	57F	No	MS	No	Positive	*Bab, Ehr, Bart*	No
Case 12	46F	No	MS	Yes	Positive	*Bab*	No

EM, erythema migrans; MD, Morgellons disease; MS, musculoskeletal; F, fatigue; N, neurological; *Bab, Babesia microti* or *Babesia duncani*; *Bart, Bartonella henselae*; *Ana, Anaplasma phagocytophilum*; *Ehr, Ehrlichia chafeensis*. Abx, on antibiotics at time of testing.

Table 2. Lyme Western Blot IgM and IgG Results in Study Patients.

Patient Number	Western Blot IgM	Western Blot IgG
1	Negative	Negative
2	Negative	Negative
3	Negative	Positive
4	Positive	Negative
5	Positive	Negative
6	Positive	Negative
7	Positive	Negative
8	Positive	Negative
9	Positive	Positive
10	Positive	Negative
11	Positive	Positive
12	Negative	Positive

Western blots were interpreted according to IGeneX criteria [60].

Control samples were obtained from two men and eight women ranging in age from 43–63 years (mean age, 50.6 years). None of the controls had symptoms of tickborne disease, and none had received antibiotic therapy. All controls were negative on Lyme IgM and IgG Western blot testing, and additional testing of controls using microscopy, histopathology and PCR techniques was negative, as outlined below.

3.1.1. Case 1

The subject is a 50-year-old native Canadian woman who resided in an area endemic for LD in eastern Canada. She did not recall an erythema migrans (EM) rash. She developed extreme fatigue and musculoskeletal pain as well as ulcerative skin lesions along with symptoms of formication. Magnification demonstrated filamentous inclusions within the lesions. The subject was seronegative for anti-Bb antibodies excepting two indeterminate IgM bands showing reactivity to the 41-kDa and the 93-kDA proteins, and a weakly positive IgG band showing reactivity to the 41-kDa protein. She was clinically diagnosed with LD by a health care provider in Canada and treated with antibiotics. The subject had discontinued antibiotics three weeks prior to the sampling period, but continued treatment with naturopathic remedies. Despite ongoing treatment with amoxicillin, the subject continues to have persistent symptoms of Lyme disease.

3.1.2. Case 2

The subject is a 54-year-old Caucasian woman who had a history of outdoor recreational activity in Western Canada including areas in British Columbia that are endemic for LD. She recalled an EM-like rash several years previously, and she did not receive treatment. She developed significant joint pains, muscle aches, headaches, memory loss, fatigue and skin lesions, and she initially tested negative for Lyme disease. She was clinically diagnosed by a Canadian health care provider, and the diagnosis was confirmed later by an American health care provider. She also had positive serological tests for *Babesia* and *Bartonella*. She did not have prior knowledge of Morgellons disease, but she did have ulcerative lesions on her face and torso consistent in appearance with the condition. Upon examination with a 50× handheld microscope, filamentous inclusions were observed in her lesions. She has been aggressively treated over the last few years with antibiotic combinations including intravenous ceftriaxone, metronidazole, telithromycin, doxycycline, amoxicillin, ciprofloxacin, tinidazole and atovaquone with little benefit.

3.1.3. Case 3

The subject is a 63-year-old Caucasian man who had a history of outdoor recreational activity in endemic areas for Lyme disease, including Europe, Western Canada, and the USA (Connecticut and Rhode Island). Although he recalls tick bites, he did not recall an EM rash. The subject developed musculoskeletal pain and extreme fatigue. His wife (Case 4) had an EM rash and a LD diagnosis that prompted him to get tested for LD. He was seroreactive for anti-Bb antibodies, and Bb DNA was detected in serum using PCR technology. He tested serologically positive for *Babesia microti* and *Anaplasma phagocytophylum*. He had received ongoing treatment with antibiotics, including doxycycline, clarithromycin, cefdinir, tinidazole, atovaquone, clindamycin and hydroxychloroquine. He was symptomatic and taking doxycycline at the time of sampling. His condition has since improved, but he still suffers from musculoskeletal pain.

3.1.4. Case 4

The subject is a 53-year-old Caucasian woman and the wife of Case 3. She had a history of outdoor recreational activity in Lyme endemic areas of the USA and Canada. She has a history of tick bites and recalled an EM rash after visiting both Connecticut and Rhode Island. Her symptoms included seizures, neuropathy, palpitations and musculoskeletal pain. She had serological testing for Bb and was initially negative, but she became seropositive after taking antibiotics. She also had positive serological testing for *Babesia microti* and *Anaplasma phagocytophylum*. She was symptomatic and taking antibiotics during the time of sample collection. Antibiotics taken included doxycycline, telithromycin, minocycline, clindamycin, clarithromycin, metronidazole, tinidazole, rifampicin, atovaquone, hydroxychloroquine and mefloquine. The subject was taking clarithromycin and cefdinir at the time of sample collection. She is currently asymptomatic.

3.1.5. Case 5

The subject is a 40-year-old Caucasian woman living in Calgary, Canada, and the partner of Case 6. She is a veterinarian and had a history of work exposure to ticks, and she had also travelled to areas endemic for LD in Europe. She did not recall an EM rash. Her symptoms were primarily musculoskeletal and severe headaches. She was seropositive for Bb and *Babesia*, and she had been treated with the following antibiotics: doxycycline, clarithromycin, metronidazole and atovaquone. She had been taking doxycycline for one month at the time of sample collection.

3.1.6. Case 6

The subject is a 42-year-old Caucasian man living in Calgary, Canada, and the partner of Case 5. He is a veterinarian and had a history of work exposure to ticks. He had also travelled to areas endemic for LD in Europe. He did not recall an EM rash. His symptoms were primarily musculoskeletal, severe headaches, memory loss, vision problems and extreme fatigue. He was seropositive for Bb and *Babesia*, and he had been treated with the following antibiotics: doxycycline, clarithromycin, metronidazole and atovaquone. He had been taking doxycycline for one month at the time of sample collection.

3.1.7. Case 7

The subject is a 36-year-old Caucasian woman living in Calgary, Canada. She was bitten by many ticks while working as a tree planter in the mountains, but she does not recall an EM rash. In September 1997 she developed profound fatigue, migratory joint pains, peripheral neuropathy and personality changes consistent with depression. She was seropositive for Bb, and she was eventually treated with intramuscular penicillin, amoxicillin, and minocycline over two years. She remains symptomatic despite antibiotic treatment.

3.1.8. Case 8

The subject is a 39-year-old Caucasian man residing in Calgary, Canada. He has a history of hiking, camping and other outdoor activities in Alberta and Manitoba, Canada, but no known tick bites or EM rash. He complains of joint pain, low back pain and headaches, and he has been treated for sciatica, depression, insomnia, and anxiety. He also has an extensive history of periodontal disease with recurrent gingival infections, and he has received multiple courses of penicillin and amoxicillin over many years. He had positive serological testing for Lyme disease, and he has not been tested for tickborne coinfections.

3.1.9. Case 9

The subject is a 71-year-old Caucasian woman living in Ontario, Canada and the partner of Case 10. She was 40 years old when she became ill in 1986 with severe flu-like symptoms, fatigue, severe pelvic pain, blurred vision, rib soreness and night sweats. She did not recall a tick bite or an EM rash. The patient had not knowingly visited a Lyme disease endemic area. She consulted six different physicians over a period of four years before being treated with six weeks of doxycycline for what was diagnosed as pelvic inflammatory disease in 1988, and her symptoms transiently improved. She was clinically diagnosed with Lyme disease in 1990 by a physician in Ontario, as the Ontario government's ELISA test was "negative" for Lyme disease. Over the next 20 years the subject was intermittently treated with doxycycline and her symptoms improved, but never completely resolved, and other symptoms developed such as muscle aches, joint pains, sleep disturbances, bladder and urethral pain, and cognitive impairment. These symptoms waxed and waned over the years. She experienced multiple Jarisch–Herxheimer reactions with repeated doxycycline treatment. The subject's two children were treated for congenital Lyme disease between 1990 and 2004 and are asymptomatic today. In May 2011, the subject was tested by a CLIA-approved laboratory in the USA and was found to be serologically positive for Lyme disease.

3.1.10. Case 10

The subject is a 72-year-old Caucasian man living in Ontario, Canada and the partner of Case 9. He was 41 years old at the onset of symptoms in 1986 with flu-like muscle aches, joint pains and unrelenting fatigue. He did not recall a tick bite or an EM rash. The subject had not knowingly visited a Lyme disease endemic area. He had consulted 12 different doctors over a period of four years before getting a confirmed diagnosis of Lyme disease, at which point he had developed severe arthritic symptoms, significant neurological symptoms including encephalopathy and dementia with brain magnetic resonance imaging (MRI) showing hyperintense white matter lesions. His antibiotic regimens over 20 years included: tetracycline, amoxicillin plus probenecid, doxycycline, clarithromycin, intravenous ceftriaxone, and intramuscular benzathine penicillin G. When the subject was on antibiotics he had relief of many symptoms, but he was never completely free of symptoms associated with Lyme disease. He had multiple Jarisch-Herxheimer reactions when new antibiotic regimens were initiated. The two-tiered Lyme disease serology test performed in Canada failed to show positivity for Lyme disease, but the subject subsequently sent blood to a CLIA-approved laboratory in the United States and was found to be seropositive for Lyme disease.

3.1.11. Case 11

The subject is a 57-year-old Caucasian woman living in Calgary, Canada. She had exposure to ticks while hiking and camping in Canada, but she did not recall an EM rash. She developed musculoskeletal and neuropsychiatric symptoms and was diagnosed with LD after testing serologically positive. She also had positive testing for *Babesia*, *Ehrlichia* and *Bartonella*. She received intermittent antibiotic therapy with multiple oral, intramuscular and intravenous antibiotics, and her symptoms improved while on antibiotics but relapsed when the antibiotics were discontinued. She remains symptomatic after five years of antibiotic treatment.

3.1.12. Case 12

The subject is a 46-year-old Caucasian woman living in Alberta, Canada who did not have a history of tick bite or EM rash. She has suffered with skin lesions consistent with Morgellons disease for more than a decade and was diagnosed with Lyme disease in the USA after testing serologically positive for Bb. She has had severe gastrointestinal problems that have necessitated frequent hospitalizations. The gastrointestinal difficulties began after she had gastric bypass surgery. Her intestines form lesions that fuse together, causing blockages. She has been treated aggressively with antibiotics before and after this study by doctors both in the USA and Canada with only minimal benefit. Antibiotic therapy included multiple treatments with intravenous ceftriaxone, doxycycline, clarithromycin and amoxicillin.

3.2. Microscopy and Histopathology

Case 1. Whole calluses were submitted for sectioning, Dieterle and anti-Bb immunostaining. Spirochetes were visible in both Dieterle and anti-Bb immunostains. Blood culture was performed and fluid from the culture demonstrated spherical bodies under darkfield microscopy. Dieterle staining and anti-Bb immunostaining was not performed.

Case 2. Blood culture was performed and fluid from the culture demonstrated spherical bodies under darkfield microscopy. Dieterle staining and anti-Bb immunostains demonstrated spherical bodies. Anti-Bb immunostaining was positive. Vaginal culture was performed and fluid from the culture demonstrated spirochetes and biofilm under darkfield microscopy. Dieterle staining and anti-Bb immunostaining demonstrated spirochetes and biofilm. Skin specimens were not submitted for staining or culture. Repeat blood and vaginal cultures were positive for *Borrelia* by immunostaining and PCR (see Tables 3–5).

Case 3. Blood culture was performed and fluid from the culture demonstrated spherical bodies and occasional spirochetes under darkfield microscopy. Dieterle staining and anti-Bb immunostains demonstrated spherical bodies and occasional spirochetes. Anti-Bb immunostaining was positive. Seminal culture was performed and fluid from the culture demonstrated spirochetes under darkfield microscopy. Dieterle staining and anti-Bb immunostaining demonstrated spirochetes. Repeat blood culture was positive for *Borrelia* by immunostaining and PCR (see Tables 3–5).

Table 3. Summary of Microscopy Results from Patient Culture Samples.

Case #	Sample Type	Darkfield	Dieterle	Bb Immunostain
Case 1	whole callus blood culture	N/A spirochetes	spirochetes N/A	positive, spirochetes N/A
Case 2	blood culture vaginal culture	spherules spirochetes	spherules spirochetes	positive, spherules positive, spirochetes, biofilm
Case 3	blood culture seminal culture	spirochetes/spherules spirochetes	spirochetes/spherules spirochetes	positive spirochetes/spherules positive, spirochetes
Case 4	blood culture vaginal culture	spirochetes/spherules spirochetes	spirochetes/spherules spirochetes	positive spirochetes/spherules positive, spirochetes
Case 5	blood culture vaginal culture	spherules spirochetes	spherules spirochetes	positive, spherules positive, spirochetes
Case 6	blood culture seminal culture	spherules spirochetes	spherules spirochetes	positive, spherules positive, spirochetes
Case 7	vaginal culture	spirochetes	spirochetes	positive, spirochetes
Case 8	seminal culture	spirochetes	spirochetes	positive, spirochetes
Case 9	vaginal culture	spirochetes	spirochetes	positive, spirochetes
Case 10	seminal culture	spirochetes	spirochetes	positive, spirochetes
Case 11	vaginal culture	spirochetes	spirochetes	positive, spirochetes
Case 12	blood culture skin culture	spherules spirochetes	spherules spirochetes	positive, spherules positive, spirochetes

N/A, not available.

Table 4. Summary of PCR Results from Patient Culture Samples.

Case #	Sample Type	University of New Haven	Australian Biologics	UC-Irvine
1	whole callus blood culture	16S rRNA (N), pyrG (N) *, fla (N) * pyrG (N), fla (N) *	N/A N/A	N/A N/A
2	blood culture vaginal culture	16S rRNA (N) pyrG (N) *, fla (N)	16S rRNA (RT), rpoC (E) * 16S rRNA (RT) *	N/A qPCR 16S-23S intergenic spacer
3	blood culture seminal culture	16S rRNA (N) * 16S rRNA (RT), 16S rRNA (N) *, fla (N)	16S rRNA (RT) 16S rRNA (RT), rpoC (E) *	N/A N/A
4	blood culture vaginal culture	16S rRNA (N), pyrG (N) 16S rRNA (RT), 16S rRNA (N), pyrG (N), fla (N)	16S rRNA (RT), rpoC (E) * 16S rRNA (RT), rpoC (E) *	N/A N/A
5	blood culture vaginal culture	16S rRNA (RT), 16S rRNA (N), pyrG (N) 16S rRNA (N)	16S rRNA (RT) 16S rRNA (RT), rpoC (E) *	N/A N/A
6	blood culture seminal culture	16S rRNA (RT), 16S rRNA (N), pyrG (N) 16S rRNA (RT), 16S rRNA (N)	16S rRNA (RT) 16S rRNA (RT)	N/A N/A
7	vaginal culture	16S rRNA (N) *	N/A	N/A
8	seminal culture	16S rRNA (N) *	N/A	N/A
9	vaginal culture	pyrG (N)	16S rRNA (RT)	N/A
10	seminal culture	pyrG (N)	16S rRNA (RT)	(+/−) qPCR16S-23S intergenic spacer
11	vaginal culture	16S rRNA (N)	16S rRNA (RT), rpoC (E) *	N/A
12	whole callus blood culture	uvrA (N) * pyrG	N/A 16S rRNA (RT)	N/A N/A

* Sequenced; RT, real time PCR; N, nested PCR; E, endpoint PCR; N/A not available; (+/−) One specimen was positive for Bb DNA, one specimen was negative (different collection dates).

Table 5. Summary of BLAST Sequence Analysis of Patient PCR Samples.

Case #	Culture Specimen	Sequence	Length	E-Value	BLAST Match Bbss	LAB
1	callus	pyrG	680	0.0	100%	UNH
	callus	fla	367	2e-172	100%	UNH
	blood	fla F	364	2e-176	99%	UNH
	blood	fla R	367	2e-172	99%	UNH
2	vaginal	pyrG F	656	0.0	99%	UNH
	vaginal	pyrG R	659	0.0	99%	UNH
	vaginal	rpoC	79	4e-32	100%	AB
	vaginal	16S-23S Intergenic spacer	474	0.0	100%	UCI
3	blood	16S rRNA F	415	0.0	99%	UNH
	blood	16S rRNA R	415	0.0	99%	UNH
	seminal	16S rRNA	388	0.0	99%	UNH
	blood 1 month Abx	rpoC	103	0.11	96%	AB
	seminal 1 month Abx	rpoC	146	9e-57	100%	AB
	seminal 4 months Abx	rpoC	158	3e-52	98%	AB
4	vaginal	rpoC	118	1e-51	99%	AB
5	vaginal	rpoC	109	6e-47	99%	AB
7	vaginal	16S rRNA	396	0.0	99%	UNH
8	seminal	16S rRNA	221	7e-10	100%	UNH
10	seminal	16S-23S Intergenic spacer	474	0.0	99%	UCI
11	vaginal	rpoC	156	1e-25	100%	AB
12	callus	uvrA F	653	0.0	99%	UNH
	callus	uvrA R	651	0.0	99%	UNH

UNH, University of New Haven; AB, Australian Biologics; UCI, University of California Irvine. F, forward sequence; R, reverse sequence; Bbss, *B. burgdorferi* sensu stricto; Abx, antibiotics.

Case 4. Blood culture was performed and fluid from the culture demonstrated spherical bodies and occasional spirochetes under darkfield microscopy. Dieterle staining and anti-Bb immunostains demonstrated spherical bodies and occasional spirochetes. Anti-Bb immunostaining was positive. Vaginal culture was performed and fluid from the culture demonstrated spirochetes under darkfield microscopy. Dieterle staining and anti-Bb immunostaining demonstrated spirochetes. Repeat blood culture was positive for *Borrelia* by immunostaining and PCR (see Tables 3–5).

Case 5. Blood culture was performed and fluid from the culture demonstrated spherical bodies under darkfield microscopy. Dieterle staining and anti-Bb immunostaining demonstrated spherical bodies. Vaginal culture was performed and fluid from the culture demonstrated spirochetes under darkfield microscopy. Dieterle staining and anti-Bb immunostaining demonstrated spirochetes. Repeat blood culture was positive for *Borrelia* by immunostaining and PCR (see Tables 3–5).

Case 6. Blood culture was performed and fluid from the culture demonstrated spherical bodies under darkfield microscopy. Dieterle staining and anti-Bb immunostains demonstrated spherical bodies. Anti-Bb immunostaining was positive. Seminal culture was performed and fluid from the culture demonstrated spirochetes under darkfield microscopy. Dieterle staining and anti-Bb immunostaining demonstrated spirochetes. Repeat blood culture was positive for *Borrelia* by immunostaining and PCR (see Tables 3–5).

Case 7. Vaginal culture was performed and fluid from the culture demonstrated spirochetes under darkfield microscopy. Dieterle staining and anti-Bb immunostaining demonstrated spirochetes.

Case 8. Seminal culture was performed and fluid from the culture demonstrated spirochetes under darkfield microscopy. Dieterle staining and anti-Bb immunostaining demonstrated spirochetes.

Case 9. Vaginal culture was performed and fluid from the culture demonstrated spirochetes, including one that was quite actively motile, under darkfield microscopy. Dieterle staining and anti-Bb immunostaining demonstrated spirochetes.

Case 10. Seminal culture was performed and fluid from the culture demonstrated spirochetes under darkfield microscopy. Dieterle staining and anti-Bb immunostaining demonstrated spirochetes. Repeat seminal culture was positive for *Borrelia* by immunostaining and PCR (see Tables 3–5).

Case 11. Vaginal culture was performed and fluid from the culture demonstrated spirochetes, including one that was quite actively motile, under darkfield microscopy. Dieterle staining and anti-Bb immunostaining demonstrated spirochetes.

Case 12. Blood culture was performed and fluid from the culture demonstrated spherical bodies under darkfield microscopy. Dieterle staining and anti-Bb immunostains demonstrated spherical bodies. Anti-Bb immunostaining was positive. Skin culture was performed and fluid from the culture demonstrated spirochetes under darkfield microscopy. Dieterle staining and anti-Bb immunostaining demonstrated spirochetes.

The results of darkfield microscopy, Dieterle silver stains and anti-Bb immunostaining from Cases 1–12 are summarized in Table 3. Examples of these spirochete detection methods are shown in Figure 1A–C. All controls tested negative using these techniques (data not shown).

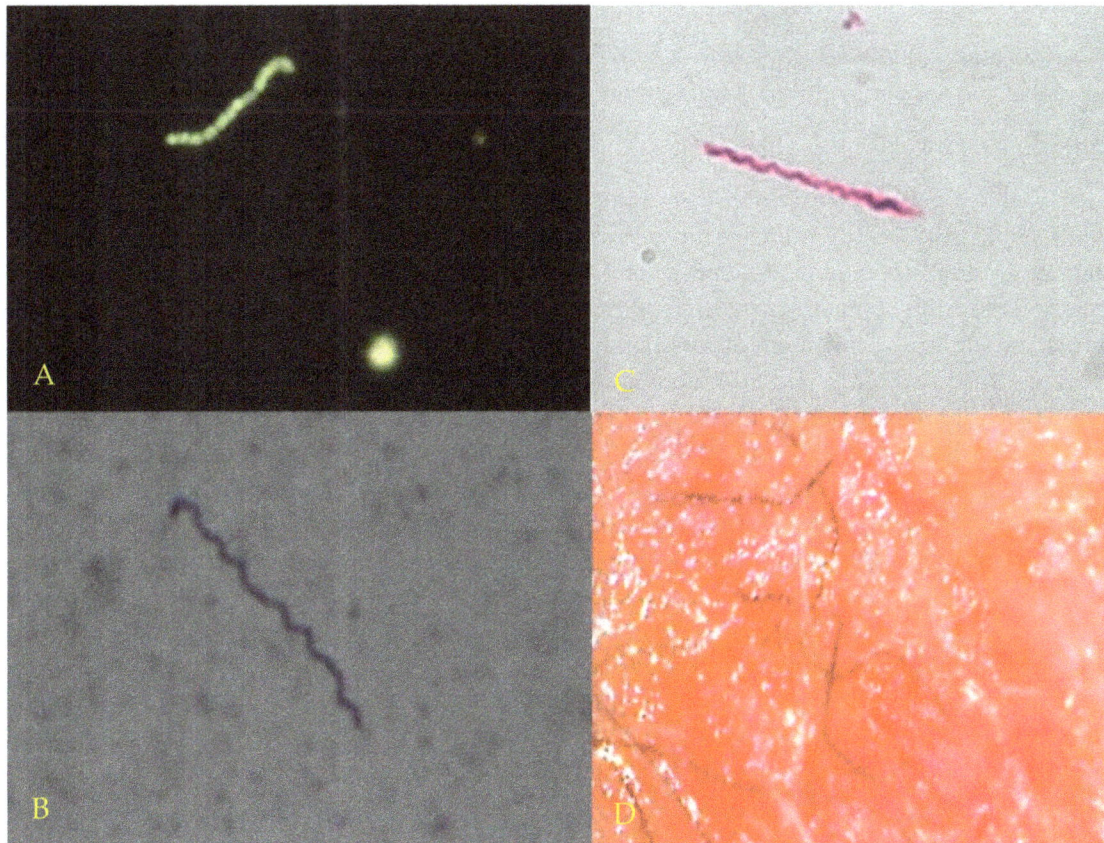

Figure 1. (**A**) (Top left): Darkfield microscopy of blood culture showing live spirochete and spherules. Magnification 400×. (**B**) (Bottom left): Dieterle silver stain of culture fluid from Case 10 showing live spirochetes. Magnification 1000×. (**C**) (Top right): *Borrelia* immunostain of culture fluid from Case 9 showing live spirochetes. Magnification 1000×. (**D**) (Bottom right). Typical dermal filaments from patient with Morgellons disease. Magnification 100×.

3.3. Molecular Testing

PCR Detection of *Borrelia*

Samples (whole dermatological calluses, blood culture, vaginal cultures, and seminal cultures) from the study patients were submitted for PCR detection and sequencing of *Borrelia* DNA at both the University of New Haven, CT, and Australian Biologics, Sydney, Australia in a blinded manner. *Borrelia* DNA was detected by at least one laboratory for all 12 patients, and amplicon sequences consistent with Bb DNA were obtained for 10/12 patients. Blinded negative cultures from healthy, seronegative subjects along with the blinded suspected positive cultures from LD patients were sent to University of New Haven and Australian Biologics.

Australian Biologics performed PCR for the detection of *Treponema denticola* and *Treponema pallidum* on all study samples and blinded controls. Treponemal DNA was not detected in any samples. For Cases #2 and #10, additional PCR and sequencing on genital cultures was performed at the University of California, Irvine, in the laboratory of Dr. Alan Barbour. In these samples, *Borrelia* DNA was detected with qPCR and then confirmed as Bb sensu stricto by sequence of the 16S-23S intergenic spacer.

Positive PCR results are summarized in Table 4, and positive sequencing results are summarized in Table 5. PCR sequences and BLAST analyses are shown in Supplemental File. All negative controls were PCR-negative for *Borrelia* species (data not shown).

4. Discussion

In this pilot study, we cultured live *Borrelia* organisms from 12 antibiotic-treated subjects with persistent Lyme disease symptoms, thus showing that viable spirochetes can be found in LD patients despite antibiotic therapy. Half of these subjects were taking antibiotics at the time of sampling. Patient cultures showed *Borrelia* spiral forms and spherical bodies, as described in other publications (Figure 1A–C) [7,59,66]. We demonstrated the presence of *Borrelia* infection in cultures from these patients using corroborative microscopy, histopathology and PCR techniques, and we obtained sequences for amplicons from 10/12 patients. Repeat cultures of blood, semen and vaginal secretions were positive for Bb by microscopy, histopathology and PCR in six patients tested by four different laboratories. Cultures from healthy *Borrelia*-seronegative controls were consistently negative using microscopy, histopathology and PCR techniques, making the possibility of *Borrelia* contamination in LD patient samples extremely unlikely.

Persistent *Borrelia* infection may result in part from the wide variety of tissues and fluids that support spirochetal growth [16–37]. The tissues susceptible to *Borrelia* infection include fibroblasts, skin, synovial tissue, ligaments, cardiac tissue, glial cells, neurons, endothelial cells, lymphoid tissue and hepatic tissue [5,48,59,71–81]. The pleotropic nature of *Borrelia* infection may allow the spirochete to evade the host immune system and antibiotic therapy, as outlined below.

The role of round body cysts and biofilms in persistent *Borrelia* infection is controversial [10,82,83]. Ongoing Lyme disease symptoms may arise from spirochetes hidden in biofilms or surviving as round body cysts or cell wall-deficient L-forms, by intracellular *Borrelia* sequestration or by sequestration within privileged sites where antibiotics do not attain therapeutic levels [13,37,84–86]. Regardless of the mechanism by which *Borrelia* spirochetes persist in tissues, persistent *Borrelia* infection requires treatment, and options at present are limited and controversial [10,13,83]. The controversy is fueled by disagreement over viability of the spirochetes, as described below.

Although there is evidence of post-treatment *Borrelia* infection in animals and humans, some researchers speculate that *Borrelia* antigens and DNA detected in studies are merely spirochetal "debris" [36,87–89]. Wormser et al. offered an "amber" hypothesis as a possible explanation for persistent symptoms, namely that persistent Lyme arthritis is caused by non-viable spirochetes enmeshed in joints within host-derived fibrinous or collagenous matrices [88]. Bockenstedt et al. proposed that the inflammation seen in mice described in their study following antibiotic treatment was caused by *Borrelia* DNA and proteins representing non-infectious spirochetal "debris" deposited in tissues [36].

In contrast, those who support the idea that active infection is responsible for persisting Lyme disease symptoms propose that there are various protective mechanisms providing spirochetal resistance or tolerance to antibiotics, including intracellular invasion and formation of cell-wall deficient L-forms, round body cysts, biofilms and persister cells [78,84–86]. Furthermore the "amber" and "debris" hypotheses of symptom persistence are difficult to support because *Borrelia* DNA is rapidly cleared from murine tissues after prompt antibiotic treatment [21], and the DNA of non-viable spirochetes is cleared from mouse tissue within several hours [90]. The present study confirms the presence of live *Borrelia* spirochetes in patients who had been treated with antibiotics for persistent Lyme disease symptoms.

Recent studies have focused on "persister cells" and "sleeper cells" as spirochetal agents of persistence in Lyme disease [91–93]. The concept involves organisms that are tolerant to antibiotics and can downregulate their metabolic needs via a "stringent response" to survive in a hostile environment, only to reemerge when the environment becomes more favorable. A similar mechanism of persistent infection has been described in *E. coli*, *Mycobacteria* and *Salmonella* [93]. The survival of metabolically tolerant spirochetes in privileged sites would explain our findings of viable *Borrelia* in antibiotic-treated patients once the antibiotics are withdrawn and culture conditions are optimized. The factors that influence viability of "persister cells" and "sleeper cells" in patients with persistent Lyme disease symptoms merit further study.

Three of our study subjects had a controversial skin condition commonly called Morgellons disease (MD) [61,94–98]. The distinguishing feature of this skin condition is the presence of white, black, or brightly colored filaments that lie under, are embedded in, or project from skin lesions (see Figure 1D). While some medical practitioners erroneously consider MD to be a purely delusional disorder, MD appears to be a *Borrelia*-associated filamentous dermatitis [94,95]. MD patients exhibit symptoms that resemble those of Lyme disease such as fatigue, joint pain, and neuropathy, and the skin condition has been shown to be associated with *Borrelia* infection [94–98]. Spirochetes from different *Borrelia* species have been detected in MD patient specimens [61,94,99,100]. We obtained positive *Borrelia* cultures from all three of our MD subjects.

The mechanism of MD filament evolution has not been resolved, but as collagen and keratin filaments arise from proliferative keratinocytes and fibroblasts in human epithelial tissue, we speculate that *Borrelia* infection alters keratin and collagen gene regulation [99,100]. *Borrelia* bacteria can invade fibroblasts and keratinocytes where they survive and replicate intracellularly [74,76,101]. As shown by in vitro studies, *Borrelia* spirochetes can be isolated from keratinocyte and fibroblast monolayers despite treatment with antibiotics [74,76]. Persistent refractory infection in MD patients may therefore result in part from sequestration of live *Borrelia* spirochetes within keratinocytes and fibroblasts.

Borrelia spirochetes have been detected in vaginal and seminal secretions [13,100]. We cultured *Borrelia* spirochetes in genital secretions from ten of our study subjects who had taken or were currently taking antibiotic therapy. Bb is a complex organism that is related to the spirochetal agent of syphilis, and therefore may have similar infectious capabilities [13,100,102]. As outlined above, *Borrelia* spirochetes penetrate tissues, can form cystic structures and L-forms, hide in biofilms, become intracellular, and sequester in privileged sites (brain, eye and synovium) [9,10,13,83,103–105]. These specialized abilities of the *Borrelia* spirochete suggest that the genital tract could harbor infection. The vagina and the seminal vesicles are privileged sites, and that may explain why the organism can persist in the genital tract despite antimicrobial therapy in a manner similar to syphilis, chlamydia, human immunodeficiency virus (HIV), Ebola and Zika virus [102,106–110].

5. Conclusions

In summary, in this pilot study we demonstrated persistent infection despite antibiotic therapy in 12 North American patients with ongoing symptoms of LD. Cultures were positive in all 12 patients in our study, indicating that the *Borrelia* spirochetes were replicating and therefore alive. The spirochetes were genetically identified as Bb in a blinded fashion using PCR and gene sequencing in three separate laboratories. In contrast, cultures from control subjects without Lyme disease were negative for *Borrelia* spirochetes. Our findings provide evidence that persistent infection rather than spirochetal "debris" was at least in part responsible for ongoing symptoms in these cases of Lyme disease, and the results mirror recent observations in a non-human primate model of treated Lyme disease [37]. Larger clinical studies using corroborative techniques are needed to confirm the findings in this pilot study.

Acknowledgments: The authors thank Alan Barbour for providing independent evaluation of our samples and for giving permission to publish his results. We are grateful to our patients and control subjects for providing samples for the study. Funding is supported in part by a grant from the Lindorf Family Foundation, Newark, OH. The funders had no role in study design, data collection and analysis, decision to publish, or preparation of the manuscript.

Author Contributions: Marianne J. Middelveen conceived the study, recruited patients, performed cultures, tabulated data and wrote the manuscript. Eva Sapi, Jennie Burke, Katherine R. Filush and Agustin Franco performed molecular detection studies, tabulated data and edited the manuscript. Melissa C. Fesler recruited patients, tabulated data and edited the manuscript. Raphael B. Stricker conceived the study, recruited patients, tabulated data and edited the manuscript.

References

1.   Steere, A.C.; Malawista, S.E.; Snydman, D.R.; Shope, R.E.; Andiman, W.A.; Ross, M.R.; Steele, F.M. Lyme arthritis: An epidemic of oligoarticular arthritis in children and adults in three Connecticut Communities. *Arthritis Rheum.* **1977**, *20*, 7–17. [CrossRef] [PubMed]

2.   Stanek, G.; Reiter, M. The expanding Lyme Borrelia complex—Clinical significance of genomic species? *Clin. Microbiol. Infect.* **2011**, *17*, 487–493. [CrossRef] [PubMed]

3.   Cutler, S.J.; Ruzic-Sabljic, E.; Potkonjak, A. Emerging borreliae—Expanding beyond Lyme borreliosis. *Mol. Cell. Probes* **2017**, *31*, 22–27. [CrossRef] [PubMed]

4.   Rudenko, N.; Golovchenko, M.; Vancova, M.; Clark, K.; Grubhoffer, L.; Oliver, J.H., Jr. Isolation of live *Borrelia burgdorferi* sensu lato spirochaetes from patients with undefined disorders and symptoms not typical for Lyme borreliosis. *Clin. Microbiol. Infect.* **2016**, *22*, 267.e9–267.e15. [CrossRef] [PubMed]

5.   Dorward, D.W.; Fischer, E.R.; Brooks, D.M. Invasion and cytopathic killing of human lymphocytes by spirochetes causing Lyme disease. *Clin. Infect. Dis.* **1997**, *25*, S2–S8. [CrossRef] [PubMed]

6.   Cameron, D.; Johnson, L.B.; Maloney, E.L. Evidence assessments and guideline recommendations in Lyme disease: The clinical management of known tick bites, erythema migrans rashes and persistent disease. *Expert Rev. Anti Infect. Ther.* **2014**, *12*, 1103–1135. [CrossRef] [PubMed]

7.   Meriläinen, L.; Brander, H.; Herranen, A.; Schwarzbach, A.; Gilbert, L. Pleomorphic forms of *Borrelia burgdorferi* induce distinct immune responses. *Microbes Infect.* **2016**, *18*, 484–495. [CrossRef] [PubMed]

8.   Miklossy, J. Bacterial amyloid and DNA are important constituents of senile plaques: Further evidence of the spirochetal and biofilm nature of senile plaques. *J. Alzheimers Dis.* **2016**, *53*, 1459–1473. [CrossRef] [PubMed]

9.   Stricker, R.B.; Johnson, L. Lyme disease diagnosis and treatment: Lessons from the AIDS epidemic. *Minerva Med.* **2010**, *101*, 419–425. [PubMed]

10. Stricker, R.B.; Johnson, L. Lyme disease: The next decade. *Infect. Drug Resist.* **2011**, *4*, 1–9. [CrossRef] [PubMed]

11. Caruso, V.G. Facial paralysis from Lyme disease. *Otolaryngol. Head Neck Surg.* **1985**, *93*, 550–553. [PubMed]

12. Habicht, G.S.; Beck, G.; Benach, J.L. Lyme disease. *Sci. Am.* **1987**, *257*, 78–83. [CrossRef] [PubMed]

13. Stricker, R.B.; Middelveen, M.J. Sexual transmission of Lyme disease: Challenging the tickborne disease paradigm. *Expert Rev. Anti Infect. Ther.* **2015**, *13*, 1303–1306. [CrossRef] [PubMed]

14. Feder, H.M.; Johnson, B.J.B.; O'Connell, S.; Shapiro, E.D.; Steere, A.C.; Wormser, G.P. Ad Hoc International Lyme Disease Group. A critical appraisal of "chronic Lyme disease". *N. Engl. J. Med.* **2007**, *357*, 1422–1430. [CrossRef] [PubMed]

15. Stricker, R.B.; Johnson, L. Spirochetal 'debris' versus persistent infection in chronic Lyme disease: From semantics to science. *Fut. Microbiol.* **2012**, *7*, 1243–1246. [CrossRef] [PubMed]

16. Duray, P.H.; Johnson, R.C. The histopathology of experimentally infected hamsters with the Lyme disease spirochete *Borrelia burgdorferi. Proc. Soc. Exp. Biol. Med.* **1986**, *181*, 263–269. [CrossRef] [PubMed]

17. Moody, K.D.; Barthold, S.W.; Terwilliger, G.A. Lyme borreliosis in laboratory animals: Effect of host species and in vitro passage *Borrelia burgdorferi*. *Am. J. Trop. Med. Hyg.* **1990**, *43*, 87–92. [CrossRef] [PubMed]

18. Preac Mursic, V.; Patsouris, E.; Wilske, B.; Reinhardt, S.; Gross, B.; Mehraein, P. Persistence of *Borrelia burgdorferi* and histopathological alterations in experimentally infected animals. A comparison with histopathological findings in human Lyme disease. *Infection* **1990**, *18*, 332–341. [CrossRef] [PubMed]

19. Goodman, J.L.; Jurkovich, P.; Kodner, C.; Johnson, R.C. Persistent cardiac and urinary tract infections with *Borrelia burgdorferi* in experimentally infected Syrian hamsters. *J. Clin. Microbiol.* **1991**, *29*, 894–896. [PubMed]

20. Schmitz, J.L.; Schell, R.F.; Lovrich, S.D.; Callister, S.M.; Coe, J.E. Characterization of the protective antibody response to *Borrelia burgdorferi* in experimentally infected LSH hamsters. *Infect. Immun.* **1991**, *59*, 1916–1921. [PubMed]

21. Malawista, S.E.; Barthold, S.W.; Persing, D.H. Fate of *Borrelia burgdorferi* DNA in tissues of infected mice after antibiotic treatment. *J. Infect. Dis.* **1994**, *170*, 1312–1316. [CrossRef] [PubMed]

22. Moody, K.D.; Adams, R.L.; Barthold, S.W. Effectiveness of antimicrobial treatment against *Borrelia burgdorferi* infection in mice. *Antimicrob. Agents Chemother.* **1994**, *38*, 1567–1572. [CrossRef] [PubMed]

23. Sonnesyn, S.W.; Manivel, J.C.; Johnson, R.C.; Goodman, J.L. A guinea pig model for Lyme disease. *Infect. Immun.* **1993**, *61*, 4777–4784. [PubMed]

24. Roberts, E.D.; Bohm, R.P., Jr.; Cogswell, F.B.; Lanners, H.N.; Lowrie, R.C., Jr.; Povinelli, L.; Piesman, J.; Philipp, M.T. Chronic Lyme disease in the rhesus monkey. *Lab. Invest.* **1995**, *72*, 146–160. [PubMed]

25. Straubinger, R.K.; Summers, B.A.; Chang, Y.F.; Appel, M.J. Persistence of *Borrelia burgdorferi* in experimentally infected dogs after antibiotic treatment. *J. Clin. Microbiol.* **1997**, *35*, 111–116. [PubMed]

26. Straubinger, R.K. PCR-Based quantification of *Borrelia burgdorferi* organisms in canine tissues over a 500-Day postinfection period. *J. Clin. Microbiol.* **2000**, *38*, 2191–2199. [PubMed]

27. Pachner, A.R.; Cadavid, D.; Shu, G.; Dail, D.; Pachner, S.; Hodzic, E.; Barthold, S.W. Central and peripheral nervous system infection, immunity, and inflammation in the NHP model of Lyme borreliosis. *Ann. Neurol.* **2001**, *50*, 330–338. [CrossRef] [PubMed]

28. Cadavid, D.; Bai, Y.; Hodzic, E.; Narayan, K.; Barthold, S.W.; Pachner, A.R. Cardiac involvement in non-human primates infected with the Lyme disease spirochete *Borrelia burgdorferi*. *Lab. Invest.* **2004**, *84*, 1439–1450. [CrossRef] [PubMed]

29. Chang, Y.F.; Ku, Y.W.; Chang, C.F.; Chang, C.D.; McDonough, S.P.; Divers, T.; Pough, M.; Torres, A. Antibiotic treatment of experimentally *Borrelia burgdorferi*-infected ponies. *Vet. Microbiol.* **2005**, *107*, 285–294. [CrossRef] [PubMed]

30. Miller, J.C.; Narayan, K.; Stevenson, B.; Pachner, A.R. Expression of *Borrelia burgdorferi* erp genes during infection of non-human primates. *Microb. Pathog.* **2005**, *39*, 27–33. [CrossRef] [PubMed]

31. Bockenstedt, L.K.; Mao, J.; Hodzic, E.; Barthold, S.W.; Fish, D. Detection of attenuated, noninfectious spirochetes in *Borrelia burgdorferi*-infected mice after antibiotic treatment. *J. Infect. Dis.* **2002**, *186*, 1430–1437. [CrossRef] [PubMed]

32. Hodzic, E.; Feng, S.; Holden, K.; Freet, K.J.; Barthold, S.W. Persistence of *Borrelia burgdorferi* following antibiotic treatment in mice. *Antimicrob. Agents Chemother.* **2008**, *52*, 1728–1736. [CrossRef] [PubMed]

33. Barthold, S.W.; Hodzic, E.; Imai, D.M.; Feng, S.; Yang, X.; Luft, B.J. Ineffectiveness of tigecycline against persistent *Borrelia burgdorferi*. *Antimicrob. Agents Chemother.* **2010**, *54*, 643–651. [CrossRef] [PubMed]

34. Yrjänäinen, H.; Hytönen, J.; Hartiala, P.; Oski, J.; Vijanen, M.K. Persistence of borrelial DNA in the joints of *Borrelia burgdorferi*-infected mice after ceftriaxone treatment. *APMIS* **2010**, *118*, 665–673. [CrossRef] [PubMed]

35. Imai, D.M.; Barr, B.C.; Daft, B.; Bertone, J.J.; Feng, S.; Hodzic, E.; Johnston, J.M.; Olsen, K.J.; Barthold, S.W. Lyme neuroborreliosis in 2 horses. *Vet. Pathol.* **2011**, *48*, 1151–1157. [CrossRef] [PubMed]

36. Bockenstedt, L.K.; Gonzales, D.G.; Haberman, A.M.; Belperron, A.A. Spirochete antigens persist near cartilage after murine Lyme borreliosis therapy. *J. Clin. Investig.* **2012**, *122*, 2652–2660. [CrossRef] [PubMed]

37. Embers, M.E.; Hasenkampf, N.R.; Jacobs, M.B.; Tardo, A.C.; Doyle-Meyers, L.A.; Philipp, M.T.; Hodzic, E. Variable manifestations, diverse seroreactivity and post-treatment persistence in non-human primates exposed to *Borrelia burgdorferi* by tick feeding. *PLoS ONE* **2017**, *12*, e0189071. [CrossRef] [PubMed]

38. Craft, J.E.; Fischer, D.K.; Shimamoto, G.T.; Steere, A.C. Antigens of *Borrelia burgdorferi* recognized during Lyme disease. Appearance of a new immunoglobulin M response and expansion of the immunoglobulin G response late in the illness. *J. Clin. Investig.* **1986**, *78*, 934–939. [CrossRef] [PubMed]

39. Cimmino, M.A.; Azzolini, A.; Tobia, F.; Pesce, C.M. Spirochetes in the spleen of a patient with chronic Lyme disease. *Am. J. Clin. Pathol.* **1989**, *91*, 95–97. [CrossRef] [PubMed]

40. De Koning, J.; Hoogkamp-Korstanje, J.A.; van der Linde, M.R.; Crijns, H.J. Demonstration of spirochetes in cardiac biopsies of patients with Lyme disease. *J. Infect. Dis.* **1989**, *160*, 150–153. [CrossRef] [PubMed]

41. Preac-Mursic, V.; Weber, K.; Pfister, H.W.; Wilske, B.; Gross, B.; Baumann, A.; Prokop, J. Survival of *Borrelia burgdorferi* in antibiotically treated patients with Lyme borreliosis. *Infection* **1989**, *17*, 355–359. [CrossRef] [PubMed]

42. Fraser, D.D.; Kong, L.I.; Miller, F.W. Molecular detection of persistent *Borrelia burgdorferi* in a man with dermatomyositis. *Clin. Exp. Rheumatol.* **1992**, *10*, 387–390. [PubMed]

43. Battafarano, D.F.; Combs, J.A.; Enzenauer, R.J.; Fitxpatrick, J.E. Chronic septic arthritis caused by *Borrelia burgdorferi*. *Clin. Orthop. Relat. Res.* **1993**, *279*, 238–241.

44. Liegner, K.B.; Shapiro, J.R.; Ramsay, D.; Halperin, A.J.; Hogrefe, W.; Kong, L. Recurrent erythema migrans despite extended antibiotic treatment with minocycline in a patient with persisting *Borrelia burgdorferi* infection. *J. Am. Acad. Dermatol.* **1993**, *28*, 312–314. [CrossRef]

45. Asch, E.S.; Bujak, D.I.; Weiss, M.; Peterson, M.G.; Weinstein, A. Lyme disease: An infectious and postinfectious syndrome. *J. Rheumatol.* **1994**, *21*, 454–461. [PubMed]

46. Nocton, J.J.; Dressler, F.; Rutledge, B.J.; Rys, P.N.; Persing, D.H.; Steere, A.C. Detection of *Borrelia burgdorferi* DNA by polymerase chain reaction in synovial fluid from patients with Lyme arthritis. *N. Engl. J. Med.* **1994**, *330*, 229–234. [CrossRef] [PubMed]

47. Bayer, M.E.; Zhang, L.; Bayer, M.H. *Borrelia burgdorferi* DNA in the urine of treated patients with chronic Lyme disease symptoms. A PCR study of 97 cases. *Infection* **1996**, *24*, 347–353. [CrossRef] [PubMed]

48. Valesova, M.; Trnavský, K.; Hulínská, D.; Alusík, S.; Janousek, J.; Jirous, J. Detection of Borrelia in the synovial tissue from a patient with Lyme borreliosis by electron microscopy. *J. Rheumatol.* **1989**, *16*, 1502–1505. [PubMed]

49. Donta, S.T. Tetracycline therapy for chronic Lyme disease. *Clin. Infect. Dis.* **1997**, *25*, S52–S56. [CrossRef] [PubMed]

50. Priem, S.; Burmester, G.R.; Kamradt, T.; Wolbart, K.; Rittig, M.G.; Krause, A. Detection of *Borrelia burgdorferi* by polymerase chain reaction in synovial membrane, but not in synovial fluid from patients with persisting Lyme arthritis after antibiotic therapy. *Ann. Rheum. Dis.* **1998**, *57*, 118–121. [CrossRef] [PubMed]

51. Hudson, B.J.; Stewart, M.; Lennox, V.A.; Fukunaga, M.; Yabuki, M.; Macorison, H.; Kitchener-Smith, J. Culture-positive Lyme borreliosis. *Med. J. Aust.* **1998**, *168*, 500–502. [PubMed]

52. Oksi, J.; Nikoskelainen, J.; Vilajanen, M.K. Comparison of oral cefixime and intravenous ceftriaxone followed by oral amoxicillin in disseminated Lyme borreliosis. *Eur. J. Clin. Microbiol. Infect. Dis.* **1998**, *17*, 715–719. [CrossRef] [PubMed]

53. Oksi, J.; Marjamäki, M.; Nikoskelainen, J.; Vilajanen, M.K. *Borrelia burgdorferi* detected by culture and PCR in clinical relapse of disseminated Lyme borreliosis. *Ann. Med.* **1999**, *31*, 225–232. [CrossRef] [PubMed]

54. Berglund, J.; Stjernberg, L.; Ornstein, K.; Tykesson-Joelsson, K.; Walter, H. Follow-up study of patients with neuroborreliosis. *Scand. J. Infect. Dis.* **2002**, *34*, 421–425. [CrossRef] [PubMed]

55. Kaiser, R. Clinical courses of acute and chronic neuroborreliosis following treatment with ceftriaxone. *Nervenarzt* **2004**, *75*, 553–557. [PubMed]

56. Cameron, D. Severity of Lyme disease with persistent symptoms. Insights from a double-blind placebo-controlled clinical trial. *Minerva Med.* **2008**, *99*, 489–496. [PubMed]

57. Fallon, B.A.; Keilp, J.G.; Corbera, K.M.; Petkova, E.; Britton, C.B.; Dwyer, E.; Slavov, I.; Cheng, J.; Dobkin, J.; Nelson, D.R.; et al. A randomized, placebo-controlled trial of repeated IV antibiotic therapy for Lyme encephalopathy. *Neurology* **2008**, *70*, 992–1003. [CrossRef] [PubMed]

58. Stricker, R.B.; Delong, A.K.; Green, C.L.; Savely, V.R.; Chamallas, S.N.; Johnson, L. Benefit of intravenous antibiotic therapy in patients referred for treatment of neurologic Lyme disease. *Int. J. Gen. Med.* **2011**, *4*, 639–646. [CrossRef] [PubMed]

59. Middelveen, M.J.; McClain, S.A.; Bandoski, C.; Israel, J.R.; Burke, J.; MacDonald, A.B.; Timmaraju, A.; Sapi, E.; Wang, Y.; Franco, A.; et al. Granulomatous hepatitis associated with chronic *Borrelia burgdorferi* infection: A case report. *Res. Open Access.* **2014**, *1*, 875. [CrossRef]

60. Shah, J.S.; Du Cruz, I.; Narciso, W.; Lo, W.; Harris, N.S. Improved sensitivity of Lyme disease Western blots prepared with a mixture of *Borrelia burgdorferi* strains 297 and B31. *Chronic Dis. Int.* **2014**, *1*, 7.

61. Middelveen, M.J.; Bandowski, C.; Burke, J.; Sapi, E.; Filush, K.R.; Wang, Y. Exploring the association between Morgellons disease and Lyme disease: Identification of *Borrelia burgdorferi* in Morgellons disease patients. *BMC Dermatol.* **2015**, *15*, 1. [CrossRef] [PubMed]

62. Bankhead, T.; Chaconas, G. The role of VlsE antigenic variation in the Lyme disease spirochete: Persistence through a mechanism that differs from other pathogens. *Mol. Microbiol.* **2007**, *65*, 1547–1558. [CrossRef] [PubMed]

63. O'Rourke, M.; Traweger, A.; Lusa, L.; Stupica, D.; Maraspin, V.; Barrett, P.N.; Strle, F.; Livey, I. Quantitative detection of *Borrelia burgdorferi* sensu lato in erythema migrans skin lesions using internally controlled duplex real time PCR. *PLoS ONE* **2013**, *8*, e63968. [CrossRef] [PubMed]

64. Margos, G.; Hojgaard, A.; Lane, R.S.; Cornet, M.; Fingerle, V.; Rudenko, N.; Ogden, N.; Aanensen, D.M.; Fish, D.; Piesman, J. Multilocus sequence analysis of *Borrelia bissettii* strains from North America reveals a new Borrelia species, *Borrelia kurtenbachii*. *Ticks Tick Borne Dis.* **2010**, *1*, 151–158. [CrossRef] [PubMed]

65. Clark, K.L.; Leydet, B.; Hartman, S. Lyme borreliosis in human patients in Florida and Georgia, USA. *Int. J. Med. Sci.* **2013**, *10*, 915–931. [CrossRef] [PubMed]

66. Sapi, E.; Pabbati, N.; Datar, A.; Davies, E.M.; Rattelle, A.; Kuo, B.A. Improved culture conditions for the growth and detection of Borrelia from human serum. *Int. J. Med. Sci.* **2013**, *10*, 362–376. [CrossRef] [PubMed]

67. Mayne, P.J. Investigation of *Borrelia burgdorferi* genotypes in Australia obtained from erythema migrans tissue. *Clin. Cosmet. Investig. Dermatol.* **2012**, *5*, 69–78. [CrossRef] [PubMed]

68. Mayne, P. Clinical determinants of Lyme borreliosis, babesiosis, bartonellosis, anaplasmosis, and ehrlichiosis in an Australian cohort. *Int. J. Gen. Med.* **2014**, *8*, 15–26. [CrossRef] [PubMed]

69. Bunikis, J.; Tsao, J.; Garpmo, U.; Berglund, J.; Fish, D.; Barbour, A.G. Sequence typing reveals extensive strain diversity of the Lyme borreliosis agents *Borrelia burgdorferi* in North America and *Borrelia afzelii* in Europe. *Microbiology* **2004**, *150*, 1741–1755. [CrossRef] [PubMed]

70. Travinsky, B.; Bunikis, J.; Barbour, A.G. Geographic differences in genetic locus linkages for *Borrelia burgdorferi*. *Emerg. Infect. Dis.* **2010**, *16*, 1147–1150. [CrossRef] [PubMed]

71. Snydman, D.R.; Schenkein, D.P.; Berardi, V.P.; Lastavica, C.C.; Pariser, K.M. *Borrelia burgdorferi* in joint fluid in chronic Lyme arthritis. *Ann. Intern. Med.* **1986**, *104*, 798–800. [CrossRef] [PubMed]

72. Stanek, G.; Klein, J.; Bittner, R.; Glogar, D. Isolation of *Borrelia burgdorferi* from the myocardium of a patient with longstanding cardiomyopathy. *N. Engl. J. Med.* **1990**, *322*, 249–252. [CrossRef] [PubMed]

73. Ma, Y.; Sturrock, A.; Weis, J.J. Intracellular localization of *Borrelia burgdorferi* within human endothelial cells. *Infect. Immun.* **1991**, *59*, 671–678. [PubMed]

74. Georgilis, K.; Peacocke, M.; Klempner, M.S. Fibroblasts protect the Lyme disease spirochete, *Borrelia burgdorferi*, from ceftriaxone in vitro. *J. Infect. Dis.* **1992**, *166*, 440–444. [CrossRef] [PubMed]

75. Haupl, T.; Hahn, G.; Rittig, M.; Krause, A.; Schoerner, C.; Schönherr, U.; Kalden, J.R.; Burmester, G.R. Persistence of *Borrelia burgdorferi* in ligamentous tissue from a patient with chronic Lyme borreliosis. *Arthritis Rheum.* **1993**, *36*, 1621–1626. [CrossRef] [PubMed]

76. Klempner, M.S.; Noring, R.; Rogers, R.A. Invasion of human skin fibroblasts by the Lyme disease spirochete, *Borrelia burgdorferi*. *J. Infect. Dis.* **1993**, *167*, 1074–1081. [CrossRef] [PubMed]

77. Aberer, E.; Kersten, A.; Klade, H.; Poitschek, C.; Jurecka, W. Heterogeneity of *Borrelia burgdorferi* in the skin. *Am. J. Dermatopathol.* **1996**, *18*, 571–579. [CrossRef] [PubMed]

78. Girschick, H.J.; Huppertz, H.I.; Rüssmann, H.; Krenn, V.; Karch, H. Intracellular persistence of *Borrelia burgdorferi* in human synovial cells. *Rheumatol. Int.* **1996**, *16*, 125–132. [CrossRef] [PubMed]

79. Nanagara, R.; Duray, P.H.; Schumacher, H.R. Ultrastructural demonstration of spirochetal antigens in synovial uid and synovial membrane in chronic Lyme disease: Possible factors contributing to persistence of organisms. *Hum. Pathol.* **1996**, *27*, 1025–1034. [CrossRef]

80. Hastey, C.J.; Elsner, R.A.; Barthold, S.W.; Baumgarth, N. Delays and diversions mark the development of B cell responses to Borrelia burgdorferi infection. *J. Immunol.* **2012**, *188*, 5612–5622. [CrossRef] [PubMed]

81. Livengood, J.A.; Gilmore, R.D. Invasion of human neuronal and glial cells by an infectious strain of *Borrelia burgdorferi*. *Microbes Infect.* **2006**, *8*, 2832–2840. [CrossRef] [PubMed]

82. Wormser, G.P.; Dattwyler, R.J.; Shapiro, E.D.; Halperin, J.J.; Steere, A.C.; Klempner, M.S.; Krause, P.J.; Bakken, J.S.; Strle, F.; Stanek, G.; et al. The clinical assessment, treatment, and prevention of lyme disease, human granulocytic anaplasmosis, and babesiosis: Clinical practice guidelines by the Infectious Diseases Society of America. *Clin. Infect. Dis.* **2006**, *43*, 1089–1134. [CrossRef] [PubMed]

83. Stricker, R.B.; Johnson, L. *Borrelia burgdorferi* aggrecanase activity: More evidence for persistent infection in Lyme disease. *Front. Cell Infect. Microbiol.* **2013**, *3*, 40. [CrossRef] [PubMed]

84. Wu, J.; Weening, E.H.; Faske, J.B.; Höök, M.; Skare, J.T. Invasion of eukaryotic cells by *Borrelia burgdorferi* requires β(1) integrins and Src kinase activity. *Infect. Immun.* **2011**, *79*, 1338–1348. [CrossRef] [PubMed]

85. Sapi, E.; Balasubramanian, K.; Poruri, A.; Maghsoudlou, J.S.; Socarras, K.M.; Timmaraju, A.V.; Filush, K.R.; Gupta, K.; Shaikh, S.; Theophilus, P.A.; et al. Evidence of in vivo existence of Borrelia biofilm in Borrelial lymphocytomas. *Eur. J. Microbiol. Immunol.* **2016**, *6*, 9–24. [CrossRef] [PubMed]

86. Feng, J.; Zhang, S.; Shi, W.; Zhang, Y. Ceftriaxone pulse dosing fails to eradicate biofilm-like microcolony *B. burgdorferi* persisters which are sterilized by daptomycin/doxycycline/cefuroxime without pulse dosing. *Front. Microbiol.* **2016**, *7*, 1744. [CrossRef] [PubMed]

87. Klempner, M.S.; Hu, L.T.; Evans, J.; Schmid, C.H.; Johnson, G.M.; Trevino, R.P.; Trevino, B.S.; DeLona Norton, M.P.H.; Lois Levy, M.S.W.; Diane Wall, R.N.; et al. Two controlled trials of antibiotic treatment in patients with persistent symptoms and a history of Lyme disease. *N. Engl. J. Med.* **2001**, *345*, 85–92. [CrossRef] [PubMed]

88. Wormser, G.P.; Nadelman, R.B.; Schwartz, I. The amber theory of Lyme arthritis: Initial description and clinical implications. *Clin. Rheumatol.* **2012**, *31*, 989–994. [CrossRef] [PubMed]

89. Aucott, J.N. Post-treatment Lyme disease syndrome. *Infect. Dis. Clin. N. Am.* **2015**, *29*, 309–323. [CrossRef] [PubMed]

90. Lazarus, J.J.; McCarter, A.L.; Neifer-Sadhwani, K.; Wooten, R.M. ELISA-based measurement of antibody responses and PCR-based detection profiles can distinguish between active infection and early clearance of *Borrelia burgdorferi*. *Clin. Dev. Immunol.* **2012**, *2012*, 138069. [CrossRef] [PubMed]

91. Feng, J.; Shi, W.; Zhang, S.; Zhang, Y. Persister mechanisms in *Borrelia burgdorferi*: Implications for improved intervention. *Emerg. Microbes Infect.* **2015**, *4*, e51. [CrossRef] [PubMed]

92. Sharma, B.; Brown, A.V.; Matluck, N.E.; Hu, L.T.; Lewis, K. *Borrelia burgdorferi*, the causative agent of Lyme disease, forms drug-tolerant persister cells. *Antimicrob. Agents Chemother.* **2015**, *59*, 4616–4624. [CrossRef] [PubMed]

93. Cabello, F.C.; Godfrey, H.P.; Bugrysheva, J.; Newman, S.A. Sleeper cells: The stringent response and persistence in the *Borreliella (Borrelia) burgdorferi* enzootic cycle. *Environ. Microbiol.* **2017**, *19*, 3846–3862. [CrossRef] [PubMed]

94. Middelveen, M.J.; Stricker, R.B. Morgellons disease: A filamentous borrelial dermatitis. *Int. J. Gen. Med.* **2016**, *9*, 349–354. [CrossRef] [PubMed]

95. Middelveen, M.J.; Fesler, M.C.; Stricker, R.B. History of Morgellons disease: From delusion to definition. *Clin. Cosmet. Investig. Dermatol.* **2018**, *11*, 71–90. [CrossRef] [PubMed]

96. Savely, V.R.; Stricker, R.B. Morgellons disease: The mystery unfolds. *Expert Rev. Dermatol.* **2007**, *2*, 585–591. [CrossRef]

97. Savely, V.R.; Stricker, R.B. Morgellons disease: Analysis of a population with clinically confirmed microscopic subcutaneous fibers of unknown etiology. *Clin. Cosmet. Investig. Dermatol.* **2010**, *3*, 67–78. [PubMed]

98. Middelveen, M.J.; Stricker, R.B. Filament formation associated with spirochetal infection: A comparative approach to Morgellons disease. *Clin. Cosmet. Investig. Dermatol.* **2011**, *4*, 167–177. [PubMed]

99. Middelveen, M.J.; Mayne, P.J.; Kahn, D.G.; Stricker, R.B. Characterization and evolution of dermal filaments from patients with Morgellons disease. *Clin. Cosmet. Investig. Dermatol.* **2013**, *6*, 1–21. [PubMed]

100. Middelveen, M.J.; Burugu, D.; Poruri, A.; Burke, J.; Mayne, P.J.; Sapi, E.; Kahn, D.G.; Stricker, R.B. Association of spirochetal infection with Morgellons disease. *F1000Res* **2013**, *2*, 25. [CrossRef] [PubMed]

101. Chmielewski, T.; Tylewska-Wierzbanowska, S. Interactions between *Borrelia burgdorferi* and mouse fibroblasts. *Pol. J. Microbiol.* **2010**, *59*, 157–160. [PubMed]

102. Radolf, J.D.; Deka, R.K.; Anand, A.; Šmajs, D.; Norgard, M.V.; Yang, X.F. *Treponema pallidum*, the syphilis spirochete: Making a living as a stealth pathogen. *Nat. Rev. Microbiol.* **2016**, *14*, 744–759. [CrossRef] [PubMed]

103. Brorson, Ø.; Brorson, S.H. Transformation of cystic forms of Borrelia burgdorferi to normal mobile spirochetes. *Infection* **1997**, *25*, 240–246. [CrossRef] [PubMed]

104. Murgia, R.; Cinco, M. Induction of cystic forms by different stress conditions in *Borrelia burgdorferi*. *APMIS* **2004**, *112*, 57–62. [CrossRef] [PubMed]

105. MacDonald, A.B. *Borrelia burgdorferi* tissue morphologies and imaging methodologies. *Eur. J. Clin. Microbiol. Infect. Dis.* **2013**, *32*, 1077–1082. [CrossRef] [PubMed]

106. Mestecky, J.; Moldoveanu, Z.; Russell, M.W. Immunologic uniqueness of the genital tract: Challenge for vaccine development. *Am. J. Reprod. Immunol.* **2005**, *53*, 208–214. [CrossRef] [PubMed]

107. Cu-Uvin, S.; DeLong, A.K.; Venkatesh, K.K.; Hogan, J.W.; Ingersoll, J.; Kurpewski, J.; De Pasquale, M.P.; D'Aquila, R.; Caliendo, A.M. Genital tract HIV-1 RNA shedding among women with below detectable plasma viral load. *AIDS* **2010**, *24*, 2489–2497. [CrossRef] [PubMed]

108. Mzingwane, M.L.; Tiemessen, C.T. Mechanisms of HIV persistence in HIV reservoirs. *Rev. Med. Virol.* **2017**, *27*, e1924. [CrossRef] [PubMed]

109. Vetter, P.; Fischer, W.A., II; Schibler, M.; Jacobs, M.; Bausch, D.G.; Kaiser, L. Ebola virus shedding and transmission: Review of current evidence. *J. Infect. Dis.* **2016**, *214*, S177–S184. [CrossRef] [PubMed]

110. Moreira, J.; Peixoto, T.M.; Siqueira, A.M.; Lamas, C.C. Sexually acquired Zika virus: A systematic review. *Clin. Microbiol. Infect.* **2017**, *23*, 296–305. [CrossRef] [PubMed]

How a Communication Intervention in Zambia Re-Oriented Health Services to the Needs of the Least-Supported

Tony Klouda [1],*[ID], Cathy Green [2], Miniratu Soyoola [3], Paula Quigley [3], Tendayi Kureya [4], Caroline Barber [5] and Kenneth Mubuyaeta [6]

[1]   Freelance Consultant, 71A Lady Margaret Road, London NW5 2NN, UK
[2]   Freelance Consultant, 28/4 Royal William Yard, Plymouth, Devon PL1 3GD, UK; cathygreenhpi@gmail.com
[3]   DAI Global Health, Waterside Centre, North Street, Lewes, East Sussex BN7 2PE, UK; Miniratu_Soyoola@dai.com (M.S.); Paula_Quigley@dai.com (P.Q.)
[4]   Development Data, Plot 4 B, Lunzua Road, Off Addis Ababa, Rhodespark, Lusaka, Zambia; tendayi@developmentdata.info
[5]   Transaid, 137 Euston Rd, Kings Cross, London NW1 2AA, UK; barberc@transaid.org
[6]   Disacare, Plot # 11305, Off Chilimbulu Road, behind Libala High School, P.O. Box 50091 Lusaka, Zambia; kennymubuyaeta@gmail.com
*   Correspondence: tonyklouda@gmail.com

Abstract: Despite decades of training health workers in communication, complaints from clients and communities about poor health worker attitudes abound. This was found to be so in Zambia where the More Mobilizing Access to Maternal Health Services in Zambia (MORE MAMaZ) program was trying to ensure the inclusion of under-supported women in a community-based maternal and newborn health program in five intervention districts. Under-supported women suffer a disproportionate burden of child mortality and are poor users of health services. An exploratory small-scale qualitative survey involving nurses from training schools and health facilities found that nurses knew how to communicate well, but were selective with whom and in what circumstances they did this. In general, those who received the worst communication were under-supported and had low confidence—the very people who needed the best communication. An experiential training program was started to help health workers reflect on the reasons for their poor communication. The training was evaluated after 14 months using semi-structured interviews and focus group discussions with staff at participating health facilities. The results showed improved inclusion of under-supported women but also increased attendance generally for ante-natal clinics, deliveries and under-five clinics. Another outcome was improved communication between, and a sense of job satisfaction among, the health workers themselves. The program demonstrated an effective way to improve the inclusion and involvement of the least-supported women and girls. There are important lessons for other health programs that aim to operationalize the goals of the Global Strategy for Women's, Children's and Adolescent's Health, which include an emphasis on reaching every woman.

Keywords: health communication; reaching every woman; social inclusion; universal health coverage; Zambia; maternal and newborn health; training; health workers

1. Introduction

Concerns about poor health worker communication are reflected in the recent call for respectful maternity care as part of the bid to improve maternal health [1,2]. Another important policy orientation is the current global commitment to reaching every woman, child and adolescent, ensuring that scarce health resources are targeted to where they are needed the most [3]. Against this backdrop, it is important to consider how health worker communication and the availability of respectful care facilitate or undermine efforts to reach the least-supported women and girls.

It is widely understood that women who feel they are not respected or supported by their families or communities are less likely to care for themselves or their children—partly as a result of the lack of support, but also because of associated depression, anxiety and frustration [4–8]. They are also less likely to communicate well, and to remain silent or unquestioning when confronted with people who they perceive to be more powerful. This has important implications for health care access and a patient's capacity to effectively communicate their needs or act on treatment and other advice when seeking health care. A recent study in northern Nigeria was pivotal in exposing the relationship between the burden of mortality and women's lack of social support and voice, with important implications for health programs that are concerned with targeting resources to where they are needed the most [9].

In 2014, the Government of Zambia requested that an intervention to improve communication for nurses and other front-line health workers be included in a maternal and newborn health program called More Mobilizing Access to Maternal Health Services in Zambia (MORE MAMaZ). Operational from 2014 to 2016, the program was primarily a demand-side intervention focused on improving maternal and newborn health care access. Integrating the learning from the earlier study in Nigeria, the program placed significant emphasis on reaching the least-supported women in intervention communities. The request from the Ministry of Health (MOH) to design and implement a communications training intervention targeted to health workers was appropriate in a context where negative health worker attitudes were known to undermine community confidence in health services [10].

The communication training was implemented as a pilot and within an operations research framework with the intention of generating evidence to inform policy. The overall research objective was to assess the impact of the training on health workers' awareness of how a lack of individual social support can be a key factor driving the skewed burden of ill-health. It also focused on health workers' attitudes towards and capacity and willingness to support under-supported women in their catchment communities. Other objectives were to assess the impact of the training on the relationships between health workers within a health facility and on the linkages between health facilities and communities. This paper describes the development and implementation of the communications training and assesses its effectiveness in changing health workers' understanding of the need to provide respectful care to all patients, whatever their background or situation.

2. Methods

In Zambia, the immediate impetus to train nurses and other front-line health workers in communication skills in the MORE MAMaZ intervention sites arose from persistent complaints from community members and health managers concerning the poor attitudes of health workers to clinic attenders. The concern was that this gap in the quality of care would impact negatively on the demand creation efforts that were underway at community level. Before beginning the training intervention, an effectiveness review of current communication training programs and a perspectives survey with health care workers were conducted. It was found that the Zambian nurse training program emphasized communication theory and practical applications similar to other programs around the world without taking into account the possibility that communication can be selective [11–13]. The underpinning assumptions were that not all health workers communicated badly; and those that did, communicated badly with all of their clients. However, there were no long-term evaluations of program effectiveness. Conversely, the pilot survey with Zambian healthcare workers found that while they knew how to communicate well, they applied these skills selectively. These findings challenged some long-standing assumptions about health worker communication skills.

2.1. Development of Communication Training

The understanding gained from the survey of nurse communication practices was used to plan a three-day training of health staff working in 64 health facilities in the program's five intervention districts. The districts were Chama district in Muchinga Province; Mkushi, Serenje and Chitambo districts in Central Province; and Mongu district in Western Province. Curricula for core trainers (District Health Management Team (DHMT) members and nurse tutors) and for step-down training were devised with nurse tutors and Zambian consultants. The step-down training was designed to be delivered in two stages: first, a training of selected front-line health workers in participating health facilities, and, second, an orientation by the latter of other health workers in the facility, and also of Community Health Volunteers (CHVs) and other community members. The second group received a one-day step-down training. The training of CHVs and community members was important not only to help with the local identification of the least-supported women, but also to encourage those women to attend health services and to join groups. It also helped to better integrate the social inclusion work of the CHVs with that of the clinic-based health workers.

The program used an experiential training approach in which health workers reviewed themselves and developed insights into why they chose to communicate badly in some instances, whilst communicating well in others. The idea was that they would then be able to review how to manage and control the factors that led to instances of poor communication in their work setting. A starting point for reflection and discussion was the notion that the very people with whom health workers were most likely to communicate badly were those most likely to suffer ill health, or to have children who suffered ill health. The results of the nurse survey indicated that the use of general categories for targeting (e.g., 'poverty' or 'lack of education') was less useful than having an understanding of a client's social situation at home. In other words, health workers needed to understand more about the underlying factors that led to a client presenting as poorly dressed, unwilling to communicate or shy. Health workers were also encouraged to think about the impact of poor communication on patients and on their colleagues—a topic not generally covered in formal health worker communication training. The need to improve communication between staff had not featured among the concerns cited by district health managers. This appeared to be a neglected area in supervision and management systems generally. The essential steps in the three-day training were:

- Reviewing the links between clinic use, mortality, deliveries and the support given to women.
- Exploring how social situations affect health.
- Analyzing why communication goes wrong with some people.
- Reflecting on how to guard against the temptation to be rude or dismissive.
- How to manage poor communication in the health facility as a team.
- Strategies for working with communities to promote the involvement of the least-supported women and girls through inclusive policies and participation in groups.

2.2. Training Evaluation

An evaluation of the training was undertaken in November 2015, 14 months after the first training input. The evaluation included 61 percent of participating health facilities (20 of 33 health facilities) in three of the five program districts: Chitambo, Serenje and Mkushi, all in Central Province. The evaluation was conducted with the full participation and involvement of the respective DHMTs.

Due to the staggered nature of the step-down training, health center staff, CHVs and community members received their training between seven and 12 months prior to the evaluation. A total of 20 health centers participated in the evaluation (eight in Chitambo, four in Serenje and eight in Mkushi). Semi-structured interviews were conducted with staff at the health centers, members of the DHMTs and the trainers. Focus group discussions were also carried out with CHVs and community representatives who were members of Neighborhood Health Committees. In each district, two teams of three interviewers conducted the interviews. A member of the DHMT was included on the interview team to improve relevance. In the health centers, 35 staff who had been trained (or oriented by other staff) were interviewed in addition to 22 CHVs. For 19 of the 20 health centers, a selection of community members (10–12 in each group) was also interviewed.

The interview questionnaires were designed separately for core trainers, health facility staff, CHVs, and community members. Each questionnaire had two components. The first set of questions was asked directly of interview respondents. These were fully open-ended to prevent bias towards a positive response. The answers were analyzed and coded by the evaluator for the main categories of response in relation to changes in communication, focus on under-supported women and changes in community support of the under-supported. The second set of questions was answered by the interviewer directly after the interview. These allowed the interviewer to check whether specific aspects of the training or experience had been mentioned, were implicit in the answers given by a respondent, or not mentioned. The answers were then appropriately coded. For this category of questions, the interviewer's answers were checked against the respondent's answers at the data analysis stage.

The teams of interviewers were given a one-day orientation on how to ask open-ended questions without giving any intimation of an expected answer. They also learnt how to assess what was implied in an answer, how to probe for fuller answers without directing them, and how to use the questionnaires. At the end of every day of interviewing, each team met to review the answers, and to provide their own feedback on what they had seen and heard.

Data was entered into Excel spreadsheets. Coded data was analyzed using the SPSS statistical package. A wide selection of the interviewee responses was provided in the evaluation. In order to contextualize the findings, the training evaluation examined in detail the government health statistics for each of the clinics visited, and compared these with areas where no training had taken place. For each area, the answers from the different types of respondents were cross-checked for consistency (e.g., the responses of clinic staff were checked against the perceptions of community members and CHVs).

The DHMTs from all intervention districts were invited to perform their own assessments of the training intervention before the evaluation. They were also invited to present these, together with their recommendations for future work, in a dissemination workshop involving donors, government representatives and other organizations.

Ethical approval was obtained as part of the overall approval given by the Zambian Ministry of Health for the operations research study as a whole.

There were few methodological limitations to the measurement of the impact of communications training to staff in clinics as the correlation between the answers of different staff (interviewed separately) at any particular clinic was very high. The clinics had been given no previous warning of the evaluation team visits, nor of the types of questions they would be asked. However, a failure to separate CHVs from other community representatives during focus group discussions meant that it was difficult to avoid positive bias in the answers as there was a tendency for the CHVs to answer in advance of others. This was dealt with by asking community members to answer first. However, this was not always successful.

3. Results

Thirteen core trainers were trained in September 2014. The core trainers trained 71 front-line health workers during September and October 2014. Over the next six months, front-line health workers oriented other health staff in their facility. The training was then extended to CHVs and other community representatives in the catchment area of participating health facilities. All training inputs were completed by April 2015.

The evaluation found that the communication training intervention was perceived to be successful in all but one health facility (a hospital outpatient clinic where staff turnover was very high) in relation to the improvement of communication in terms of: staff–staff relationships in health centers;

communication between staff and their clients in general; a stronger, more nuanced and supportive focus on under-supported women in clinics; and improved linkages between health center staff, volunteers, community workers and communities. These improvements were described at every level (by DHMTs, health center staff, CHVs, community leaders and other representatives).

Almost all trainees who had received the three-day version of the training described how transformative the process had been for them as individuals. In general, they reported that it changed the way in which they understood people and approached their work. The majority of respondents amongst the clinic staff mentioned specifically that the training impacted them personally and significantly in terms of their understanding of why they communicated badly only with some people, and the realization that it was important to hide their frustrations from clients. In terms of improved communication within facility teams, one health worker explained:

"The training has helped very much. It gave us an opportunity to think together as a team. Now people are happy to go to any staff rather than preferring to see only one. The way people interact, if we're not on good terms, the client suffers. So we talk together."

Health workers reported that reviewing their experiences with other staff made communication easier.

Sensitivity to the social factors that affected women's and girls' health seeking behavior and responsiveness to treatment advice was also reported as having increased. As one health worker argued:

"Before the training we did not bother to pay attention to the reasons for women's circumstances, like looking dirty, unkempt and late for clinic. After the training we became more aware—we began to pay attention to these people to identify their situation better."

Overall, the general feedback from health workers was that the three-day communications training made their work more satisfactory and valued.

The communication training had a complementary and strengthening effect on the program overall. The work carried out by the program's District Program Officers, who were embedded within the District Health Offices together with the District Mother and Child Health Coordinators, was seen to be invaluable in this regard. In many health facilities (with the backing of the DHMTs), health workers reported increased access to services by single pregnant women over and above that already achieved by the program. Although at first many clinic staff were wary of accepting pregnant women who had no partner because of the strong local antipathy to pregnancy outside of marriage, the awareness given by the training helped considerably in their acceptance of such women. In addition, clinic staff reported that, as a result of the training, they made more effort to improve the extent to which men accompanied such women to the health center. This resulted from their probing of women's social situations and the fact that they then took time to find and interview partners (in instances where they had obtained the client's consent).

Almost all the health facilities involved in the evaluation reported that attendance increased as a result of the training. It was reported that within the general increase in clinic attendance for institutional delivery, antenatal care and family planning services attendance by under-supported women also increased, as well as their attendance at general out-patients and under-five clinics.

The evaluation also identified a general increase in awareness of, and sensitivity to, the needs of under-supported women in the program intervention communities. Specific examples of improved support for women were given by 58 percent of community respondents. CHVs reported that their increased understanding of problems in their communication had further improved their ability to work with, assess and support the families of under-supported women.

Staff at the majority of the clinics reported that their training encouraged them to increase their probing of clients when they appeared to lack confidence, or when a client communicated badly. They reported that this encouraged many more women to talk frankly about their situations at home.

They felt, in turn, that they were able to provide better advice to the women, and felt that this translated into a greater willingness to attend clinics, and better relations with the communities on social matters. It was reported in several of the health facilities that increased probing also helped women to talk about intimate partner violence. Although health staff were supposed to refer these cases to the police, after the training they reported that they spent more time counseling women, trying to interview domestic partners, and suggesting other forms of community support for the women.

4. Discussion

Much of the training given to health workers to date has been based on the assumption that health workers do not necessarily know how to communicate well, and that explaining the principles of communication will make them better communicators. The training intervention developed by MORE MAMaZ in Zambia was an attempt to approach the improvement of communication by other means—notably through internalization of the fact that people already know how to communicate well but choose when, and with whom, they communicate badly. The major success of the training was improved control of communication by health workers. This resulted not only from greater awareness of their choices, but also from the understanding that they could receive support from colleagues when trying to improve communication. The particular route chosen for this orientation was through demonstration of the impact of poor communication on those most likely to need good communication—notably the least supported women and girls in communities, those less likely to frequent health services as a result of that poor communication, and those most likely to neglect themselves and their children, and to suffer the highest mortality of their children.

Many of the headline results of the training evaluation were confirmed by the program's statistical endline household survey, which was carried out in five intervention districts in 2016. The endline survey found that 73 percent of women and 70 percent of men in intervention communities were aware of efforts to include socially excluded women and girls in maternal and newborn health group activities. This was considerably more than in control sites (51 percent women and 61 percent of men) [14]. The endline survey also confirmed that intimate partner violence was perceived to have decreased across the program sites by 89 percent of male and 88 percent of female respondents [14]. The increase in facility attendance reported in the training evaluation was also confirmed. The endline survey identified a 25 percent increase in institutional delivery (from 64 percent to 89 percent), a 25 percent increase in antenatal care (ANC) attendance in the first trimester (from 37 percent to 62 percent), and a 14 percent increase in use of modern family planning methods (from 24 percent to 38 percent) [14]. The increases in service uptake were expected in relation to ANC and institutional deliveries, which had been major focal issues for the MORE MAMaZ program. Verbal reports by clinic-based staff and CHVs made clear their strong belief that more under-supported women were using health services as a result of the training. This appeared to be consistent with the evidence from the endline survey that first-time clinic attendance had increased. However, the lack of a reliable baseline that identified under-supported women separately from other women meant that there was no completely objective system of measurement of the increased attendance by under-supported women. It was also difficult to determine whether the work of CHVs, who had been trained by the program to seek out socially excluded women and girls and include them in maternal and newborn health group activities, or the work of health workers was more or less important in increasing facility attendance by individuals perceived locally to be under-supported. What can be said, however, is that the training intervention complemented other program activities to improve access by the least-supported women and girls. It is also likely that the focus on under-supported women within the program more generally, in combination with the communication training, increased the proportion of under-supported women using health services. Such difficulties in attributing change to a single intervention that is part of a broad-ranging, multi-focal program are not unusual, though they do point to the need to put in place robust monitoring and evaluation systems for pilot initiatives such as these if the aim is to prove their significance as an 'innovation'.

The three-day training provided to clinic staff had considerable impact. By contrast, the one-day step-down training provided by clinic staff to colleagues and to CHVs and other community representatives in catchment communities proved to be less effective. Whilst the step-down short courses clearly improved communication, the short duration of such training and orientation inevitably meant that full understanding of the complexity and reasons for the training was compromised. The evaluation found that some of the beneficiaries of this shorter training showed a lack of understanding of the term 'under-supported' in that they referred only to 'those who don't go to clinics', or to people who fell into categories such as 'disabled, mentally ill, widows, orphans, or women beaten by husbands'. Whilst it is true that such categories may include women who are under-supported, individuals in these categories may also be well-supported, limiting their usefulness as a means of targeting resources to where they are needed the most. These challenges reinforce the importance of a longer orientation and subsequent reinforcement and follow-up. They also reflect the more general challenges related to the effective provision of in-service training in contexts where health facilities are affected by challenging staffing shortages.

A key feature of the MORE MAMaZ communication training was the reliance not so much on individual training, but rather on the training of teams of staff at the health facilities. This enabled mutual reinforcement and helped to increase staff morale, as health workers began to believe that their supervisors listened to their ideas and concerns. It would be of great benefit if all health workers were oriented in the same way in pre-service training. This is especially important in contexts where health facilities operate in low-resource environments and are affected by high staff turnover.

Despite the clear benefits of the communications training intervention (such as better health worker morale, greater trust in services, a positive impact on domestic social situations, better balance between community services and clinic-based services), the problems facing the development, establishment and maintenance of such an approach are the same as those faced by many health systems. In Zambia, there are inadequate funds available for in-service training and for follow-up supervision and management. Districts are highly dependent on taking advantage of externally funded programs to do what little training they can provide. The majority of in-service training conducted by District Health Teams is piggy-backed on to training funded by external donors. During the implementation timeframe of MORE MAMaZ, despite considerable interest in, and support for, the communications training within the respective DHMTs, none of the districts were able to provide any additional support or expanded training other than that provided within the context of the program itself. During the evaluation process however, possibilities for extending the training were explored with the DHMTs. They also signaled their commitment to using their regular monitoring of clinics and of staff through the staff appraisal process to embed some sort of follow-up of the training. With just a few adjustments to existing staff monitoring mechanisms, they acknowledged that it should be possible to establish some form of on-going assessment of the extent of good communication both among health workers and between health workers and their clients.

The evaluation of the communication training revealed some side-effects that were not fully expected. The increase in the number of women who were willing to talk about domestic social issues in clinic consultations showed that it is possible to contribute through this route to on-going efforts to reduce intimate partner violence. Listening to women and girls affected by violence and giving them confidence to communicate about their problems is a first step, especially in cases where they lack other opportunities to communicate about the difficulties they are facing.

The MORE MAMaZ communications training design was strongly influenced by a study that investigated the relationship between child mortality and lack of support among women within the context of a large health systems strengthening program focused on improving maternal, newborn and child health in northern Nigeria between 2006 and 2014 [9]. Implemented in a context where study populations were generally very poor, had few resources, similar employment opportunities, and the overall culture within which the entire population operated, the study identified a skew of child mortality where 20 percent of survey households had experienced 80 percent of the child deaths.

This type of skew has been recognized by demographers for well over one hundred years [15–25]. However, the standard variables used in studies that have explored this skew (e.g., health service availability, birth spacing, availability of services, poverty, education, resources, etc.) have failed to provide sufficient explanation. Responding to this gap in understanding, the Nigeria study tested the hypothesis that social variables relating to the support of women were important in determining the skew of mortality. The hypothesis was that those women who felt least respected and supported by their husbands or families would be the most likely to neglect themselves and their children. This was found to be the case. Health seeking behavior, child mortality, and lack of delivery by trained midwives were all strongly linked to the support the woman received from their husbands or families [9]. The Nigeria study strongly influenced the design of the communications training. Wider implications of this approach are that health programs that aim to reach every woman, adolescent and child need to disaggregate beyond poverty (and other standard variables such as level of education), and place more emphasis on understanding the social factors that influence poor health. Perhaps one of the most important implications is the need to move from a focus on individual women and children, towards a focus on the family unit, as it is the situation of the family and its interactions that have the most significant impact on the health (including the mental health) of each and every family member.

5. Conclusions

The impact of the MORE MAMaZ communications training intervention could be seen through improved clinic attendance; improved relevance of clinical diagnosis, treatment, support and referral of under-supported women; improved morale of staff and fewer complaints about staff; and a decrease in intimate partner violence, with a concomitant improvement in the participation and voice of women affected by violence. The fact that a short communications training stimulated Zambian health workers to explore, try to understand and respond to clients' social situations, indicates that it is possible to operationalize the social determinants of health perspectives in clinical settings. The way in which the communications training was perceived by health workers, DHMTs and community members to have contributed to an increase in poorly-supported women and girls using maternal health services is significant in a context where there is as yet inadequate understanding of how to effectively reach the least-supported individuals. Further testing of the efficacy of this training is warranted in the Zambian context, including in a pre-service training scenario. Should this approach to communications training and inclusion of under-supported women prove to be useful in other contexts, it will provide a valuable contribution to the goals of the Global Strategy for Women's, Children's and Adolescent's Health, with its emphasis on reaching every woman, adolescent and child.

Author Contributions: Conceptualization, T.K. (Tony Klouda), M.S., C.G.; Writing-Original Draft Preparation, T.K. (Tony Klouda) and C.G.; Writing-Review & Editing, P.Q., T.K. (Tendayi Kureya), M.S., C.B. and K.M.

Funding: This work was supported by Comic Relief under Grant number ID 308183.

Acknowledgments: The authors would like to acknowledge the enormous contributions of the Ministry of Health and the five District Health Management Teams in the program's intervention districts in supporting the design and implementation of the training approach outlined in this paper. In addition, the results outlined in this article would not have been possible without the dedicated contributions of the program's Senior Program Officer, Esnart Banda, four District Program Officers, Ruth Nyirendra, Ernest Chanda, Likando Mundia and Daniel Malambo, and national consultant, Maureen Syanzila.

References

1.   White Ribbon Alliance. *Respectful Maternity Care Charter: The Universal Rights of Childbearing Women [Internet]*; WRA: Washington, DC, USA, 2011. Available online: http://whiteribbonalliance.org/wp-content/uploads/2013/10/Final_RMC_Charter.pdf (accessed on 2 May 2018).

2.   World Health Organization. *The Prevention and Elimination of Disrespect and Abuse during Facility-Based Childbirth [Internet]*; WHO: Geneva, Switzerland, 2014. Available online: http://apps.who.int/iris/bitstream/10665/134588/1/WHO_RHR_14.23_eng.pdf?ua=1&ua=1 (accessed on 2 May 2018).

3.   Every Woman Every Child. *Global Strategy for Women's, Children's and Adolescents' Health (2016–2030)*; Every Woman Every Child: New York, NY, USA, 2015.

4.   De Silva, M.J.; McKenzie, K.; Harpham, T.; Huttly, S.R. Social capital and mental illness: A systematic review. *J. Epidemiol. Community Health* **2005**, *59*, 619–627. [CrossRef] [PubMed]

5.   Lund, C.; Breen, A.; Fisher, A.J.; Kakuma, R.; Corrigall, J.; Joska, J.A.; Swartz, L.; Patel, V. Poverty and common mental disorders in low and middle income countries: A systematic review. *Soc. Sci. Med.* **2010**, *71*, 517–528. [CrossRef] [PubMed]

6.   Patel, V. Poverty, inequality, and mental health in developing countries. In *Poverty, Inequality and Health: An International Perspective*; Leon, D.A., Walt, G., Eds.; Oxford University Press: Oxford, UK, 2001; pp. 247–262.

7.   Mindes, E.J.; Ingram, K.M.; Kliewer, W.; James, C.A. Longitudinal analyses of the relationship between unsupportive social interactions and psychological adjustment among women with fertility problems. *Soc. Sci. Med.* **2003**, *56*, 2165–2180. [CrossRef]

8.   Rahman, A.; Iqbal, Z.; Bunn, J.; Harrington, R. Impact of Maternal Depression on Infant Nutritional Status and Illness. *Arch. Gen. Psychiatry* **2004**, *61*, 946–952. [CrossRef] [PubMed]

9.   PRRINN-MNCH. *Adjusting Health Strategies to Include Women and Children with the Least Social Support*; Health Partners International: Sussex, UK, 2014.

10.   Central Statistical Office [Zambia]; Ministry of Health [Zambia]; ICF International. *Zambia Demographic and Health Survey 2013–14*; Central Statistical Office, Ministry of Health, and ICF International: Rockville, MD, USA, 2015.

11.   Zimbabwe Ministry of Health and Child Welfare (Health Education Unit). *Interpersonal Communication: Manual for Trainers of Health Service Providers*; Zimbabwe Ministry of Health and Child Welfare: Harare, Zimbabwe, 1998.

12.   Partnership for Transforming Health Systems Programme. *An Interpersonal Communication and Counselling (IPC & C) Skills Training Manual for Health Care Providers*; PATHS: Abuja, Nigeria, 2004.

13.   Bramhall, E. Effective communication skills in nursing practice. *Nurs. Stand.* **2014**, *29*, 53–59. [CrossRef] [PubMed]

14.   Kureya, T.; Green, C.; Soyoola, M. *MORE MAMaZ Endline Survey Report*; Development Data: Lusaka, Zambia, 2016.

15.   Meegama, S.A. *Socio-Economic Determinants of Infant and Child Mortality in Sri Lanka: An Analysis of Post-War Experience*; Scientific Report; World Fertility Survey: Princeton, NJ, USA, 1980.

16.   Arulampalam, W.; Bhalotra, S. *Sibling Death Clustering in India: Genuine Scarring vs Unobserved Heterogeneity*; Discussion Paper; Department of Economics, University of Bristol: Bristol, UK, 2003.

17.   Barthélémy, K.D.; Diallo, K. Geography of child mortality clustering within African families. *Health Place* **2002**, *8*, 93–117.

18.   Das Gupta, M. Death clustering, mother's education and the determinants of child mortality in rural Punjab, India. In *What We Know about Health Transition: The Cultural, Social and Behavioural Determinants of Health: The Proceedings of an International Workshop, Canberra, May 1989*; Health Transition Series No. 2; Australian National University: Canberra, Australia, 1990; pp. 441–461.

19.   Das Gupta, M. Socio-economic status and clustering of child deaths in rural Punjab. *Popul. Stud.* **1997**, *51*, 191–202. [CrossRef]

20.   Edvinsson, S.; Brändström, A.; Rogers, J.; Broström, G. High-risk families: The unequal distribution of infant mortality in nineteenth-century Sweden. *Popul. Stud.* **2005**, *59*, 321–337. [CrossRef] [PubMed]

21.   Guo, G. Use of sibling data to estimate family mortality effects in Guatemala. *Demography* **1993**, *30*, 15–32. [CrossRef] [PubMed]

22.   Madise, N.J.; Diamond, I. Determinants of infant mortality in Malawi: An analysis to control for death clustering within families. *J. Biosoc. Sci.* **1995**, *27*, 95–106. [CrossRef] [PubMed]

23.   Omariba, D.W.R. *Levels, Trends and Correlates of Child Mortality in Kenya: An Exploration into the Phenomenon of Death Clustering*; University of Western Ontario: London, ON, Canada, 2005.

24.   Ronsmans, C. Patterns of Clustering of Child Mortality in a Rural Area of Senegal. *Popul. Stud.* **2005**, *49*, 443–461. [CrossRef]

25.   Vandezande, M.; Moreels, S.; Koen, M. *Explaining Death Clustering: Intergenerational Patterns in Infant Mortality Antwerp 1846–1905*; Working paper of the Scientific Research Community Historical Demography; Centre for Sociological Research: Leuven, Belgium, 2010.

22. Madise, N.J.; Diamond, I. Determinants of infant mortality in Malawi: An analysis to control for death clustering within families. *J. Biosoc. Sci.* **1995**, *27*, 95–106. [CrossRef] [PubMed]
23. Omariba, D.W.R. *Levels, Trends and Correlates of Child Mortality in Kenya: An Exploration into the Phenomenon of Death Clustering*; University of Western Ontario: London, ON, Canada, 2005.
24. Ronsmans, C. Patterns of Clustering of Child Mortality in a Rural Area of Senegal. *Popul. Stud.* **2005**, *49*, 443–461. [CrossRef]
25. Vandezande, M.; Moreels, S.; Koen, M. *Explaining Death Clustering: Intergenerational Patterns in Infant Mortality Antwerp 1846–1905*; Working paper of the Scientific Research Community Historical Demography; Centre for Sociological Research: Leuven, Belgium, 2010.

3

Harmonizing Outcomes for Genomic Medicine: Comparison of eMERGE Outcomes to ClinGen Outcome/Intervention Pairs

Janet L. Williams [1], Wendy K. Chung [2], Alex Fedotov [3], Krzysztof Kiryluk [4], Chunhua Weng [5], John J. Connolly [6], Margaret Harr [6], Hakon Hakonarson [6,7], Kathleen A. Leppig [8], Eric B. Larson [9], Gail P. Jarvik [10], David L. Veenstra [11], Christin Hoell [12], Maureen E. Smith [12], Ingrid A. Holm [13], Josh F. Peterson [14] and Marc S. Williams [1,*]

[1] Genomic Medicine Institute, Geisinger, Danville, PA 17822, USA; Jlwilliams3@geisinger.edu
[2] Departments of Pediatrics and Medicine, Columbia University, New York, NY 10025, USA; wkc15@cumc.columbia.edu
[3] Irving Institute for Clinical and Translational Research, Columbia University, New York, NY 10025, USA; avf2117@cumc.columbia.edu
[4] Department of Medicine, Division of Nephrology, Columbia University, New York, NY 10025, USA; kk473@cumc.columbia.edu
[5] Department of Biomedical Informatics, Columbia University, New York, NY 10025, USA; chunhua@columbia.edu
[6] Children's Hospital of Philadelphia, Philadelphia, PA 19104, USA; connollyj1@chop.edu (J.J.C.); harrm@email.chop.edu (M.H.); hakonarson@email.chop.edu (H.H.)
[7] Perelman School of Medicine, University of Pennsylvania, Philadelphia, PA 19104, USA
[8] Genetic Services, Kaiser Permanente of Washington, Seattle, WA 98101, USA; leppig.k@ghc.org
[9] Kaiser Permanente Washington Health Research Institute, Seattle, WA 98101, USA; larson.e@ghc.org
[10] Departments of Medicine (Medical Genetics) and Genome Sciences, University of Washington, Seattle, WA 98195, USA; gjarvik@medicine.washington.edu
[11] Department Pharmacy, University of Washington, Seattle, WA 98195, USA; veenstra@uw.edu
[12] Center for Genetic Medicine, Northwestern University, Chicago, IL 60611, USA; christin.hoell@northwestern.edu (C.H.); m-smith6@northwestern.edu (M.E.S.)
[13] Division of Genetics and Genomics, Boston Children's Hospital, and Department of Pediatrics, Harvard Medical School, Boston, MA 02115, USA; Ingrid.Holm@childrens.harvard.edu
[14] Departments of Biomedical Informatics and Medicine, School of Medicine, Vanderbilt University, Nashville, TN 37232, USA; josh.peterson@Vanderbilt.Edu
* Correspondence: mswilliams1@geisinger.edu

Abstract: Genomic medicine is moving from research to the clinic. There is a lack of evidence about the impact of genomic medicine interventions on health outcomes. This is due in part to a lack of standardized outcome measures that can be used across different programs to evaluate the impact of interventions targeted to specific genetic conditions. The eMERGE Outcomes working group (OWG) developed measures to collect information on outcomes following the return of genomic results to participants for several genetic disorders. These outcomes were compared to outcome intervention pairs for genetic disorders developed independently by the ClinGen Actionability working group (AWG). In general, there was concordance between the defined outcomes between the two groups. The ClinGen outcomes tended to be from a higher level and the AWG scored outcomes represented a subset of outcomes referenced in the accompanying AWG evidence review. eMERGE OWG outcomes were more detailed and discrete, facilitating a collection of relevant information from the health records. This paper demonstrates that common outcomes for genomic medicine interventions can be identified. Further work is needed to standardize outcomes across genomic medicine implementation projects and to make these publicly available to enhance dissemination and assist in making precision public health a reality.

Keywords: genomics; genomic medicine; health outcomes; evidence; standards; eMERGE; ClinGen; precision public health

---

1. Introduction

Genomic medicine is defined by the National Human Genome Research Institute (NHGRI) as, "an emerging medical discipline that involves using genomic information about an individual as part of their clinical care (e.g., for diagnostic or therapeutic decision-making) and the health outcomes and policy implications of that clinical use" [1]. Prior research has demonstrated that genomic medicine has promise for improving health outcomes. As a result, it is beginning to emerge into the clinical practice for selected indications including pharmacogenomics [2], precision oncology [3], and diagnosis of complex conditions suspected be genetic [4]. Large-scale research programs such as the All of Us program funded by the United States National Institutes of Health (NIH) [5] and smaller private clinical research programs [6,7] are beginning to explore the integration of genomic information with other health information to assess the impact on patient outcomes that, it is hoped, will ultimately result in more programs in precision public health.

Several barriers to the implementation of genomic medicine have been identified [8]. One of the most important of these is the lack of evidence of the clinical utility of the interventions. Stated another way, while there is strong evidence about the association of genomic variation with genetic disorders, there is, with few exceptions, inadequate information about the impact on outcomes (both positive and negative) of implementing genomic medicine into clinical care [9,10]. This lack of evidence results in a reluctance of healthcare systems to invest in and payers to reimburse for genomic medicine interventions. There is a general agreement that evidence of the impact of genomic medicine on health outcomes must be generated. There are many barriers to the generation of evidence [9,10], one of which is the lack of agreed-upon outcomes to measure the impact of conditions of interest.

The NHGRI has funded several large collaborations to study genomic medicine in clinical care. These include, but are not limited to, the Implementing Genomics in Practice (IGNITE) network [11], the Clinical Sequencing Evidence-Generating Research (CSER) consortium [12], and the Electronic Medical Records and Genomics (eMERGE) network [13]. All three of these groups have a workgroup tasked to develop outcomes for site-specific and network projects. While these groups have worked to harmonize outcomes within each project, it was not until 2017 that an effort started to try to harmonize outcomes across these and potentially other NHGRI-funded projects. This was initially accomplished by creating formal liaisons between each of the respective outcomes groups, and by holding joint meetings between the networks/consortium [14]. While this has resulted in some convergence, the differences between the projects and the lack of alignment of the project timelines have hindered the agreement on a standard set of outcomes across the three networks.

eMERGE is in its third phase of funding. The focus of this phase is the return of genomic results to participants [15]. A total of just over 25,000 participants will be sequenced on a next-generation sequencing platform, eMERGEseq, that contains 109 genes and a number of single nucleotide variants, including pharmacogenomic variants that may also be returned to participants [16]. The eMERGE Outcomes Working Group (OWG) was tasked to develop outcome measures for a set of genetic disorders for which the associated genes would be interrogated by sequencing. The OWG identified another NHGRI-funded project, the Clinical Genome Resource (ClinGen) [17] that had a relevant activity that could be used to move outcomes harmonization forward. Herein we report the results of a comparison between the eMERGE-defined outcomes and the ClinGen outcome intervention pairs.

2. Materials and Methods

eMERGE network sites represented on the OWG selected a disorder(s) for which their site developed clinical outcome measures. The outcomes were organized into three categories, process outcomes, intermediate outcomes, and health outcomes (Table 1). While health outcomes are of the greatest interest, the relatively short project timeline necessitated reliance on the process and intermediate outcomes for which a chain of evidence exists relating them to health outcomes of interest. Sites developed outcomes using their own approach, with the expectation that any proposed outcomes would have evidence of its relevance to clinical care. Emphasis was given to outcomes that were related to published clinical and practice guidelines where available. Once the draft outcomes were developed, they were presented to the OWG for discussion and revisions. The penultimate draft was submitted to the eMERGE coordinating center that, under the direction of one of the OWG co-chairs (JP), was tasked to develop the outcomes into a collection tool that could be created in REDCap [18] using a standard format. The coordinating center worked with the individual sites to create the final version of the outcomes.

Table 1. The framework of outcomes for clinical implementation.

Outcome Type	Description	Examples
Process	The specific steps in a process that lead—either positively or negatively—to a particular health outcome	Lipid profile performed after the return of a pathogenic variant in *LDLR*, a gene associated with familial hypercholesterolemia
Intermediate	A biomarker associated—either positively or negatively—to a particular health outcome	An LDL cholesterol level at or below the target level of 100 mg/dL in response to interventions recommended based on presences of a pathogenic variant in *LDLR*
Health	Change in the health of an individual, group of people or population which is attributable to an intervention or series of interventions	Decrease in myocardial infarction, or cardiac revascularization procedures in response to interventions recommended based on presences of a pathogenic variant in *LDLR*

The ClinGen Actionability Working Group (AWG) was tasked to assess the relative actionability of returning a genomic variant identified in an asymptomatic patient undergoing next-generation sequencing [19]. This was to be accomplished through four activities:

1. Develop rigorous and standardized procedures for categorically defining "clinical actionability"; a concept that includes a known ability to intervene and thereby avert a poor outcome due to a previously unsuspected high risk of disease
2. Nominate genes and diseases to score for "clinical actionability"
3. Produce evidence-based reports and semi-quantitative metric scores using a standardized method for nominated gene-disease pairs
4. Make these reports and actionability scores publicly available to aid broad efforts for prioritizing those human genes with the greatest relevance for clinical intervention.

The AWG has developed a set of outcome intervention pairs [20] that have been scored using a standardized approach informed by evidence-based summaries as described in a methods paper from 2016 [21]. The published outcome intervention pairs table represents those that have been scored by the AWG. The evidence summary also contains interventions and outcomes that were not formally scored. Both the table and the associated evidence summary were reviewed to completely ascertain the interventions and outcomes that had been reviewed by the AWG.

For the comparison, each site participating in the exercise compared the set of outcomes developed for the disorder in eMERGE to the corresponding outcome intervention pair published on the AWG website. If the eMERGE outcome was represented in the scored AWG outcome intervention pair, it was categorized as concordant. If it was not represented in the scored AWG outcome intervention pair, but was noted in the evidence summary, it was also categorized as concordant with the annotation that it did not cross the threshold for scoring by the AWG. If the outcome was not present in either the scored list or evidence summary, it was categorized as discordant. Conversely, if an outcome intervention was present on the AWG scored list, but not represented as an eMERGE outcome, it was also categorized as discordant. The evidence summaries were not comprehensively reviewed for outcomes to compare to eMERGE outcomes.

The sites' comparisons were compiled and reviewed by one of the authors (MSW) who also independently compared the eMERGE outcomes to the AWG outcome intervention pairs. No differences were noted between the sites' scores and the second review for the AWG outcome intervention pairs. A few outcomes were identified in the evidence summaries that had not been scored by the sites, and these were added to the comparison table. The final comparison table was reviewed and approved by all the authors.

3. Results

A total of 12 disorders were scored (Tables 2 and 3). The full comparison table with all defined eMERGE outcomes for each disorder is provided in the supplemental materials. Three gene/variant disorder pairs with outcomes defined by eMERGE do not have an AWG actionability score or evidence summary. *CFTR*/Cystic Fibrosis is being returned by eMERGE but has not yet been evaluated by the ClinGen AWG. While adult familial hypercholesterolemia (FH associated with the genes *LDLR*, *APOB*, and *PCSK9*) has been evaluated by both the OWG and AWG, FH in the pediatric population has only been evaluated by the OWG. This is because ClinGen initially focused on conditions in the adult population. However, this year, a pediatric AWG is being convened by ClinGen and one of their first conditions to evaluate will be pediatric FH. Finally, eMERGE is studying a large, well-characterized copy number variant (CNV) at chromosome 22q11.2 that encompasses many genes. The AWG is only looking at single gene-disorder associations at present.

Of the remaining nine gene(s)-disorder pairs defined by eMERGE, five had equivalent definitions from the AWG, while four had some differences which raised interesting issues that impacted the comparison. These two groups will be discussed separately.

The five disorders with equivalent definitions from both groups and the associated genes are presented in Table 2. It should be noted that the eMERGE project is only returning results from two genes that are associated with breast and/or ovarian cancer risk (*BRCA1* and *BRCA2*). Three genes with evidence for association with breast cancer are on the eMERGEseq platform (*ATM*, *CHEK2*, *PALB2*), but were not used to develop outcomes. These have been scored by the AWG but had much lower actionability scores than *BRCA1* and *BRCA2*; therefore, they were excluded from the comparison for the purposes of this study.

Comparing AWG scoring to the eMERGE outcomes list demonstrates significant concordance. Only two of the outcome intervention pairs scored by AWG was not present in the eMERGE outcomes. Both of these represented health outcomes (diagnosis of tumors and/or lymphangioleiomyomatosis (LAM) in the tuberous sclerosis complex (TSC) and high cholesterol in adult FH. For the latter, lipid values will be obtained from EHR review so a determination can be made as to whether a participant who has been tested is at a goal. Thus, while this is not explicitly represented in the eMERGE outcomes, it should be added given the robust association between low-density lipoprotein cholesterol (LDLC) and cardiovascular events [22–24]. For the TSC health outcomes, eMERGE will be capturing information about the prior diagnosis of sub-ependymal giant astrocytoma (SEGA), other TSC-associated non-SEGA tumors, and LAM. It is also possible that the diagnostic evaluation prompted by the genomic result could lead to a diagnosis of one of the conditions. However, given the short time period of the eMERGE project, a long-term longitudinal follow-up is not feasible, in contrast to the AWG score, which is meant to inform interventions over a patient's lifetime.

While most of the eMERGE outcomes are not represented in the AWG scored outcome intervention pairs, most are discussed in the evidence review that accompanies the scored pairs. The AWG methodology does not score all possible outcome intervention pairs, rather it focuses on those interventions that have the strongest impact on the most important health outcomes of interest.

Table 2. Disorders with equivalent definitions from eMERGE and ClinGen.

Disorder	Genes	eMERGE Outcomes	AWG Scored O/I Pair	AWG Evidence Review
		Process		
		Metabolic Testing	No	Yes
		Metabolic Crisis Plan in EHR	No	No
OTC Deficiency	*OTC*	**Intermediate**		
		Low Protein Diet	Yes	
		Prescription for Nitrogen Scavenger	Yes	
		Health		
		Metabolic protocol applied during illness	Yes (Hyperammonemic encephalopathy)	
		Process		
		Imaging studies	Yes	
		Assessment for LAM	Yes	
		Intermediate		
Tuberous Sclerosis	*TSC1, TSC2*	Discontinuation of estrogen containing medications (F)	No	Yes
		Use of inhibitor of renin-aldosterone-angiotensin system as first line therapy for hypertension	No	No
		Avoid ACE inhibitor	No	No
		No	Use of mTOR inhibitor	
		Health		
		No	Development of SEGA, non-SEGA tumors, LAM	
		Process		
		Breast Self-exam	Yes	
		Breast Imaging	Yes	
		Specialty Referral	No	Yes
HBOC (Breast)	*BRCA1, BRCA2*	**Intermediate**		
		Risk reducing mastectomy	Yes	Yes
		Selective estrogen receptor modulator	No	No
		Aromatase Inhibitor	No	No
		Discontinuation HRT	No	
		Health		
		Breast Cancer	Yes	Yes
		Vital Status	No	

Table 2. *Cont.*

Disorder	Genes	eMERGE Outcomes	AWG Scored O/I Pair	AWG Evidence Review
HBOC (Ovarian)	*BRCA1, BRCA2*	**Process**		
		Pelvic US	No	Yes
		CA 125	No	No
		Specialty Referral	No	Yes
		Intermediate		
		Prophylactic BSO or TAH/BSO	Yes	No
		Oral Contraceptives	No	
		Health		
		Ovarian, Fallopian, Peritoneal or Endometrial Cancer	Yes	
		Vital Status	No	Yes
		Process		
		Laboratory testing (lipid, CRP)	No	Yes
		Coronary CT angiogram	No	Yes
		Echocardiogram	No	Yes
		ECG	No	No
		Stress test	No	No
		Specialty Referral	No	No
		No		Cardiac Catheterization
Adult FH	*LDLR, APOB, PCSK9*	**Intermediate**		
		Lipid Lowering Therapy	Yes (statins)	High-intensity statins
		Aspirin	No	Yes
		Coronary revascularization	No	No
		No	High Cholesterol	
		Health		

Table 3. Disorders with differing definitions between eMERGE and ClinGen.

Disorder	Genes	eMERGE Outcomes	ClinGen Actionability Working Group			
			Lynch syndrome (*MLH1, MSH2, MSH6, PMS2*)		Familial Adenomatous Polyposis (*FAP*)	
		Process	**Scored O/I Pair**	**Evidence Review**	**Scored O/I Pair**	**Evidence Review**
Colorectal Cancer	*MLH1, MSH2, MSH6, PMS2, FAP*	Specialist Referral	No	No	No	Yes (Gastroenterology)
		Intermediate				
		CRC Screening	Yes		No	No
		Other cancer screening	Yes	Yes	No	Yes
		Familial Cascade Testing	No		Colectomy	Yes
		Health				
		CRC (Polyps, Hospitalization, Death)	Yes		Yes	
		Gynecologic cancer (endometrial, ovarian)	Yes		N/A	N/A

Disorder	Genes	eMERGE Outcomes	ClinGen Actionability Working Group			
			Arterial Tortuosity Syndrome (*SLC2A10*)		FTAAD (*FBN1, TGFBR1/2, SMAD3, ACTA2, MYLK, MYH11*)	
		Process	**Scored O/I Pair**	**Evidence Review**	**Scored O/I Pair**	**Evidence Review**
Aortopathies	*FBN1, TGFBR1/2, SMAD3, ACTA2, MYLK, MYH11*	Aortic Imaging	Yes		Yes	
		Magnetic Resonance Angiography	Yes		Yes	
		High risk pregnancy management	Yes		Yes	
		Recommendation to avoid contact sports	No		No	Yes
		Ophthalmologic eval	No		No	Yes
		Intermediate				
		Medication (beta-blocker, ARB)	Yes (both)		Yes (beta-blocker)	
		Prophylactic surgical intervention	No	Yes	No	Yes

Table 3. Cont.

Disorder	Genes	eMERGE Outcomes	ClinGen Actionability Working Group					
			Dilated Cardiomyopathy (TNNT2, LMNA, DMD)		Hypertrophic Cardiomyopathy (ACTC1, CSRP3, MYBPC3, MYH7, MYL2, MYL3, PRKAG2, TNNI3, TNNT2, TPM1)		Arrhythmogenic Right Ventricular Cardiomyopathy (DSC2, DSG2, DSP, PKP2, TMEM43)	
		Process	Scored O/I Pair	Evidence Review	Scored O/I Pair	Evidence Review	Scored O/I Pair	Evidence Review
Cardiomyopathies	ACTC1, DSC2, DSG2, DSP, LMNA, MYCH7, MYBPC3, MYL2, MYL3, PKP2, TMEM43, TNNI3, TNNT2, TPM1	EKG	Yes		No	Yes	No	Yes
		Echocardiogram	Yes		No	Yes	No	Yes
		Holter Monitor	No	No	No	Yes	No	Yes
		Loop recorder	No	No	No	Yes	No	No
		Stress Test	No	No	No	Yes	No	No
		Electrophysiology Study	No	No	No	No	No	Yes
		Cardiac MRI	No	No	No	No	No	Yes
		Intermediate						
		Specialty Referral	Yes		No	Yes	No	No
		Medications	Yes		No	Yes	Yes	
		Implantable Defibrillator	Yes		Yes		Yes	
		Documentation of Activity Restriction	No	No	No	Yes	No	Yes
		Health						
		Sudden Cardiac Death	Yes		Yes		Yes	
		Reduce Heart Failure	Yes		No	No	No	

Disorder	Genes	eMERGE Outcomes	ClinGen Actionability Working Group					
			Brugada syndrome (SCN5A)		Catecholaminergic polymorphic ventricular tachycardia (RYR2)		Romano-Ward Long QT syndromes (KCNH2, KCNQ1, SCN5A)	
		Process	Scored O/I Pair	Evidence Review	Scored O/I Pair	Evidence Review	Scored O/I Pair	Evidence Review
Inherited arrhythmias	KCNH2, KCNQ1, RYR2, SCN5A	EKG	No	Yes	No	Yes	No	Yes
		Echocardiogram	No	No	No	No	No	No
		Holter Monitor	No	No	No	Yes	No	No
		Loop recorder	No	Yes	No	No	No	No
		Stress Test	No	No	No	Yes	No	No
		Electrophysiology Study	No	No	No	No	No	No
		Cardiac MRI	No	No	No	No	No	No
		Trial Sodium Channel Blocker	No	Yes	No	No	No	No
		Personal history of arrhythmias	No	Yes	No	Yes	No	Yes
		Specialty referral	No	Yes	No	No	No	No
		Intermediate						
		Symptoms suggestive of arrhythmia	No	Yes	No	Yes	No	Yes
		Medications	No	Yes (quinidine)	Yes	Yes	Yes (beta-blockers are ineffective for LQT3)	
		Activity restriction	Yes		No	Yes	No	Yes
		ICD	Yes		No	No	Yes	No
		Health						
		Sudden Cardiac Death	Yes		Yes	Yes	Yes	

Hereditary breast and ovarian cancer syndrome (HBOC), associated with *BRCA1/2*, illustrates an interesting difference in the OWG and AWG approaches. The eMERGE OWG developed outcomes for HBOC as a whole, while the AWG has organized this around the two primary cancer types, breast, and ovarian and associated gynecologic cancers. This is logical as the outcome intervention pairs for the two types of cancers are quite different. This is not incompatible with the eMERGE outcomes, and Table 2 reflects how the outcomes can be separated to allow comparison.

A more important difference in the approach between the two groups is illustrated in Table 3. The four disorders represented, cardiomyopathy, inherited arrhythmogenic disorders, aortopathies, and colorectal cancer (CRC) predisposition illustrate the tension between pragmatic decisions to reduce the burden to collect outcomes of interest at the expense of capturing outcomes that are specific to individual disorders lumped within the overarching category of disorders. Some of these differences are clinically significant as discussed below.

3.1. Colorectal Cancer Predisposition

The eMERGE outcomes combine two disorders, Lynch syndrome (LS) and the rarer familial adenomatous polyposis (FAP), while these are scored separately by the ClinGen AWG. There is good concordance between eMERGE and the AWG scored intervention outcome pairs. One significant difference is in FAP, for which the AWG does not score CRC surveillance. Review of the evidence summary presents the rationale that the polyp burden reduces the effectiveness of surveillance. The outcome intervention pair scored by the AWG for FAP is colectomy to prevent CRC. This is consistent with the clinical guidelines for FAP [25], although this recommendation may not be as relevant for patients with attenuated FAP, as they have fewer polyps than FAP (hundreds vs. thousands). Colectomy is listed as an option for reducing the risk of CRC in patients with LS, but is generally not indicated due to the effectiveness of routine colonoscopy in prevention. Another difference between FAP and LS is that the non-CRC tumors differ and occur at a higher frequency in LS. This necessitates different screening approaches which are detailed in the AWG evidence reports. Finally, the AWG evidence reports also discuss the use of aspirin (LS) and non-steroidal anti-inflammatory drugs other than aspirin (FAP) to reduce the CRC risk. These should be considered for inclusion in the eMERGE outcomes.

3.2. Aortopathies

The OWG developed outcomes to accommodate all disorders that could result in aortic root dilation and other arteriopathies. The AWG divided these into arterial tortuosity syndrome (associated with variants in *SLC2A10*), and Familial Thoracic Aortic Aneurysms and Dissections (FTAAD associated with seven genes-Table 3). The AWG scored each of these FTAAD genes separately, although the evidence summary was the same for all seven genes. The actionability scores for the seven gene-disorder pairs were identical. As with CRC, there was very good concordance between the eMERGE outcomes and the AWG scored outcome intervention pairs. Indeed, the only discrepancies were recommendations for avoidance of contact sports and evaluation by an ophthalmologist, both present as a scored recommendation for arterial tortuosity syndrome, present in the evidence summary for FTAAD but not scored, and absent from eMERGE. Given that many of these disorders have associated ophthalmologic findings, this should be considered as an outcome by the eMERGE OWG. Recommendations to avoid activities such as contact sports are difficult to extract from medical records, so they were not considered for practical considerations.

There is one other issue with the aortopathies that complicates outcome development. There are two multiple malformation syndromes that can be seen in patients with variants in some of these genes, the Marfan and Loeys-Dietz syndromes. This complexity was acknowledged by the ClinGen AWG, as both disorders have been scored as separate entities. These syndromes are associated with many other medical issues; however, the scored outcome intervention pairs are concordant with the recommendations for aortic root dilation represented in arterial tortuosity syndrome and FTAAD.

However, the evidence summary goes into much more detail about the other medical issues associated with these syndromes. The eMERGE OWG recognizes this issue and it is anticipated that a targeted clinical evaluation will occur in conjunction with the return of results.

3.3. Cardiomyopathies

The eMERGEseq platform has 14 genes associated with three forms of cardiomyopathy: dilated, hypertrophic, and arrhythmogenic right ventricular (ARVC). One form was developed to capture outcomes for all three disorders. The ClinGen AWG scored each of the three disorders separately, and further scored each of the five ARVC genes separately, although as with FTAAD, the scores were identical for each of the five genes. The major risk for all three of these disorders is sudden death, and this health outcome is common across all the conditions. Related to this, an implantable cardiac defibrillator (ICD) is also present across all conditions. Not surprisingly, given the differences in the clinical course of these three conditions, beyond sudden cardiac death and ICD, there is a considerably more difference in the other outcomes. Most of these differences appropriately reflect the clinical differences between the conditions. There is only one AWG recommendation that is not reflected in the OWG outcomes. A creatine kinase determination is recommended for dilated cardiomyopathy associated with variants in *DMD*. However, *DMD* is not included on the eMERGEseq platform, explaining this difference. One gene associated with dilated cardiomyopathy, *LMNA*, is associated with several other disorders. One of them is Emery-Dreifuss Muscular Dystrophy (EDMD), which was scored separately by the AWG. There were other outcome intervention pairs scored for EDMD in addition to those related to cardiomyopathy. The eMERGE network decided that it would only return variants in *LMNA* associated with dilated cardiomyopathy, so outcomes for the other disorders were not considered. One other issue with the cardiomyopathies reviewed by the AWG is that variants in *TNNT2* can cause either dilated or hypertrophic cardiomyopathy. This pleiotropy will be more of an issue in the next group of disorders.

3.4. Inherited Arrhythmias

The eMERGEseq platform has four genes associated with three inherited arrhythmogenic disorders: Brugada syndrome, catecholaminergic polymorphic ventricular tachycardia (CPVT), and Romano-Ward Long QT syndromes (LQT). As with the cardiomyopathies, the major risk is for sudden death. This health outcome is represented across all conditions. ICD is an AWG recommendation for two of the three conditions. CPVT is the exception given the effectiveness of the beta-blockade to prevent sudden cardiac death in this disorder. There are numerous differences between the OWG outcomes and the AWG that reflect the differences in the conditions. The most notable absence from the eMERGE outcomes were medications to avoid in each condition. The AWG evidence reports provide detailed lists of medications and other substances to avoid as they can provoke abnormal cardiac rhythms. These are important to document and should be considered in addition to the eMERGE outcomes, as the documentation of medications associated with adverse events are relatively easy to find on the chart review.

As noted with *TNNT2* previously, one gene (*SCN5A*) is associated with two different arrhythmogenic disorders: Brugada syndrome and LQT3. There are several unique aspects to disorders associated with variants in *SCN5A*. For patients with Brugada syndrome, a trial of therapy with sodium channel blockers is indicated. The recommended anti-arrhythmic drug is quinidine. Both recommendations are specific only for the arrhythmogenic disorders associated with variants in *SCN5A*. For LQT3, the treatment with beta-blockers is not indicated as these have been shown to be ineffective in this condition. These findings argue persuasively for outcomes that are not only condition specific but gene and potentially even variant specific when appropriate.

4. Discussion

The results of this study show that it is possible to compare outcomes from two projects despite differences in the project objectives and methods. The important finding is that outcomes that are represented across multiple projects can be prioritized to harmonize the outcome definitions and develop guidance for their collection. This will facilitate the collection of prioritized outcomes from a wider set of research projects and clinical implementations, allowing evidence to accumulate at a faster rate to support clinical use. An example of the power of this type of approach for a genetic condition is cystic fibrosis (CF). Certified CF centers who receive funding from the CF Foundation are required to collect and submit many standard outcome measures. The outcomes are compared across sites and opportunities to improve care are identified, followed by implementation at the centers. This approach, which is also being used in other settings, has resulted in a dramatic improvement in multiple outcomes of interest for patients with CF [26]. The hope is that similar improvements in care could be realized across the many conditions for which genomic information can be used to inform care.

While there was generally good agreement for the high-level outcomes across the various conditions, there are some significant differences—the highlighting of which could inform further efforts to harmonize outcomes. eMERGE and ClinGen have very different objectives. The eMERGE network is studying the impact of implementation of genomic information into clinical care. To fully understand this impact, the outcomes are much more granular and detailed to allow chart abstractors to identify relevant information from the EHR. For example, in the cardiomyopathies (Table 3), process outcomes include five different interventions that assess the cardiac conduction system and two imaging modalities. The ClinGen scored outcome/intervention pairs only list one assessment of the cardiac conduction system and one imaging modality, and that was only for dilated cardiomyopathy. This is understandable as the scored pairs represent the results of the evidence synthesis that identifies the interventions and outcomes that drive clinical actionability, the key objective for ClinGen—a much different objective compared to eMERGE. Nonetheless, most of the eMERGE outcomes were identified in the ClinGen evidence reviews, although the reviews identified a few outcomes not included in the eMERGE OWG outcomes that are worthy of consideration for inclusion. Additionally, the AWG scored some gene-disorder pairs that, while on the eMERGEseq platform, are not being routinely returned. If the OWG proceeds with outcomes development for these genes, the AWG outcome intervention pairs and evidence summary will be used to inform the process.

A more complex issue is illustrated by the conditions in Tables 2 and 3, that is, how best to map outcomes for separate but related disorders. While it may be desirable to create outcomes specific for each disorder within a category, the time and effort required to do this are significant. Therefore, the eMERGE OWG opted to develop one outcome form for an overarching disorder category that encompasses multiple conditions. While this reduces the resources needed to create the outcome forms and simplifies the work for the chart abstractor, it will require more effort by the OWG after the abstraction to map the outcomes that are specific to the relevant disorder in order to determine whether appropriate condition-specific management goals were achieved. Challenges with this issue are also evident in the ClinGen AWG scoring as some conditions lump all genes under one disorder (e.g., familial hypertrophic cardiomyopathy), while others have a separate score for each gene (e.g., FTAAD, ARVC). In these examples the scored outcome intervention pairs are identical across the different genes, raising the question as to the value added from this approach. In contrast, the three LQT disorders have different interventions based on the causal gene, supporting separate scoring of the outcome intervention pair. A further complication involves a pleiotropy of disorders associated with variants in the same gene. The issues with *SCN5A* and *LMNA* described previously illustrate the challenges of developing outcomes for disorders associated with variants in these genes. The most precise solution would be to develop outcomes based on the established genotype-phenotype correlations, but this further increases the complexity. This issue has led to the creation within ClinGen of the Lumping and Splitting Working Group (LSWG) [27]. The goal of the LSWG is to engage with a broad range of stakeholders to gather input " ... to coordinate disease classification and categorization in order to harmonize disease categorization and classification for the greater community". The work product from this group will be incorporated into the ongoing efforts for outcomes harmonization.

Chromosome 22q11.2 deletion syndrome (22q11.2DS) is the most common chromosomal microdeletion disorder with approximately 3.0 million base pairs deleted (ranging from 0.7–3.0 Mb) resulting in a loss of ~90 known or predicted genes, including 46 protein-coding genes and 7 microRNAs, 10 non-coding RNAs, and 27 pseudogenes (Figure 1) [28]. The 22q11.2DS results most commonly from de novo non-homologous meiotic recombination events occurring in approximately 1 in every 1000 fetuses and 1 in 2000 live births. About 4% of infants with 22q11.2DS succumb to it, while cardiac defects, hypocalcemia, and airways disease are risk factors for early death, with the median age of death at 3–4 months. However, most individuals with 22q11.2DS survive well into adulthood, at which time approximately 50% of them develop schizophrenia.

While ClinGen (currently) makes no recommendations with respect to 22q11.2DS we note the syndrome has become a model for understanding rare and frequent congenital anomalies such as heart defects, medical conditions including immunodeficiency, allergies, asthma, and psychiatric and developmental differences, which may provide a platform into better understanding these phenotypes, while affording opportunities for translational strategies across the lifespan for both patients with 22q11.2DS and for those with these associated features in the general population. The diverse phenotype and outcomes of nearly every organ system make this population valuable for understanding the variables that impact on the manifestations of the deletion, which is relatively consistent from person to person.

The eMERGESeq panel captures six SNPs (five in the *COMT* gene and one flanking the region), which can be used to capture 22q11.2DS, while existing genotype data can be readily used to detect the syndrome. Current efforts aim at assessing the prevalence of 22q11.2DS in respective eMERGE cohorts, and to determine a health outcome across multiple organ systems and outcome measures as available.

We are using PennCNV and XHMM to derive CNVs from eMERGESeq data, as well as existing array data. Data will be returned to participating sites for outcome evaluation of relevant phenotypes (e.g., heart defects, immunodeficiency, allergy, asthma, psychiatric, and developmental differences) and for additional validation, if required.

This study represents a pilot to assess the feasibility of harmonizing outcomes across two notable research projects. As such the results are descriptive and limited to the two projects assessed. The study did not include the evaluation of outcomes for any clinical genomic medicine implementation projects. However, one eMERGE site reports the genomic results on a large scale in a clinical research setting [7]. Institutional authors (MSW, JLW), in conjunction with the Genetic Screening and Counseling Program at the institution, have aligned the eMERGE and institutional outcomes for the disorders shared in common between the two efforts (data not shown). The availability of the outcomes from eMERGE aided in the prioritization of the institutional outcomes, while input from the authors, both of whom are members of the eMERGE OWG, influenced the outcome definitions for the OWG. This illustrates that the harmonization of outcomes is not only feasible but may represent a generalizable approach. Mapping outcomes to standardized, structured terminologies such as the International Classifications of Disease (ICD) or the Systematized Nomenclature of Medicine-Clinical Terms (SNOMED-CT) would facilitate generalizability and reduce the reliance on manual collection, although it is important to note that many critical outcomes are not currently represented as structured data so some manual review will be required. It is possible that outcome "algorithms" could be developed. These would be similar to phenotyping algorithms that eMERGE has developed, disseminated across multiple healthcare and electronic health record systems and made publicly available through the Phenotype Knowledgebase-PheKB. [29] This could further reduce, although not eliminate, the burden of manual review.

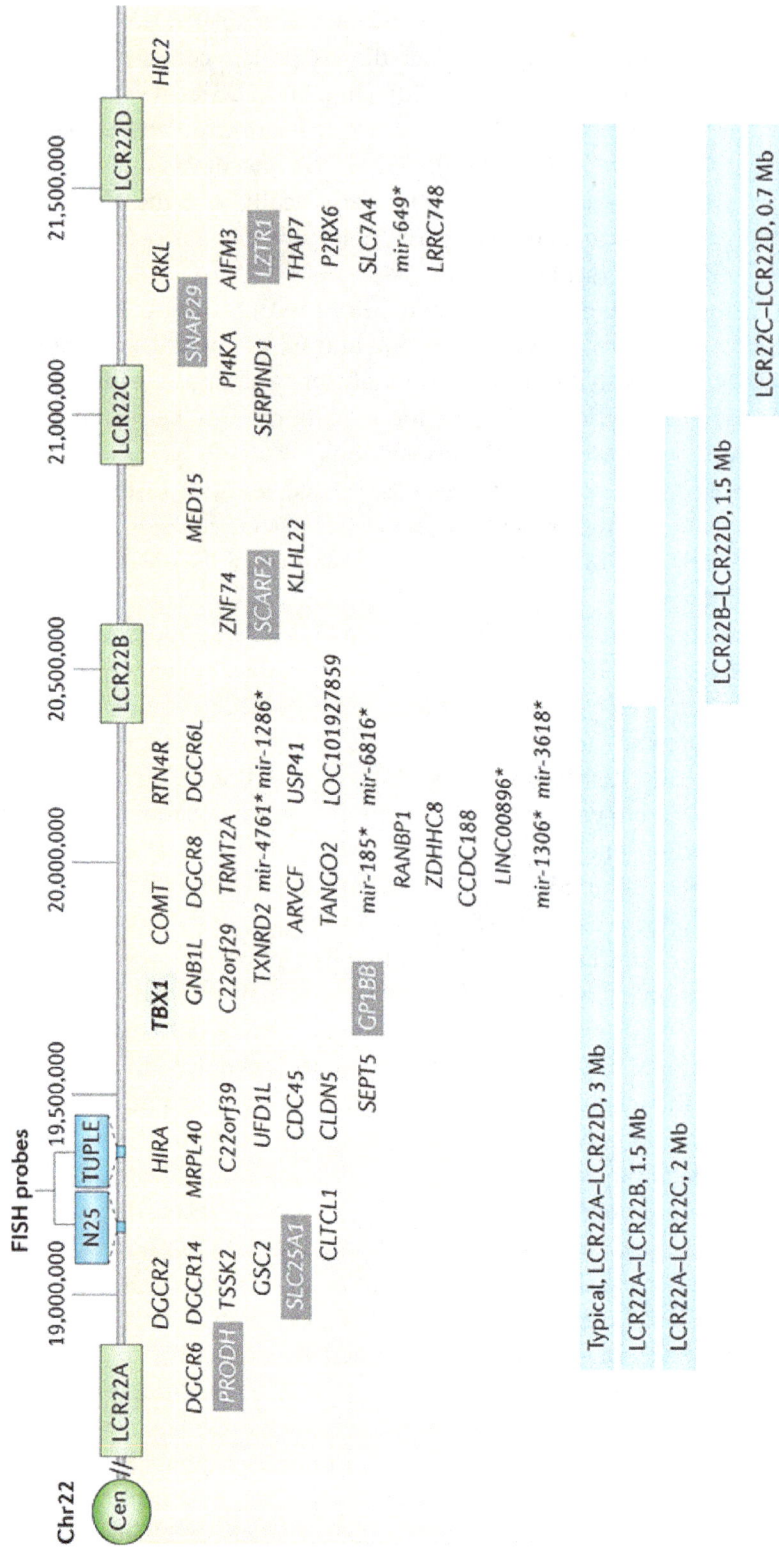

Figure 1. The depiction of the chromosome 22q11.2 deletion including the deleted genes and variations of the common deletions reported.

Another limitation of this study was the outcomes and process measures such as cost, reimbursement, institutional visibility, access, etc., which also play a role in decisions about implementation were not assessed. We also did not focus on patient-centered outcomes, which are not always aligned with health or other outcomes. Measuring outcomes from the perspective of the patient has been identified as a deficiency in much medical research as evidenced by the creation of the Patient-centered Outcomes Research Institute (PCORI) in 2010 [30]. The PCORI vision statement ("patients and the public have the information they can use to make decisions that reflect their desired health outcomes") emphasizes that part of precision medicine is understanding what outcomes the patient desires, which will vary from patient to patient. Patient engagement is a key part of the All of Us project [5], therefore, developing and harmonizing patient-centered outcomes for genomic medicine is important. Of interest, the NIH funded the development and harmonization of a large set of patient-centered outcome measures now included in the Patient-Reported Outcomes Measurement Information System (PROMIS®) [31] made available through the Department of Health and Human Services. These measures can be reviewed and revised as necessary to develop patient-reported outcomes for genomic medicine. This also illustrates that a process led by the NIH to collect and harmonize outcome measures across its portfolio of projects is a successful approach and can promote the use of standardized measures going forward.

5. Conclusions

The definition and harmonization of common outcomes to develop evidence and assess the value of genomic medicine implementation are needed to further the goals embodied in precision public health. The approach proposed in this study will be applied to other NHGRI-funded genomic implementation projects. The resulting outcomes will be made publicly available and their use will be encouraged for outcome measurement, collection, and research to accelerate the implementation of those interventions that demonstrate improved value.

Author Contributions: Conceptualization and Methodology, M.S.W., J.L.W., D.L.V., J.F.P., H.H.; Validation, M.S.W.; Formal Analysis, All authors; Data Curation, M.S.W., G.P.J., J.F.P., W.K.C., I.A.H., C.H., H.H., J.J.C.; Writing—Original Draft Preparation, M.S.W.; Writing—Review & Editing, All authors; Supervision, M.S.W.; Project Administration, M.S.W., G.P.J., M.E.S.; Funding Acquisition, G.P.J., E.B.L., H.H., J.F.P., M.E.S., W.K.C., K.K., C.W., M.S.W.

Funding: This work was supported by U01HG8657 (Group Health Cooperative/University of Washington); U01HG8685 (Brigham and Women's Hospital); U01HG8672 (Vanderbilt University Medical Center); U01HG8679 (Geisinger Clinic); U01HG8680 (Columbia University Health Sciences); U01HG8684 (Children's Hospital of Philadelphia); U01HG8673 (Northwestern University); U01HG8701 (Vanderbilt University Medical Center serving as the Coordinating Center).

Acknowledgments: Northwestern University—Laura Rasmussen-Torvik, Lisa Castillo for creating the cardiomyopathy outcome forms; Vanderbilt—Brittany City for coordinating and editing eMERGE outcomes forms, Department of Medicine, Columbia University—Katherine Crew for creating the breast cancer outcomes form.

References

1. Definition Genomic Medicine NHGRI. Available online: https://www.genome.gov/27552451/what-is-genomic-medicine/ (accessed on 26 May 2018).
2. Relling, M.V.; Evan, W.E. Pharmacogenomics in the Clinic. *Nature* **2015**, *526*, 343–350. [CrossRef] [PubMed]
3. Haslem, D.S.; Van Norman, S.B.; Fulde, G.; Knighton, A.J.; Belnap, T.; Butler, A.M.; Rhagunath, S.; Newman, D.; Gilbert, H.; Tudor, B.P.; et al. A retrospective analysis of precision medicine outcomes in patients with advanced cancer reveals improved progression-free survival without increased health care costs. *J. Oncol. Pract.* **2017**, *13*, e108–e119. [CrossRef] [PubMed]
4. Stark, Z.; Schofield, D.; Martyn, M.; Rynehart, L.; Shrestha, R.; Alam, K.; Lunke, S.; Tan, T.Y.; Gaff, C.L.; White, S.M. Does genomic sequencing early in the diagnostic trajectory make a difference? A follow-up study of clinical outcomes and cost-effectiveness. *Genet. Med.* **2018**, *15*. [CrossRef] [PubMed]
5. All of Us. Available online: https://allofus.nih.gov/ (accessed on 26 May 2018).

6.   Inova Translational Medicine Institute. Available online: https://www.inova.org/itmi/home (accessed on 26 May 2018).

7.   Williams, M.S.; Buchanan, A.H.; Davis, F.D.; Faucett, W.A.; Hallquist, M.L.G.; Leader, J.B.; Martin, C.L.; McCormick, C.Z.; Meyer, M.N.; Murray, M.F.; et al. Patient-Centered precision health in a learning health care system: Geisinger's Genomic medicine experience. *Health Aff.* **2018**, *37*, 757–764. [CrossRef] [PubMed]

8.   Manolio, T.A.; Chisolm, R.L.; Ozenberger, B.; Roden, D.M.; Williams, M.S.; Wilson, R.; Bick, D.; Bottinger, E.; Brilliant, M.H.; Eng, C.; et al. Implementing Genomic Medicine in the Clinic: The Future is Here. *Genet. Med.* **2013**, *15*, 258–267. [CrossRef] [PubMed]

9.   Phillips, K.A.; Deverka, P.A.; Sox, H.C.; Khoury, M.J.; Sandy, L.G.; Ginsburg, G.S.; Tunis, S.R.; Orlando, L.A.; Douglas, M.P. Making genomic medicine evidence-based and patient-centered: A structured review and landscape analysis of comparative effectiveness research. *Genet. Med.* **2017**, *19*, 1081–1091. [CrossRef] [PubMed]

10. Horgan, D.; Jansen, M.; Leyens, L.; Lal, J.A.; Sudbrak, R.; Hackenitz, E.; Bußhoff, U.; Ballensiefen, W.; Brand, A. An index of barriers for the implementation of personalised medicine and pharmacogenomics in Europe. *Public Health Genom.* **2014**, *17*, 287–298. [CrossRef] [PubMed]

11. IGNITE Network. Available online: https://ignite-genomics.org/ (accessed on 26 May 2018).

12. CSER Consortium. Available online: https://cser-consortium.org/ (accessed on 26 May 2018).

13. eMERGE Network. Available online: https://emerge.mc.vanderbilt.edu/ (accessed on 26 May 2018).

14. eMERGE and CSER Joint Meeting. Available online: https://www.genome.gov/27567557/emerge--cser-the-convergence-of-genomics-and-medicine/ (accessed on 26 May 2018).

15. eMERGE Phase 3. Available online: https://www.genome.gov/27540473/electronic-medical-records-and-genomics-emerge-network/ (accessed on 26 May 2018).

16. eMERGEseq Platform. Available online: https://emerge.mc.vanderbilt.edu/the-emergeseq-platform/ (accessed on 26 May 2018).

17. Clinical Genome Resource. Available online: https://www.clinicalgenome.org/ (accessed on 26 May 2018).

18. REDCap. Available online: https://www.project-redcap.org/ (accessed on 26 May 2018).

19. ClinGen Actionability Working Group. Available online: https://www.clinicalgenome.org/working-groups/actionability/ (accessed on 26 May 2018).

20. Actionability Outcome Intervention Pairs. Available online: https://www.clinicalgenome.org/working-groups/actionability/projects-initiatives/actionability-evidence-based-summaries/ (accessed on 26 May 2018).

21. Hunter, J.E.; Irving, S.A.; Biesecker, L.G.; Buchanan, A.; Jensen, B.; Lee, K.; Martin, C.L.; Milko, L.; Muessig, K.; Niehaus, A.D.; et al. A standardized, evidence-based protocol to assess clinical actionability of genetic disorders associated with genomic variation. *Genet. Med.* **2016**, *18*, 1258–1268. [CrossRef] [PubMed]

22. Stamler, J.; Wentworth, D.; Neaton, J.D. Is relationship between serum cholesterol and risk of premature death from coronary heart disease continuous and graded? Findings in 356,222 primary screenees of the Multiple Risk Factor Intervention Trial (MRFIT). *JAMA* **1986**, *256*, 2823–2828. [CrossRef] [PubMed]

23. Castelli, W.P.; Anderson, K.; Wilson, P.W.; Levy, D. Lipids and risk of coronary heart disease. The Framingham Study. *Ann. Epidemiol.* **1992**, *2*, 23–28. [CrossRef]

24. Levinson, S.S. Critical review of 2016 ACC guidelines on therapies for cholesterol lowering with reference to laboratory testing. *Clin. Chim. Acta* **2017**. [CrossRef] [PubMed]

25. Kohlmann, W.; Gruber, S.B. Lynch Syndrome. In *GeneReviews®*; Adam, M.P., Ardinger, H.H., Pagon, R.A., Eds.; University of Washington: Seattle, WA, USA, 2018. Available online: https://www.ncbi.nlm.nih.gov/books/NBK1211/ (accessed on 26 May 2018).

26. Khan, A.A.; Nash, E.F.; Whitehouse, J.; Rashid, R. Improving the care of patients with cystic fibrosis (CF). *BMJ Open Qual.* **2017**, *6*, e000020. [CrossRef] [PubMed]

27. ClinGen Lumping and Splitting Working Group. Available online: https://www.clinicalgenome.org/working-groups/lumping-and-splitting/ (accessed on 26 May 2018).

28. McDonald-McGinn, D.M.; Emanuel, B.S.; Zackai, E.H. 22q11.2 Deletion Syndrome. In *GeneReviews®*; Adam, M.P., Ardinger, H.H., Pagon, R.A., Eds.; University of Washington: Seattle, WA, USA, 2018. Available online: https://www.ncbi.nlm.nih.gov/books/NBK1523/ (accessed on 26 May 2018).

29. Phenotype Knowledgebase. Available online: https://phekb.org/ (accessed on 26 May 2018).

30. Patient Centered Outcomes Research Institute. Available online: https://www.pcori.org/about-us (accessed on 26 May 2018).
31. PROMIS®. Available online: http://www.healthmeasures.net/explore-measurement-systems/promis (accessed on 26 May 2018).

4

Impact of Quality Improvement on Care of Chronic Obstructive Pulmonary Disease Patients in an Internal Medicine Resident Clinic

Robert M. Burkes [1,*], Takudzwa Mkorombindo [1], Udit Chaddha [1], Alok Bhatt [1], Karim El-Kersh [2], Rodrigo Cavallazzi [2] and Nancy Kubiak [3] (iD)

[1]   Department of Internal Medicine, University of Louisville, 550 S. Jackson Street, ACB 3rd Floor, Louisville, KY 40202, USA; tmkorombindo@uabmc.edu (T.M.); drudit@gmail.com (U.C.); Alok.Bhatt@nyumc.org (A.B.)

[2]   Division of Pulmonary, Critical Care, and Sleep Medicine Disorders, Department of Internal Medicine, University of Louisville, 550 S. Jackson Street, Pulmonary, Critical Care and Sleep Disorders Medicine Offices, ACB 3rd Floor, Louisville, KY 40202, USA; Karim.elkersh@louisville.edu (K.E.-K.); r0cava01@louisville.edu (R.C.)

[3]   Department of General Internal Medicine, University of Louisville, Palliative Care, and Medical Education, 550 S. Jackson Street, General Internal Medicine and Palliative Care Offices, ACB 3rd Floor, Louisville, KY 40202, USA; Nancy.Kubiak@louisville.edu

*   Correspondence: Robert.Burkes@unchealth.unc.edu

Abstract: Chronic obstructive pulmonary disease (COPD) is a leading cause of morbidity and mortality. Guideline-discordant care of COPD is not uncommon. Further, there is a push to incorporate quality improvement (QI) training into internal medicine (IM) residency curricula. This study compared quality of care of COPD patients in an IM residents' clinic and a pulmonary fellows' clinic and, subsequently, the results of a quality improvement program in the residents' clinic. Pre-intervention rates of quality measure adherence were compared between the IM teaching clinic ($n = 451$) and pulmonary fellows' clinic ($n = 177$). Patient encounters in the residents' teaching clinic after quality improvement intervention ($n = 119$) were reviewed and compared with pre-intervention data. Prior to intervention, fellows were significantly more likely to offer smoking cessation counseling ($p = 0.024$) and document spirometry showing airway obstruction ($p < 0.001$). Smoking cessation counseling, pneumococcal vaccination, and diagnosis of COPD by spirometry were targets for QI. A single-cycle, resident-led QI project was initiated. After, residents numerically improved in the utilization of spirometry (66.5% vs. 74.8%) and smoking cessation counseling (81.8% vs. 86.6%), and significantly improved rates of pneumococcal vaccination ($p = 0.024$). One cycle of resident-led QI significantly improved the rates of pneumococcal vaccination, with numerical improvement in other areas of COPD care.

Keywords: pulmonary diseases; quality improvement; Medical Education; vaccinations; smoking cessation

1. Introduction

Chronic obstructive pulmonary disease (COPD) is a leading cause of death worldwide, with a prevalence of 10% [1,2]. The burden of COPD and tobacco abuse falls most heavily on those in the lower socioeconomic strata [3]. Further, misdiagnosis of chronic lung conditions is common in this demographic [4]. In light of these findings, it is imperative that residents in academic medical centers that treat underserved populations diagnose COPD accurately and provide high quality care.

The Accreditation Council for Graduate Medical Education (ACGME) requires residents to obtain skills to analyze patients' outcomes and "implement changes with the goal of practice improvement" [5]. Despite barriers including time constraints and lack of sufficient faculty with quality improvement (QI) training, projects with resident involvement have been successful at enacting meaningful change in the care of chronic medical conditions [6–9].

Spirometric testing showing obstructive lung disease, which is required for the diagnosis of COPD [2], is underutilized in the primary care setting. Without the use of spirometric measures, COPD is often misdiagnosed, and patients are treated with inhalers and steroids inappropriately [10–14]. Further, smoking cessation efforts are both efficacious and cost-effective, making cessation counseling an imperative aspect of care provided to COPD patients [15,16]. Also, the reported trend towards prevention of pneumococcal pneumonia and acute exacerbation of COPD with pneumococcal vaccination makes this an important aspect of the longitudinal care of the COPD patient [2].

The goal of this investigation is to evaluate shortcomings in the care of COPD patients in a residents' clinic and attempt a brief and low-cost intervention to improve these processes of care. This study evaluates the care of COPD patients provided by internal medicine residents as it pertains to guideline-based care and compares process-of-care measures with fellows at the same institution and assesses the feasibility and efficacy of a single round of quality improvement developed by residents and directed at their peers.

2. Materials and Methods

2.1. Participants

This is a quality improvement study with two distinct phases. An initial retrospective chart review phase included 628 patients (451 seen in the internal medicine residents' clinic and 177 seen in the pulmonary medicine fellows' clinic, both at the University of Louisville). For this particular training environment, residents had completed medical school training. Fellows were in pulmonary and critical care specialty training, had completed internal medicine training, and were board eligible/certified to practice general internal medicine (but not yet pulmonary medicine) in the United States. After identifying areas of treatment deficiency, a QI initiative (described below) was implemented from June 2016 to May 2017 (the bulk of one academic year for residents of training programs in the United States). Charts of the subsequent 119 encounters that received a billing code for COPD in the residents' clinic were reviewed in a prospective fashion.

The charts of patients diagnosed with chronic bronchitis (ICD-9 Code 491), emphysema (ICD-9 Code 492), and/or chronic airway obstruction (ICD-9 Code 496) were selected for review. For the purpose of this study, those with asthma (ICD-9 Code 493) without one of the aforementioned diagnoses, patients with paper charts that were illegible or had poor quality electronic scans, patients seen only once and lost to follow-up, and patients where COPD status was not actively reflected (i.e., COPD or respiratory symptoms never being addressed by provider) in their chart were excluded. Demographics, comorbidities including heart failure and asthma, spirometric data, smoking status, inhaled COPD medications, and vaccination status were collected. Spirometry data was found in either the patient's inpatient or outpatient chart or from scans of outside records. Each patient's vaccination record was recorded from inpatient or outpatient charts. Smoking cessation was determined based on the resident clinic note documenting that he or she had provided a smoking cessation intervention to the patient.

2.2. Quality Improvement Intervention

The quality improvement intervention was targeted at all residents ($n = 72$ residents, including this study's authors, sharing roughly the same size patient panel) in the general internal medicine residency training program at the University of Louisville, using the PDSA model of quality improvement. During the planning stage, the team identified opportunities for improving care by comparing resident-to-fellow performance for COPD guidelines. They crafted a short 15 min PowerPoint-based didactic session discussing current guideline-based care of COPD, data showing the adherence of residents to studied quality measures, and the plan for the future QI intervention. They created easy-to-use index cards to guide correct pneumococcal immunization and remind residents of the need for tobacco cessation counseling and spirometry to confirm diagnosis in patients with COPD. In the Do phase, the presentation was given by a third-year internal medicine resident to both residents and staff in the clinic, and that information was also sent via e-mail correspondence to residents. Residents were also provided weekly verbal reminders of the project. Index cards with an algorithmic approach to pneumococcal vaccination, based on current guidelines, were posted on the clinic's computers where residents checked-out to attending physicians and did office note documentation. A standing order for pneumococcal immunization was implemented in the clinic, allowing medical assistants to identify and vaccinate COPD patients. In the study phase, information on the effectiveness of the interventions was collected. Since the interventions improved rates, the team opted to continue episodic reminders about the intervention during the Act phase. Because printed index cards were donated, this intervention accrued no cost. The design, presentation, and implementation of the QI initiative was carried out by a group of four internal medicine residents (first four authors).

2.3. Outcomes Measured

Our outcomes were the rate at which patients who had a diagnosis of COPD underwent spirometry or pulmonary function testing (PFTs), the rate of pneumococcal vaccination, and documentation of smoking cessation counseling. These were chosen based on perceived importance in the care of COPD patients in the outpatient setting, the wide difference between rates of application in the residents' and fellows' clinic, and because these were considered the deficiencies most readily addressable by a QI expert consultant (Kubiak). These measures were compared in the residents' clinic and the fellows' clinic retrospectively prior to QI intervention, in order to delineate what was possible in the setting and to establish a baseline for the resident performance. In response to the retrospective findings, the same outcomes were compared in the residents' clinic before and after the QI intervention in a prospective, un-blinded fashion.

2.4. Statistical Analysis

The statistical modeling strategy sought to provide enumeration of adherence to quality measures [17]. We report continuous variables as mean and standard deviation, and categorical variables as frequency and percentage. We used a chi-squared test to compare categorical data and paired t-tests for continuous data. We considered a p-value less than 0.05 as statistically significant. Because each quality measure was assessed individually and not assumed to be associated with demographic or clinical aspects of the patient cohort, multivariate modeling was not performed. Statistical analysis was performed using Stata 10 (Stata Corp., College Station, TX, USA) software. The publication of this study, including the waiver of consent, was deemed exempt by the institutional review board at the University of Louisville (IRB: 15.0243).

3. Results

Prior to QI intervention, of the 628 charts reviewed, 451 patients were seen in the residents' clinic and 177 patients in the pulmonary fellows' clinic. The charts of the subsequent 119 patients seen in the residents' clinic after QI intervention were reviewed after QI intervention. When comparing pre-intervention residents' clinic to fellows' clinic, patients seen in the fellows' clinic were more likely to be female ($p = 0.039$), have a lower forced-expiratory-volume-in-one-second to forced vital capacity ratio (FEV1/FVC) ($p < 0.001$), have a lower percent-predicted forced-expiratory-volume-in-one-second (FEV1) ($p < 0.001$), greater percent predicted residual volume ($p = 0.006$), and lower percent-predicted diffusion capacity ($p < 0.001$). Fellows' clinic patients were more likely to have been prescribed a long-acting muscarinic agent, inhaled corticosteroids, or long-acting beta agonists ($p < 0.001$ for each class of medication), and to have been prescribed home oxygen for chronic hypoxic respiratory failure ($p < 0.001$). Resident clinic patients were more likely to carry a diagnosis of heart failure ($p = 0.045$). Further, only 15.7% of resident clinic patients were seen by any pulmonologist in the year prior to their index resident clinic visit.

Patients in the post-intervention resident clinic cohort were more likely to have a lower FEV1/FVC ($p = 0.04$), lower FEV1 ($p = 0.005$), higher total lung capacity ($p = 0.001$), and more likely to be prescribed a long acting muscarinic agent ($p = 0.004$) when compared to the pre-intervention residents' clinic cohort. The baseline characteristics of these cohorts are shown in Table 1.

Table 1. Baseline clinical characteristics of cohorts.

	Fellows' Clinic, (n = 177)	Pre-Intervention Residents' Clinic, (n = 451)	Post-Intervention Residents' Clinic, (n = 119)
Age, mean (SD)	57.07 (8.23)	58.9 (9.1)	58.7 (8.6)
Female, n (%)	101 (57.06) *	216 (47.9)	55 (46.2)
Physician-documented history of asthma, n (%)	21 (11.86)	63 (14.1)	21 (17.7)
Physician-documented history of congestive heart failure, n (%)	28 (15.82) *	104 (23.2)	23 (19.3)
FEV1/FVC, mean (SD)	56.5 (16.2) *	63.4 (15.6)	60.1 (15.4) *
FEV1, % predicted, mean (SD)	54.8 (22.8) *	64.2 (23.4)	57.4 (23.1) *
Total Lung Capacity, % predicted, mean (SD)	97 (22.7)	94 (21.7)	102.3 (24.6) *
Residual Volume, % predicted, mean (SD)	128.4 (51.5) *	116 (48.8)	123.3 (48.2)
Diffusion Capacity, % predicted, mean (SD)	58.8 (20) *	65.4 (21.3)	66.5 (23.7)
Use of short acting beta-agonist, n (%)	158 (89.27) *	396 (88)	106 (89.1)
Use of long acting beta-agonist, n (%)	134 (75.71) *	260 (57.8)	75 (63)
Use of inhaled corticosteroid, n (%)	141 (79.66)*	291 (64.7)	79 (66.4)
Use of long-acting muscarinic antagonist, n (%)	92 (51.98)*	162 (36)	60 (50.4) *
Active tobacco smoker, n (%)	95 (54.9)	252 (58.3)	67 (56.3)
Home oxygen, n (%)	47 (26.2) *	64 (14.2)	21 (17.7)
Patients seen by a pulmonologist in the year prior to index visit, n (%)	177 (100) *	70 (15.7)	25 (21)

* Indicates significant ($p < 0.05$) difference when compared to pre-intervention resident's clinic.

Prior to intervention, patients with a clinical diagnosis of COPD in the residents' clinic had office spirometry or PFTs in 66.5% of cases, with 42.6% of these tests showing no airway obstruction as defined by Global Initiative for Chronic Obstructive Lung Disease (GOLD) guidelines [2]. This performance was significantly inferior to the patients seen in the fellows' clinic where 83.6% had spirometry or PFTs ($p < 0.001$) with 23.8% ($p < 0.001$) of these having no obstructive airway disease. Residents provided smoking cessation counseling to 81.8% of active smokers while fellows counseled 91.6% of active smokers ($p = 0.024$). There was no significant difference in the rate of pneumococcal vaccination between the two clinics. These results are illustrated in Table 2.

Table 2. Comparison of quality measure adherence in the pre-QI resident clinic and the fellows' clinic.

	Residents' Clinic, (n = 451)	Fellows' Clinic, (n = 177)	p Value
Smoking cessation counseling documented, n (%) *	206 (81.8)	87 (91.6)	0.024
Spirometry performed, n (%)	300 (66.5)	148 (83.6)	<0.001
Obstruction confirmed by spirometry, n (%)	166 (36.8)	109 (61.6)	<0.001
Pneumococcal vaccine, n (%)	271 (61)	110 (62.5)	0.74

* For those who are active smokers.

After QI intervention, 119 subsequent visits to the residents' clinic in a single academic year were analyzed. Active smokers received cessation counseling in 86.8% of the visits compared to 81.8% prior to QI intervention (p = 0.360). After the QI intervention, 74.8% of patients who carried a diagnosis of COPD underwent spirometry or PFTs, improved from 66.5% in the pre-intervention cohort (p = 0.085). Pneumococcal vaccination rates significantly improved to 72.3% from 61% pre-intervention (p = 0.024). These results are seen in Table 3.

Table 3. Result of QI intervention of quality measure adherence in residents' clinic.

	Pre-Intervention	Post-Intervention	p Value
Spirometry performed, n (%)	300 (66.5)	89 (74.8)	0.085
Smoking cessation counseling documented, n (%) *	207 (81.8)	58 (86.6)	0.360
Pneumococcal vaccination, n (%)	271 (61)	86 (72.3)	0.024

* For those who are active smokers.

4. Discussion

This study shows a significant improvement in the rates of pneumococcal vaccination after the implementation of a QI regimen directed at internal medicine residents by their peers. Improvements in COPD patients who had spirometry and COPD patients who received smoking cessation counseling were seen but were statistically non-significant. The initial retrospective phase suggests internal medicine residents did not perform as well as pulmonary fellows in adherence to guideline-based COPD care measures. While this finding may not be true across all United States-based training programs, it is consistent with studies showing more inconsistent COPD guideline adherence among primary care providers when compared to pulmonary specialists [18–21]. Rates of smoking cessation counseling and the utilization of spirometry in diagnosis of COPD improved in a non-significant fashion, as well.

Successfully using residents as vehicles for QI has been reported elsewhere [22]. Our three specific quality improvement measures, namely smoking cessation in active tobacco users, pneumococcal vaccination, and diagnosis by spirometry, were chosen based on clinical importance, poor adherence noted in our residents' clinic compared to the pulmonology fellows' clinic, and the feasibility of improvement in a single QI cycle. Our resident-led strategy involved a multifaceted approach of a short presentation during a weekly resident didactic session, ongoing dissemination of study results to keep residents aware of the study and informed on deficiencies, posting index cards noting pneumococcal vaccination guidelines at each workstation in the clinic, and implementing a standing order for pneumococcal vaccination for patients with a diagnosis of COPD. This strategy was chosen because they were seen as the most efficient means by which the residents performing the QI study could reach their peers with the limited resources available.

Several QI strategies in the literature have been described to improve the rates of pneumococcal vaccinations [23–25]. One study described a simple physician reminder document as sufficient to produce a significant improvement in pneumococcal vaccination in ambulatory rheumatology clinics.

This particular trial quoted an improvement from a 67.6% to 80% vaccination rate, which was similar to our improvement from 61% to 72.3% post-intervention [23]. Our use of reminder cards mirrored the intervention in this study [23], and demonstrates simplistic interventions are useful at creating meaningful, statistically significant change. Further, involving clinic staff by means of a standing order decreased the chance of pneumococcal vaccination being forgotten during a clinic encounter.

Our intervention focused primarily on improving resident knowledge of guidelines as they pertain to spirometry being used in the diagnosis of COPD [2]. It has been suggested that a "chronic care model" that involves both the patient and non-physician staff members actively seeking to improve access to spirometry may be the most effective approach to improve rates of spirometry in patients with COPD symptoms [12]. Educational endeavors directed at providers (similar to our didactic talk and e-mail correspondence with residents) have been shown to improve appropriate application of spirometry in clinical practice [26]. While we do not demonstrate a significant improvement, the trend towards improvement in this facet of care may suggest a promising switch in clinic culture toward a guideline-based, objective assessment of pulmonary symptoms. To improve further, we would involve non-physician staff (e.g., nursing to identify who would benefit from bedside spirometry) as targets of QI intervention similar to the model purported by Joo et al. [12]. Anecdotally, the increased use of spirometry in patients with a diagnosis of COPD or pulmonary symptoms was not felt to improve the accuracy of COPD diagnosis in the residents' clinic. An interesting follow-up PDSA cycle could focus on improving the accuracy of diagnosis of COPD in our clinic and finding root cause of failure to consider alternative diagnoses.

Residents have been shown to improve their approach to smoking cessation counseling after receiving formal training on smoking cessation techniques [27,28]. Our intervention involved no formal training and was tailored to data showing that brief physician advice alone was adequate to improve the 1-year smoking quit rate [29]. Residents improved, albeit non-significantly, in rates of smoking cessation counseling after quality improvement intervention (81.8% to 86%). Larger, significant improvements have been shown in formally-trained residents taking care of smokers with and without chronic lung disease (10% to 21%) [28]. Although our demonstrated improvement is not statistically significant, we found the numerical improvement to be potentially promising for the brevity and simplicity of our intervention. Endeavors to incorporate formal training into residency didactics concerning smoking cessation counseling and therapeutic approaches is a potential future direction.

Among the limitations of our approach, we do not know the number of patients who were referred to the clinics with an incorrect diagnosis of "COPD" from a hospital admission and treated as such. Although this study was single center, internal medicine training programs in the United States may be able to implement these changes and replicate the results, due to their simplicity. However, every aspect of residency training is not uniform, which makes complete generalizability of this single-center study unlikely. Because a major goal of this QI project was to educate residents on guideline-based COPD care and improve clinician-in-training approach to patients with COPD, we elected not to have a control group who did not undergo QI intervention. Further, durability over time with this intervention is not presented, nor does the data extend beyond a single PDSA cycle. As our initial intervention only focused on spirometry being performed and not the result, a subsequent PDSA cycle focused on spirometry analysis to improve the accuracy of COPD diagnosis and adherence to treatment guidelines would be the natural next step. Calling attention to the use of spirometry could potentially lead to over-prescription of this diagnostic tool. Data is not available on the change in the clinic-wide use of spirometry based on this QI intervention. Also, prospective data in the fellows' clinic was not collected, which may introduce bias to the study. As this study was performed as an uncontrolled before-after design, a longer trial would have granted more statistical power to assess smoking quit rate, and provide more insight into COPD exacerbation rate and all-cause hospitalization, allowing for a more robust analysis of patient outcomes.

5. Conclusions

In conclusion, this study demonstrated a resident-led QI intervention directed towards peers. It illustrated a succinct and low-cost method of education that was successful at eliciting a change in approach to guideline-based care of COPD patients. Statistical improvement in the number of patients who received pneumococcal vaccination and non-significant improvement in patients diagnosed with COPD who underwent spirometry and smoking cessation was noted. Further, it demonstrated the continued educational strides needed to improve care of chronic lung disease in general internal medicine training.

Author Contributions: R.M.B. is the corresponding author and takes responsibility for the accuracy of presented data. R.M.B., T.M., A.B., U.C., K.E.-K., R.C., and N.K. designed study. R.M.B., U.C., T.M., and A.B. collected data and performed QI interventions. N.K. acted as QI expert and mentor. R.C. and R.M.B. performed the statistical analysis. R.M.B. wrote the manuscript that was reviewed by all other co-authors.

Funding: The authors of this article received no financial support, via funding or otherwise.

Acknowledgments: Special thanks to the residents and clinic faculty at the University of Louisville for their participation.

References

1.   Buist, A.S.; McBurnie, M.A.; Vollmer, W.M.; Gillespie, S.; Burney, P.; Mannino, D.M.; Menezes, A.M.; Sullivan, S.D.; Lee, T.A.; Weiss, K.B.; et al. International variation in the prevalence of COPD (the BOLD Study): A population-based prevalence study. *Lancet* **2007**, *370*, 741–750. [CrossRef]

2.   Global Initiative for Chronic Lung Disease. Global Strategy for the Diagnosis, Management, and Prevention of Chronic Obstructive Pulmonary Disease, Update 2015. Available online: www.goldcopd.org (accessed on 20 June 2018).

3.   Burney, P.; Jithoo, A.; Kato, B.; Janson, C.; Mannino, D.; Nizankowska-Mogilnicka, E.; Studnicka, M.; Tan, W.; Bateman, E.; Kocabas, A.; et al. Chronic obstructive pulmonary disease mortality and prevalence: The associations with smoking and poverty—A BOLD analysis. *Thorax* **2014**, *69*, 465–473. [CrossRef] [PubMed]

4.   Ghattas, C.; Dai, A.; Gemmel, D.J.; Awad, M.H. Over diagnosis of chronic obstructive pulmonary disease in an underserved patient population. *Int. J. Chronic Obstr. Pulm. Dis.* **2013**, *8*, 545–549. [CrossRef] [PubMed]

5.   Accreditation Counsil for Graduate Medical Education. Available online: http://www.acgme.org/what-we-do/accredidation/common-program-requirements (accessed on 20 June 2018).

6.   Coleman, M.T.; Nasraty, S.; Ostapchuk, M.; Wheeler, S.; Looney, S.; Rhodes, S. Introducing practice-based learning and improvement ACGME core competencies into a family medicine residency curriculum. *Jt. Comm. J. Qual. Saf.* **2003**, *29*, 238–247. [CrossRef]

7.   Fox, C.H.; Mahoney, M.C. Improving diabetes preventive care in a family practice residency program: A case study in continuous quality improvement. *Fam. Med.* **1998**, *30*, 441–445. [PubMed]

8.   Mohr, J.J.; Randolph, G.D.; Laughon, M.M.; Schaff, E. Integrating improvement competencies into residency education: A pilot project from a pediatric continuity clinic. *Ambul. Pediatr.* **2003**, *3*, 131–136. [CrossRef]

9.   Patow, C.A.; Karpovich, K.; Riesenberg, L.A.; Jaeger, J.; Rosenfeld, J.C.; Wittenbreer, M.; Padmore, J.S. Residents' engagement in quality improvement: A systematic review of the literature. *Acad. Med.* **2009**, *84*, 1757–1764. [CrossRef] [PubMed]

10.   Celli, B.R.; MacNee, W. Standards for the diagnosis and treatment of patients with COPD: A summary of the ATS/ERS position paper. *Eur. Respir. J.* **2004**, *23*, 932–946. [CrossRef] [PubMed]

11.   Foster, J.A.; Yawn, B.P.; Maziar, A.; Jenkins, T.; Rennard, S.I.; Casebeer, L. Enhancing COPD management in primary care settings. *Medscape Gen. Med.* **2007**, *9*, 24.

12.   Joo, M.J.; Au, D.H.; Lee, T.A. Use of spirometry in the diagnosis of chronic obstructive pulmonary disease and efforts to improve quality of care. *Transl. Res.* **2009**, *154*, 103–110. [CrossRef] [PubMed]

13. Lin, K.; Watkins, B.; Johnson, T.; Rodriguez, J.A.; Barton, M.B. U.S. Preventive Services Task Force Evidence Syntheses, formerly Systematic Evidence Reviews. In *Screening for Chronic Obstructive Pulmonary Disease Using Spirometry: Summary of the Evidence for the U.S. Preventive Services Task Force*; Agency for Healthcare Research and Quality (US): Rockville, MD, USA, 2008.

14. Yawn, B.P.; Duvall, K.; Peabody, J.; Albers, F.; Iqbal, A.; Paden, H.; Zubek, V.B.; Wadland, W.C. The impact of screening tools on diagnosis of chronic obstructive pulmonary disease in primary care. *Am. J. Prev. Med.* **2014**, *47*, 563–575. [CrossRef] [PubMed]

15. Hoogendoorn, M.; Feenstra, T.L.; Hoogenveen, R.T.; Rutten-van Molken, M.P. Long-term effectiveness and cost-effectiveness of smoking cessation interventions in patients with COPD. *Thorax* **2010**, *65*, 711–718. [CrossRef] [PubMed]

16. Thabane, M. Smoking cessation for patients with chronic obstructive pulmonary disease (COPD): An evidence-based analysis. *Ont. Health Technol. Assess. Ser.* **2012**, *12*, 1–50. [PubMed]

17. Provost, L.P. Analytical studies: A framework for quality improvement design and analysis. *BMJ Qual. Saf.* **2011**, *20* (Suppl. S1), 92–96. [CrossRef] [PubMed]

18. Lopez-Campos, J.L.; Abad Arranz, M.; Calero-Acuna, C.; Romero-Valero, F.; Ayerbe-Garcia, R.; Hidalgo-Molina, A.; Aguilar-Perez-Grovas, R.I.; Garcia-Gil, F.; Casas-Maldonado, F.; Caballero-Ballesteros, L.; et al. Guideline Adherence in Outpatient Clinics for Chronic Obstructive Pulmonary Disease: Results from a Clinical Audit. *PLoS ONE* **2016**, *11*, e0151896. [CrossRef] [PubMed]

19. Perez, X.; Wisnivesky, J.P.; Lurslurchachai, L.; Kleinman, L.C.; Kronish, I.M. Barriers to adherence to COPD guidelines among primary care providers. *Respir. Med.* **2012**, *106*, 374–381. [CrossRef] [PubMed]

20. Salinas, G.D.; Williamson, J.C.; Kalhan, R.; Thomashow, B.; Scheckermann, J.L.; Walsh, J.; Abdolrasulnia, M.; Foster, J.A. Barriers to adherence to chronic obstructive pulmonary disease guidelines by primary care physicians. *Int. J. Chronic Obstr. Pulm. Dis.* **2011**, *6*, 171–179. [CrossRef] [PubMed]

21. Sharif, R.; Cuevas, C.R.; Wang, Y.; Arora, M.; Sharma, G. Guideline adherence in management of stable chronic obstructive pulmonary disease. *Respir. Med.* **2013**, *107*, 1046–1052. [CrossRef] [PubMed]

22. Jones, A.C.; Shipman, S.A.; Ogrinc, G. Key characteristics of successful quality improvement curricula in physician education: A realist review. *BMJ Qual. Saf.* **2015**, *24*, 77–88. [CrossRef] [PubMed]

23. Desai, S.P.; Lu, B.; Szent-Gyorgyi, L.E.; Bogdanova, A.A.; Turchin, A.; Weinblatt, M.; Coblyn, J.; Greenberg, J.O.; Kachalia, A.; Solomon, D.H. Increasing pneumococcal vaccination for immunosuppressed patients: A cluster quality improvement trial. *Arthritis Rheum.* **2013**, *65*, 39–47. [CrossRef] [PubMed]

24. Parker, S.; Chambers White, L.; Spangler, C.; Rosenblum, J.; Sweeney, S.; Homan, E.; Bensen, S.P.; Levy, L.C.; Dragnev, M.C.; Moskalenko-Locke, K.; et al. A quality improvement project significantly increased the vaccination rate for immunosuppressed patients with IBD. *Inflamm. Bowel Dis.* **2013**, *19*, 1809–1814. [CrossRef] [PubMed]

25. Pennant, K.N.; Costa, J.J.; Fuhlbrigge, A.L.; Sax, P.E.; Szent-Gyorgyi, L.E.; Coblyn, J.; Desai, S.P. Improving Influenza and Pneumococcal Vaccination Rates in Ambulatory Specialty Practices. *Open Forum Infect. Dis.* **2015**, *2*, ofv119. [CrossRef] [PubMed]

26. Gupta, S.; Moosa, D.; MacPherson, A.; Allen, C.; Tamari, I.E. Effects of a 12-month multi-faceted mentoring intervention on knowledge, quality, and usage of spirometry in primary care: A before-and-after study. *BMC Pulm. Med.* **2016**, *16*, 56. [CrossRef] [PubMed]

27. Cornuz, J.; Humair, J.P.; Seematter, L.; Stoianov, R.; van Melle, G.; Stalder, H.; Pecoud, A. Efficacy of resident training in smoking cessation: A randomized, controlled trial of a program based on application of behavioral theory and practice with standardized patients. *Ann. Intern. Med.* **2002**, *136*, 429–437. [CrossRef] [PubMed]

28. Cornuz, J.; Zellweger, J.P.; Mounoud, C.; Decrey, H.; Pecoud, A.; Burnand, B. Smoking cessation counseling by residents in an outpatient clinic. *Prev. Med.* **1997**, *26*, 292–296. [CrossRef] [PubMed]

29. Stead, L.F.; Bergson, G.; Lancaster, T. Physician advice for smoking cessation. *Cochrane Database Syst. Rev.* **2008**. [CrossRef]

5

PTSD in U.S. Veterans: The Role of Social Connectedness, Combat Experience and Discharge

Sara Kintzle * [ID], Nicholas Barr [ID], Gisele Corletto and Carl A. Castro

USC Suzanne Dworak-Peck School of Social Work, University of Southern California, 1150 S. Olive Street Suite 1406, Los Angeles, CA 90015, USA; nicholub@usc.edu (N.B.); gcorlett@usc.edu (G.C.); cacastro@usc.edu (C.A.C.)
* Correspondence: kintzle@usc.edu

Abstract: Service members who transition out of the military often face substantial challenges during their transition to civilian life. Leaving military service requires establishing a new community as well as sense of connectedness to that community. Little is known about how social connectedness may be related to other prominent transition outcomes, particularly symptoms of posttraumatic stress disorder (PTSD). The purpose of this study was to explore the role of social connectedness in the development of PTSD, as well as its relationship to the known risk factors of combat exposure and discharge status. Data used were drawn from a needs assessment survey of 722 veterans. A path model was specified to test direct and indirect effects of combat experiences, non-honorable discharge status, and social connectedness on PTSD symptoms. Results demonstrated positive direct effects for combat experiences and non-honorable discharge status on PTSD symptoms while social connectedness demonstrated a negative direct effect. Both combat experiences and non-honorable discharge status demonstrated negative direct effects on social connectedness and indirect on PTSD through the social connectedness pathway. Study findings indicate social connectedness may be an important factor related to PTSD in veterans as well as an intervention point for mitigating risk related to combat exposure and discharge status.

Keywords: social connectedness; military; veterans; combat; discharge status; PTSD; mental health

1. Introduction

Serving in the U.S. military provides a substantial opportunity for a sense of community, belonging and understanding. Re-establishing a new sense of community is essential for veterans transitioning out of the military and into civilian life. However, developing a new sense of connectedness is one of many challenges separating service members may face. Little is known about the role social connectedness may play in promoting positive transition outcomes.

One such challenge transitioning veterans may encounter is unmet mental health needs, particularly posttraumatic stress disorder (PTSD). Evidence suggests that veterans are especially at risk of developing PTSD due to the potential stressors associated with combat exposure and military-related trauma. The prevalence of PTSD among veterans ranges from 11 to 30% based on the area of service [1,2]. Research indicates that an estimated 30% of Vietnam, 10% of Gulf War, 15% of Iraq veterans and 11% of veterans returning from Afghanistan struggle with PTSD [1–3]. PTSD is a result of traumatic or stressful life events, and it can interfere with social, physical and psychological functioning. PTSD is characterized by intrusive thoughts in which the trauma is re-experienced, avoidance of situations that might trigger the trauma, a state of hyperarousal or vigilance and negative alterations in cognition and mood which may cause irritability and aggression [4,5]. Veterans with trauma exposure and PTSD are more susceptible to sleep disorders, mood changes, reckless behavior, substance use and isolation which may impede a successful transition from military to civilian life [1,5].

One of the primary risk factors for the development of PTSD is combat exposure. Extensive research identifies combat exposure as a strong predictor of health and psychological complications in veterans due to the risk of physical injury, psychological trauma and other stressors related to war [6,7]. A recent study examined associations between combat exposure and physical and psychological health focusing on the physical pain, PTSD and depression in veterans. The findings indicate that veterans exposed to combat had greater pain intensity and as a result higher PTSD and depression symptoms in comparison veterans without combat exposure [7].

Another factor associated with negative outcomes during transition is non-honorable discharge status. As qualification for benefits is determined by discharge status, the roughly 16% of veterans who leave the military with non-honorable discharge status are often met with additional barriers to getting care, which can create significant transition challenges [8,9]. With limited access to services, veterans with non-honorable discharge status are at increased risk of adverse mental health outcomes including PTSD [10].

Among the challenges that military veterans encounter during their transition from military to civilian life is a loss of social connectedness. Social connectedness refers to an individual's internal sense of belongingness to the social environment [11]. Social connectedness impacts interpersonal relationships, peer affiliation, memberships, social behavior and overall social integration throughout the lifespan [12]. There are health and psychological benefits linked to social connectedness. Documented benefits to social connectedness include intimacy, sense of sharing and belonging [13]. Existing research shows that experiencing a higher sense of social connectedness may serve as a protective factor against psychological distress, depression, PTSD, low self-esteem and suicidal ideation [14,15]. The need for social connection is fundamental to the successful reintegration of veterans into civilian life. With the loss a sense of community, identity and belongingness often provided by the military, the inability to find a new sense of social connectedness may create difficulty for veterans interacting in the civilian world. This can lead to isolation and further transition challenges.

While it is well established that veterans may struggle in their transition out of the military and into civilian communities, little has been done to examine this transition in relation to social connectedness and its impact on risk factors and transition outcomes. The purpose of this study is to explore the effect of combat exposure, non-honorable discharge status, and social connectedness on PTSD symptoms in individuals who have served in the U.S. military.

2. Materials and Methods

Data used for this study were drawn from a community-based needs assessment involving veterans living in the San Francisco Bay Area [16]. Multiple recruitment strategies were utilized to achieve representativeness of the veteran population in the San Francisco Bay Area. Utilizing two methods for reaching potential participants, researchers partnered with higher-learning institutions and local agencies which serve veterans in the San Francisco Bay Area. The first method utilized an online survey approach by which the agency would send out an invitation and survey link to veterans within their database. The second method used an on-the-ground survey approach by which agencies would work with researchers to organize data-collection events within their respective organizations. Those who agreed to participate were sent either a paper survey copy or the online survey link. The final sampling strategy used print advertisements and social media to reach out to veterans within the San Francisco community. Avenues such as Facebook, Twitter, LinkedIn, mass emails and the survey website promoted the survey opportunity to potential participants. The survey took approximately 30 to 90 min to complete. All participants received a $15 gift card. All data collection procedures were approved by the University of Southern California (UP-15-00697) Institutional Review Board.

2.1. Measures

PTSD: The Posttraumatic Stress Disorder Checklist 5 (PCL-5) [17], a 20-item measure on a 0–4 Likert-type scale, was used to measure PTSD. The PCL-5 is a four-factor measure indexing disturbances in intrusive thoughts, physical arousal, cognitive, and avoidance symptoms. Responses to the 20 items result in a score from 0–80, with a cut-point score of 33 [18]. Sample items include "in the past month, how much were you been bothered by: Repeated, disturbing, and unwanted memories of the stressful experience?" and "in the past month, how much were you been bothered by: Feeling jumpy or easily startled?" Cronbach's alpha for the PCL was 0.97 in these data.

Combat experiences: The 13-item short version of the Combat Experiences Scale [19] was used to measure combat experiences. Scale items are dichotomous and capture common impactful deployment-related experiences like receiving enemy fire and seeing dead bodies. Scores range from 0–13. Cronbach's alpha for the CES was 0.90 in these data.

Discharge status: Participants reported honorable discharge or one of seven possible non-honorable discharge statuses, including general under honorable conditions, other than honorable, bad conduct discharge, dishonorable discharge, dismissal (officer), uncharacterized or other. These categories were summed to produce a dichotomous variable capturing any non-honorable discharge.

Social connectedness: The Social Connectedness Scale [20], an 8-item measure scored on a 6-point Likert scale, indexed social connectedness. The scale was developed based on the theory of self-psychology and measures feelings of belongingness. The scale was validated in a study with 626 undergraduate students and was found to have good test stability over a 2-week period (0.96) and strong internal reliability (0.91). Sample items include "I feel disconnected from the world around me" and "even around people I know, I don't feel that I really belong". Scores range from 8–48. Cronbach's alpha for the Social Connectedness Scale was 0.94 in these data.

2.2. Analyses

First, bivariate correlations were computed for study variables of interest including combat experiences, discharge status, social connectedness, and PTSD symptoms (See Table 1). Next, a path model was specified to test the direct and indirect effects of combat experiences, non-honorable discharge status, and social connectedness on PTSD symptoms. The estimator was maximum likelihood with missing data. Direct effects were modeled for each of the three predictors, and indirect effects were modeled for both combat experiences and non-honorable discharge status through the social connectedness pathway. Normality of residual distributions for continuous predictors combat experiences and social connectedness were tested using post-estimation residual plots. All analyses were conducted in Stata [21].

Table 1. Bivariate correlations for variables of interest.

Variable	Combat Experiences	Non-Honorable Discharge Status	Social Connectedness	PTSD Symptoms
Combat experiences	1			
Non-honorable discharge status	0.01	1		
Social connectedness	−0.14 *	−0.09	1	
PTSD symptoms	0.40 ***	0.26 ***	−0.40 ***	1

* $p < 0.05$, *** $p < 0.001$. Pearson's product moment correlations were computed for continuous by continuous associations. Biserial correlations were computed for non-honorable discharge status and continuous variables.

3. Results

The final sample consisted of 722 veterans who lived in the San Francisco Bay Area and completed the survey. Over half of the sample identified as white (54%) and married or with a domestic partner (51%). One-quarter of the sample was aged over 60 while 37% were between the ages of 30 and 39. Thirty percent of the sample indicated receiving a non-honorable discharge status. The sample as a whole reported high levels of PTSD symptoms ($M = 36.07$, $SD = 21.6$) and moderate levels of social connectedness ($M = 32.15$, $SD = 13.27$). Sample demographics are displayed in Table 2.

Table 2. Sample descriptive statistics.

Variable	Variable Descriptors	%	N = 722	M	SD
	18–29	8.61%	62		
	30–39	37.36%	269		
Age	40–49	16.25%	117		
	50–59	12.91%	93		
	60 and older	15.69%	179		
	70 and older	9.17%	66		
	Male	80.56%	580		
Gender	Female	19.03%	137		
	Transgender	0.40%	3		
	Single	28.02%	202		
Marital Status	Married/Domestic Partnership	51.04%	368		
	Divorced/separated	17.89%	129		
	Widowed	3.05%	22		
	American Indian/Alaska Native	2.78%	20		
	Asian	6.40%	46		
	Black	17.25%	124		
Race/Ethnicity	Hawaiian/Pacific Islander	2.50%	18		
	White	54.38%	391		
	Hispanic/Latino	11.82%	85		
	Other	4.87%	35		
	Some High School	2.22%	16		
	GED	3.47%	25		
	High school diploma	9.29%	67		
	Some college	26.49%	191		
Education	Associate degree	12.48%	90		
	Bachelor's	23.30%	168		
	Master's	18.45%	133		
	Doctorate	2.50%	18		
	Other	1.80%	13		
Non-Honorable Discharge Status		29.64%	214		
Combat Experiences				6.64	4.38
Social Connectedness				32.15	13.27
PTSD Symptoms				36.07	21.6

Combat experiences, social connectedness, and PTSD symptoms were significantly correlated at the bivariate level, as were non-honorable discharge status and PTSD symptoms. Despite the finding of a nonsignificant bivariate association between discharge status and social connectedness, theoretical and empirical considerations [22], including hypothesized indirect effects among study variables, warranted the testing of the full model.

In path analysis, the model was fully identified ($N = 722$). The final model with unstandardized direct effects is shown in Figure 1. Standardized direct, indirect, and total effects are reported below. As hypothesized, there were positive direct effects for combat experiences ($\beta = 0.36$, $p < 0.001$) and non-honorable discharge status ($\beta = 0.21$, $p < 0.001$) on PTSD symptoms. Social connectedness demonstrated a negative direct effect on PTSD symptoms ($\beta = -0.41$, $p < 0.001$). In addition, both combat experiences ($\beta = -0.13$, $p < 0.05$) and non-honorable discharge status ($\beta = -0.14$, $p < 0.05$) demonstrated negative direct effects on social connectedness. There were also significant indirect effects for both combat experiences ($\beta = 0.05$, $p < 0.05$) and non-honorable discharge status ($\beta = 0.06$, $p < 0.05$) on PTSD through the social connectedness pathway. The total effect for combat experiences on PTSD was $\beta = 0.41$, $p < 0.001$. The total effect for non-honorable discharge status on PTSD was $\beta = 0.26$, $p < 0.001$.

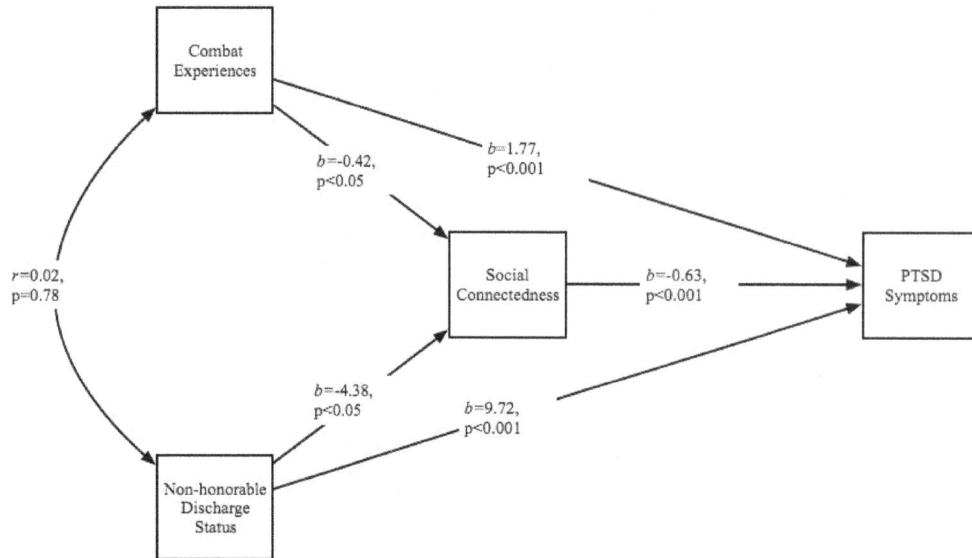

Figure 1. Path model with unstandardized direct effects.

Figure 1 displays the fully identified (N = 722) path analysis model demonstrating a direct negative effects of social connectedness on PTSD symptoms and direct positive effects of non-honorable discharge status and combat experiences on PTSD symptoms. Also demonstrated are significant indirect effects for both combat experiences and non-honorable discharge status on PTSD through the social connectedness pathway.

4. Discussion

Study findings indicate social connectedness may be an important factor related to PTSD in veterans. Social connectedness had a direct effect on PTSD symptoms, indicating the extent to which veterans in the study felt socially connected inversely impacted the level of PTSD symptoms. As expected, both combat experience and a non-honorable discharge status had a positive direct effect on PTSD, indicating higher levels of combat experience and a non-honorable discharge status to be associated with more severe PTSD symptom severity. This aligns with the body of research which has examined the traumatic impact of combat as well as emerging literature on non-honorable discharge status as a risk factor for PTSD [5,10].

Combat experiences and non-honorable discharge status were also found to have an indirect effect on PTSD symptoms through their effects on social connectedness. This means that while these factors are present, they not only act on PTSD directly but also indirectly by inhibiting social connectedness. This indicates that veterans in the study who endorsed experiencing combat, as well as those who identified as having a non-honorable discharge status, were less likely to report feeling connected to individuals and their community. This, in turn, is associated with increased severity of PTSD symptoms. Conversely, social connectedness was negatively associated with PTSD and exerted the strongest direct effect of all predictors. This finding suggests that enhancing social connectedness may provide a robust buffering effect against the risks posed by combat experiences and non-honorable discharge status.

While there is limited research examining the role of social connectedness in the mental health of veterans, these findings are similar to those that have been found in other populations. Research has demonstrated social connectedness to have a significant positive impact on the physical and mental health of older adults [23,24]. Other studies have also found important connections between social connectedness and mental health in adolescents, transgender adults and college athletes [25–27].

Study findings have significant implications for considering PTSD in veterans. Although expected, both combat experiences and a non-honorable discharge status resulted in increased risk for PTSD.

Identifying service members leaving the military with such risk factors should be identified early for intervention. This is particularly true for those with a non-honorable discharge status as these individuals may not have access to benefits that allow for mental health treatment. Results indicate social connectedness may be an important protective factor in the development of symptoms of PTSD. While researchers and practitioners often discuss the importance of reducing risk factors, combat exposure and discharge status are risk factors that occur during service. Increased social connectedness is a potential protective factor that can be targeted during and after the transition from service by assisting veterans in building a new community that provides a sense of belonging. While we know that such activities that target social connectedness are important to overall well-being, findings suggest they could be a significant contributor to positive mental health in veterans.

Further research is needed to examine social connectedness in veterans. The protective nature of social connectedness should be explored further in relation to the broad military transition experience. Early interventions during transition related to social connectedness could be an avenue for protecting veterans for negative outcomes related to suicide risk, mental and physical health. Further research should detail these relationships. It is also imperative that practitioners working with veterans take the time to explore feelings of social connectedness and encourage activities that promote a sense of connection to individuals and the community.

5. Conclusions

While transition from the military has received considerable attention as a point of intervention for promoting veteran success, little has been done to explore the role community and social connections may have in encouraging a positive transition. Findings demonstrate that facilitating the development of new social connections may serve as a protective factor in the development of PTSD symptoms. The results also indicate this may be particularly true for vulnerable veterans, such as those who have experienced combat and veterans with a non-honorable discharge status.

Author Contributions: Conceptualization, S.K. and C.A.C.; Methodology, S.K. and C.A.C.; Formal Analysis, B.B.; Investigation, S.K., C.A.C. & G.C.; Data Curation, S.K.; Writing—Original Draft Preparation, S.K., B.B. & G.C.; Writing—Review & Editing, S.K., B.B., G.C. & C.A.C.; Project Administration, S.K.; Supervision, S.K. & G.C.; Funding Acquisition, S.K. & C.A.C.; Resources, S.K. & C.A.C.

Funding: The study was funded by Wells Fargo.

References

1. Muller, J.; Ganeshamoorthy, S.; Myers, J. Risk factors associated with posttraumatic stress disorder in US veterans: A cohort study. *PLoS ONE* **2017**, *12*, e0181647.
2. Richardson, L.K.; Frueh, B.C; Acierno, R. Prevalence estimates of combat—Related post-traumatic stress disorder: Critical review. *Aust. N. Z. J. Psychiatry* **2010**, *44*, 4–19.
3. Knowles, K.A.; Sripada, R.K.; Defever, M.; Rauch, S.A.M. Comorbid mood and anxiety disorder and severity of posttraumatic stress symptoms in treatment seeking veterans. *Psychol. Trauma* **2018**. [CrossRef]
4. Sippel, L.M.; Watkins, L.E.; Pietrzak, R.H.; Hoff, R.; Harpaz-Rtem, I. The unique roles of emotional numbing and arousal symptoms in relation to social connectedness among military veterans in residential treatment for PTSD. *Psychiatry* **2018** [CrossRef]
5. Xue, C.; Ge, Y.; Tang, B.; Liu, Y.; Kang, P.; Wang, M.; Zhang, L. A meta-analysis of risk factors for combat related PTSD among military personnel and veterans. *PLoS ONE* **2015**, *10*, e0120270.
6. Amdur, D.; Batres, A.; Beslisle, J.; Brown, J.H.; Cornis-Pop, M.; Matthewson-Chapman, M.; Harms, G.; Hunt, S.C.; Kennedy, P.; Mahoney-Gleason, H.; et al. VA Integrated post-combat care: A systemic approach to caring for returning combat veterans. *Sci. Work Healthc.* **2011**, *50*, 564–575. [CrossRef] [PubMed]
7. Buttner, M.M.; Godfrey, K.M.; Floto, E.; Pittman, J.; Lindamer, L.; Afari, N. Combat exposure and pain in male and female afghanistan and iraq veterans: The role of mediators and moderators. *Psychiatr. Res.* **2017**, *257*, 7–13.

8.   Holliday, S.B.; Pedersen, E.R. The association between discharge status, mental health, and substance misuse among young adult veterans. *Psychiatr. Res.* **2017**, *256*, 428–434. [CrossRef] [PubMed]

9.   Veterans Legal Clinic. Underserved: How the VA Wrongfully Excludes Veterans with Bad Paper. Available online: https://www.swords-to-plowshares.org/wp-content/uploads/Underserved.pdf (accessed on 6 August 2018).

10.   Barr, N.; Kintzle, S.; Alday, E.; Castro, C.A. How does discharge status impact suicide risk in military veterans? *Health Soc. Work* **2018**. [CrossRef]

11.   Lee, R.M.; Draper, M.; Lee, S. Social connectedness, dysfunctional interpersonal behaviors, and psychological distress: Testing a mediator model. *J. Couns. Psychol.* **2001**, *48*, 310–318.

12.   Williams, K.L.; Galliher, R.V. Predicting depression and self-esteem from social connectedness, support and competence. *J. Soc. Clin. Psychol.* **2006**, *25*, 855–874.

13.   Satici, S.A.; Uysal, R.; Deniz, M.E. Linking Social connectedness to loneliness: The mediating role of subjective happiness. *Pers. Indiv. Differ.* **2016**, *97*, 306–310.

14.   Fanning, J.F.; Peirrzak, R.H. Suicidality among older male veterans in the United States: Results from the national health and resilience in veterans study. *J. Psychiatr. Res.* **2013**, *47*, 1766–1775. [CrossRef] [PubMed]

15.   Mauss, I.B.; Shallcross, A.J.; Troy, A.S.; John, O.P.; Ferrer, E.; Wilhelm, F.H.; Gross, J.J. Don't hide your happiness! Positive emotion dissociation, social connectedness, and psychological functioning. *J. Pers. Soc. Psychol.* **2011**, *100*, 738–748.

16.   Castro, C.A.; Kintzle, S. *The State of the American Veteran: The San Francisco Veterans Study*; USC CIR: San Francisco, CA, USA, 2017; Available online: http://cir.usc.edu/wp-content/uploads/2017/05/USC-CIR-SF-VET-2017_FINAL-Pgs.pdf (accessed on 6 August 2018).

17.   PTSD Checklist for DSM-5 (PCL-5)—PTSD: National Center for PTSD. Available online: https://www.ptsd.va.gov/professional/assessment/adult-sr/ptsd-checklist.asp (accessed on 6 August 2018).

18.   PTSD: National Center for PTSD. Treatment of PTSD: Recommended Treatments. Available online: https://www.ptsd.va.gov/public/treatment/therapy-med/treatment-ptsd.asp (accessed on 8 June 2018).

19.   Hoge, C.W.; Castro, C.A.; Messer, S.C.; McGurk, D.; Cotting, D.I.; Koffman, R.L. Combat duty in Iraq and Afghanistan, mental health problems, and barriers to care. *N. Engl. J. Med.* **2004**, *351*, 13–22. [CrossRef] [PubMed]

20.   Lee, R.M.; Robbins, S.B. Measuring belongingness: The social connectedness and the social assurance scales. *J. Couns. Psychol.* **1995**, *42*, 232–241. [CrossRef]

21.   StataCorp LLC. *Stata Data Analysis and Statistical Software*; Special Edition Release; StataCorp LLC: College Station, TX, USA, 2007; Volume 10, p. 733. Available online: https://www.stata.com/order/GS35F0108W-Rel12.pdf (accessed on 6 August 2018).

22.   Lo, S.K.; Li, I.T.; Tsou, T.S.; See, L. Non-significant in univariate but significant in multivariate analysis: A discussion with examples. *Changgeng Yi Xue Za Zhi* **1995**, *18*, 95–101. [PubMed]

23.   Ashida, S.; Heaney, C.A. Differential associations of social support and social connectedness with structural features of social networks and the health status of older adults. *J. Aging Health* **2008**, *20*, 872–893. [CrossRef] [PubMed]

24.   Cornwell, E.Y.; Waite, L.J. Social disconnectedness, perceived isolation, and health among older adults. *J. Health Soc. Behav.* **2009**, *50*, 31–48. [CrossRef] [PubMed]

25.   Bond, L.; Butler, H.; Thomas, L.; Carlin, J.; Glover, S.; Bowes, G.; Patton, G. Social and school connectedness in early secondary school as predictors of late teenage substance use, mental health, and academic outcomes. *J. Adolesc. Health* **2007**, *40*, 9–18. [CrossRef] [PubMed]

26.   Pflum, S.R.; Testa, R.J.; Balsam, K.F.; Goldblum, P.B.; Bongar, B. Social support, trans community connectedness, and mental health symptoms among transgender and gender nonconforming adults. *Psychol. Sex. Orientat. Gend. Divers.* **2015**, *2*, 281–286. [CrossRef]

27.   Armstrong, S.; Oomen-Early, J. Social connectedness, self-esteem, and depression symptomatology among collegiate athletes versus nonathletes. *J. Am. Coll. Health* **2009**, *57*, 521–526. [CrossRef] [PubMed]

6

Conversations about Death and Dying with Older People: An Ethnographic Study in Nursing Homes

Åsa Alftberg [1], Gerd Ahlström [2,*] , Per Nilsen [3], Lina Behm [2], Anna Sandgren [4] ,
Eva Benzein [4], Birgitta Wallerstedt [4] and Birgit H. Rasmussen [2,5]

[1] Department of Social Work, Faculty of Health and Society, Malmö University, SE-205 06 Malmö, Sweden;
Asa.Alftberg@mau.se

[2] Department of Health Sciences, Faculty of Medicine, Lund University, P.O. Box 157, SE-221 00 Lund,
Sweden; Lina.Behm@med.lu.se (L.B.); Birgit.Rasmussen@med.lu.se (B.H.R.)

[3] Department of Medical and Health Sciences, Division of Community Medicine, Linköping University,
SE-581 83 Linköping, Sweden; Per.Nilsen@liu.se

[4] Center for Collaborative Palliative Care, Department of Health and Caring Sciences, Faculty of Health and
Life Sciences, Linnaeus University, SE-351 95 Växjö, Sweden; Anna.Sandgren@lnu.se (A.S.);
Eva.Benzein@lnu.se (E.B.); Birgitta.Wallerstedt@lnu.se (B.W.)

[5] The Institute for Palliative Care, Region Skane and Lund University, P.O. Box 157, SE-221 00 Lund, Sweden

* Correspondence: gerd.ahlstrom@med.lu.se

Abstract: Nursing homes are often places where older persons "come to die." Despite this, death and dying are seldom articulated or talked about. The aim of this study was to explore assistant nurses' experiences of conversations about death and dying with nursing home residents. This study is part of an implementation project through a knowledge-based educational intervention based on palliative care principles. An ethnographic study design was applied in seven nursing homes, where eight assistant nurses were interviewed and followed in their daily assignments through participant observations. The assistant nurses stated that they had the knowledge and tools to conduct such conversations, even though they lacked the time and felt that emotional strain could be a hinder for conversations about death and dying. The assistant nurses used the strategies of distracting, comforting, and disregarding either when they perceived that residents' reflections on death and dying were part of their illness and disease or when there was a lack of alignment between the residents' contemplations and the concept of dying well. They indicated that ambivalence and ambiguity toward conversations about death and dying should be taken into consideration in future implementations of knowledge-based palliative care that take place in nursing homes after this project is finalized.

Keywords: auxiliary nurse; existential communication; frailty; ethnographic approach; life-limiting disease; older; aged; palliative care; residential care; end-of-life

1. Introduction

Palliative care encompasses conversations that are expected to help dying individuals prepare for death, to create a closing of what has been (life) and an opening to what is to come (death). This means that dying individuals should receive the opportunity to express their wishes, needs, and feelings, and obtain insight into their own dying [1–4]. Being able to express thoughts and feelings about death and dying is regarded as fundamental to quality of life, provided that the dying person wants to talk about these issues [5], and this can be described as a spiritual need that should be addressed by medical staff [6]. Accordingly, society's expectations of palliative care staff are that they are to facilitate such expressions and insights by encouraging nursing home residents to talk about their feelings and thoughts about death and dying. Such conversations are expected to promote a good and dignified death, which also can be regarded as a cultural concept or ideal [7].

The World Health Organization (WHO) has called for improved palliative care for older persons in general [4]. Older people dying of multiple morbidities, or merely of "old age," have until recently received far less of this type of care [8]. In several countries around the world, a high proportion of all deaths among older people over 65 years occur in residential care facilities [9]. This is the case in Sweden, where 24.5% of all deaths among those aged 70 years and older occur in nursing homes; this figure increases to 62% for people aged 90 years and older [9,10]. The Swedish policy is to support older people to live normal lives in their own homes for as long as possible [11]. This has contributed to the situation whereby the oldest and frailest persons move to nursing homes, with an average life expectancy in Swedish nursing homes of six to nine months; this time frame has reduced in recent years [12]. In addition, relatively few individuals living in nursing homes are transferred to hospitals to die there [10]. This means that the staff in nursing homes are given the role of handling death and dying and to provide "a good dying process" [1,13].

The principles of palliative care that have been developed within specialized palliative care and hospices may be lacking in nursing homes, since they traditionally have not been part of regular education or training [4,14,15] of staff in specialized palliative and oncology units. While staff in nursing homes strive to provide good care for older persons in their final stages of life, practical routines and everyday life rather than death and dying are considered more appropriate topics to discuss with the residents. Emotional and existential needs and concerns tend to be avoided due to uncertainty about how to talk about such topics [16–18]. Matters that relate to death and dying have been found to create emotional strain and even evoke fear among the staff, who are uncertain about how to face a dying person's suffering [19,20]. Previous studies have shown a lack of communication about existential issues such as death and dying between staff and older persons [21–24]. To remedy this situation, several attempts to implement palliative care in nursing homes are described in the literature, for example through education [8,17,25] and Advance Care Planning (ACP) [26–28].

In a recent publication on mapping palliative care implementation activities on the macro-, meso-, and micro levels in 29 European countries, Froggatt et al. [8] identified low levels of palliative care development and delivery in nursing homes, although there is great variation and diversity among countries. Palliative care is an integrated part of the Swedish health care system, including national guidelines for good palliative care at the end of life [29] and a national program for palliative care [30]. However, the quality of palliative care is still substandard and random for many residents living in nursing homes [12,14,31].

The Swedish system of health care and social services is financed primarily by taxes. The provision of long-term care and services for older people is within the remit of municipalities and is preceded by needs assessments. The most common staff members employed in Swedish nursing homes are assistant nurses (ANs). They generally have a shorter education (secondary school and 6–12 months of practical training for working in elder care and in the hospital) than registered nurses. They work most closely with the nursing home residents, while supervised by a few registered nurses. Many tasks are formally delegated by registered nurses to ANs, who then provide everyday care, including such conversations with the residents as studied here. At the national level, the ratio of ANs to RNs is 25:1 [32].

In agreement with ongoing efforts to improve palliative care in nursing homes, an implementation project called Implementation of Knowledge-Based Palliative Care in Nursing Homes (Swedish acronym KUPA) was performed in 2015–2017. The educational intervention was provided to nursing home staff and managers, addressing knowledge and skills of relevance to develop evidence-based palliative care [33]. The importance of context has increasingly been emphasized in implementation research [34], and conversation can be seen as one key aspect of context. This study explores conversation in the context of the ongoing implementation of palliative care in nursing homes based on education to support staff. This knowledge may contribute to increasing understanding of the outcomes of the implementation process and context in future implementation studies.

2. Aim

The aim of this paper is to explore assistant nurses' experiences of conversations about death and dying with nursing home residents within the framework of an ongoing implementation of palliative care.

3. Materials and Methods

This study is based on an ethnographic design with fieldwork. By applying an ethnographic method using both participant observations and interviews, a deeper understanding of concrete conversations about death and dying in the nursing home setting can be achieved. Following assistant nurses (ANs) in their everyday work made it possible to study their experiences in context. By the term "conversations about death and dying," we refer to situations where the residents bring up issues that somehow concern their death and how the ANs respond.

3.1. Context of the Study

The fieldwork was performed as part of the KUPA implementation project concerning palliative care for older people in nursing homes [33]. The project consists of a complex intervention through educational seminars that address the knowledge and skills required to achieve knowledge-based palliative care in nursing homes. The seminars involved 20 nursing homes over 6 months. The seminar covered the importance of talking about dying and death and the participants' own feelings and thoughts about these issues, and highlighted the significance of palliative care, support for next of kin, symptom relief, and collaborative care. The intervention was evaluated before, during, and after implementation through an experimental crossover design with intervention and control groups. The KUPA has the clinical trial registration number NCT02708498 [33].

This study was carried out in seven nursing homes in southern Sweden. The nursing homes were strategically selected from the 20 nursing homes included in the KUPA project, reflecting diversity in size and location, a mix of larger and smaller nursing homes, and between towns and the countryside. Three nursing homes were located in rural areas: with 35, 54, and 78 beds, respectively, and four nursing homes in urban areas with 26, 48, and 90 beds, respectively. The mean nursing staff to resident ratio was 0.9:1.

3.2. Participants

Eight ANs participating in ongoing seminars of the implementation project in the seven nursing homes were included. Their attention to issues of death and dying was of interest to inform the implementation process in the KUPA project, which motivated the timing of this study.

They were selected after contact with the nursing home managers. The managers forwarded a request to the ANs in the educational seminars, who then voluntarily decided to be part of the ethnographic study. In one nursing home, two ANs chose to participate. They were female, 30 to 64 years old (median 57 years), and had been working as ANs in elderly care for between 10 and 30 years (median 22 years).

3.3. Data Collection in the Ethnographic Fieldwork

The intention was to follow each of the eight ANs on four occasions (two ANs were followed on two occasions) in their daily work through participant observations by the first author on 28 occasions in total. Each period of observation lasted 3 to 4 h (about 110 h total). The observations were made at different times of day, from 7:00 a.m. to 9:00 p.m. The first author shadowed the participating ANs in every part of their work.

During the observations, informal conversations occurred between the ANs and the first author, which later were recorded as field notes together with descriptions of the situations that took place at the nursing homes [35].

On the last occasion of observation in each nursing home, semi-structured interviews with the participating ANs were performed, containing questions about their views and experiences of existential issues such as death and dying. Questions were based on the observations and the specific situations that had occurred ("How did you feel when ... ?" "What did you think when ... ?"). The eight interviews lasted around 45 min on average, were recorded digitally, and were transcribed verbatim as well as validated by the first author.

3.4. Data Analysis

A qualitative inductive thematic analysis process was applied [36] by the first, second, and last author. Field notes from the observations (which included informal conversations between the first author and ANs) and the semi-structured interviews were read as a whole to get an overall understanding of experiences and communication in the context of death and dying. Next, meaning units, i.e., text segments that related to death and dying, were identified and coded for their content, and were then sorted and grouped into clusters. Then the codes and meaning units in each cluster were reread and compared and searched for similarities and differences, forming and supporting the development of two basic themes: (1) barriers to conversations about death and dying and (2) managing conversations about death and dying in practice, i.e., in encounters between ANs and residents. The analysis continued by rereading and reflecting on the codes and meaning units, and this meant examining and recording patterns within and between the two themes, leading to the construction of six subthemes. In the group of co-authors, the interpretations made during the analysis featured a reflexive consideration, where understandings and interpretations were critically examined and discussed.

4. Ethical Considerations

The study was guided by the research ethical principles for medical research (the Declaration of Helsinki) and approved by the Regional Ethics Review Board in Lund (reference number: 2015/4).

During the fieldwork, the interactions between ANs and nursing home residents were observed, and all were informed and gave consent to be part of the research project. The residents were regarded as a vulnerable group, and the presence of the first author was guided by responsiveness towards their reactions to the observations. Any hesitation or unwillingness to participate was respected, and in some delicate situations (for instance, helping residents with intimate care or dealing with residents with severe dementia), the observations were stopped at the first author's own initiative. No personal data about staff or residents was recorded during the observations. In the account of the results, characteristics of the ANs and the residents have been changed or omitted, and they have been given assumed and neutral names to protect their identities.

5. Results

The first theme, barriers to conversations about death and dying, contains two subthemes: lacking time and feeling emotional strain. The second theme, managing conversations in practice, contains four subthemes: having tools, distracting, comforting, and disregarding. The ethnographic method designates that the subthemes are presented with extensive excerpts, which are presented as cases below, as being representative of the total dataset.

5.1. Barriers to Conversations about Death and Dying

All the ANs highlight the importance of being prepared to talk about death and dying whenever residents express their thoughts on the subject. Nevertheless, they perceive two barriers in particular, as described below. When the ANs talk about the experience of having conversations about death and dying with the residents, they describe feeling that lack of time is a difficulty. The ANs can also experience emotional strain in relation to these conversations.

5.1.1. Lacking Time

The context aspect of time is raised continuously by the ANs. They sometimes have very little time to actually pick up the thread and continue a conversation when a resident unexpectedly wants to talk about death and dying. Melissa describes how she tries to manage this:

> It may be that I don't have time to sit down and talk about it, sometimes the timing is bad. But you have to try, if you can't talk at that moment you'll have to ask, nicely, if you can come back later when things are not so busy when I really feel that I have a moment to spare, and then we can talk.

However, some of the ANs claim that one should not postpone such a conversation. Even if time is lacking, due to staff shortage, for example, one has to seize the opportunity. Elizabeth says:

> It must be when it happens, that's when I have to take the time to ... you try to, you'll have to sacrifice, well sacrifice is perhaps not the right word, but I have to take time to listen if they want to talk. Sometimes you feel you don't have the time, really. That's awful. But you try as much as you can. And everyone at work thinks the same, and we understand if someone takes their time with one of the residents, it's like "well, she's still in there, probably something is going on" and you won't disturb.

The ANs experience that lack of time may interfere with the residents' desire to talk about death and dying, and they try to manage time constraints.

5.1.2. Feeling Emotional Strain

Apart from lack of time, another barrier to conversations about death and dying is that it may cause emotional stress that can be exhausting for the ANs. Rebecca expresses that it can be difficult to come as close to another person as one does when talking about death and dying, and she occasionally wishes she did not have to: "It may sound weird I guess, but to not have to listen. Not having to know everything about that other person." Working as an AN and caring for older persons' bodies (washing, dressing, and feeding) is different than caring for existential needs, which, according to Rebecca, is much more strenuous. She describes that taking part in the residents' reflections on death and dying feels almost too intrusive. Sarah remarks on the intimate nature of care work from another perspective. She refers to how staff and residents are "feeling as one big family," but that also makes the work exhausting:

> It can drain your energy, sometimes you don't have the strength to sit and talk. ... We try to give them [the residents] so much energy, and we try to take away their negative emotions. But sometimes it's too much.

To sum up, conversations about death and dying appear to involve emotional strain for the ANs, which may act as a barrier to carrying out these conversations.

5.2. Managing Conversations in Practice

This section illustrates different strategies that ANs apply when it comes to managing conversations about death and dying with residents. The ANs point out that they have received knowledge and tools to conduct conversations about death and dying, and they give examples of strategies that they find helpful to use. However, most of the examples that were observed during the fieldwork included strategies used to circumvent conversations about death and dying. Distracting contains aspects of comfort, but it is mainly about redirecting a resident's attention to something other than death and dying. Comforting illustrates how the ANs truly focus on the residents, even though the comfort in itself may connote distraction, while disregarding is an evasive strategy, avoiding the perceived potential risk of talking about death and dying.

5.2.1. Having Tools

The ANs say that they appreciate having the opportunity to receive more knowledge by participating in the seminars of the implementation project. Sharing experiences and knowledge with colleagues working in a similar context is highly valued. They describe experiences of having acquired tools, including knowledge of how to talk about dying and death, through the seminars. Barbara gives an example of how one dying resident returned from the hospital, immediately saying, "I'm just coming home to die." Barbara says that she was a little bit surprised by this statement, but as she had recently learned to do, she asked the woman what thoughts she had about her dying. The resident replied that it felt "bright" and she was not afraid. Barbara emphasizes that it was a short conversation, but it felt nice to have support and knowledge from the seminars and tools such as asking questions about the resident's thoughts when she brought up the topic. She senses that she has learned to talk about death and dying in a way that she could not before. It is very much a question of listening and confirming, she explains. "One mustn't be afraid of these issues," she says. "Perhaps we are not so good at talking about it as we should be, but I do feel better if the residents are comfortable with their coming death."

The ANs express a wish to improve how to talk about death, which the seminars have promoted. Many of them state that death and dying usually is a topic that they mainly come in contact with when residents begin to express that they no longer have the strength to carry on. Melissa refers to a typical situation in her work:

> I think these conversations start when you have arrived at final phase, when they are really ill, not before. It happens all of a sudden; one of the residents was washing at the washbasin and suddenly she asked me: "Am I going to die here?" At first, I was surprised and didn't know what to say. I think I answered that she could stay here as long as she wanted and that maybe she was going to die here, nobody can tell. Such things can come all of a sudden. Sometimes you reply, "Oh no, don't think like that, you're healthy right now," and you try to encourage them, but I have learned now that this is wrong, you should ask another question instead: "What are you thinking now?" rather than saying "You shouldn't think about that, you're not there yet, you're healthy right now.

The ANs demonstrate an awareness of what ought to be the right response to the older person's questions and reflections. They highlight that the residents' reflections emerge in the very final stage of life, often at unexpected moments, and commonly concern more practical matters about the funeral. Overall, when the residents talk about death and dying, the ANs feel they have received more knowledge and a strategy, which is to listen and to ask questions.

5.2.2. Distracting

Even if the ANs feel more skilled and secure, there are still situations where they do not use the strategy of listening and asking questions, but rather a strategy of distraction. The following example is representative of this strategy. Mildred, a resident, is lying in bed when the AN, Rebecca, knocks on her door and enters her room. Rebecca asks Mildred if she wants some supper, but Mildred declines. Mildred says there is no use eating. "I'm not going to lie here much longer, I hope," she says. Rebecca gives a soft laugh and says "all right" while putting a blanket over Mildred in her bed. Mildred then says that she wishes she had died when she had a fall and injured herself badly, something that happened several years ago. "But think of all you would have missed. All your great-grandchildren," Rebecca replies. "Yes," Mildred says, and tells a story of one of her great-grandchildren.

Rebecca later explains that Mildred talks a great deal about death. According to Rebecca, Mildred is ready to die, but at the same time she is afraid. She is in pain and wants more medication, but Rebecca believes that she may suffer from spiritual angst rather than physical pain, with the medications intended to reduce her anxiety. Mildred's greatest fear is to be buried alive before being completely dead, and Rebecca has promised to make sure that Mildred is dead by sticking her finger with a needle or knife when that time comes. They have also talked about other aspects of dying. For example, Rebecca has explained what will happen to Mildred after she dies: the staff will wash her gently, dress her in fine clothes, and make her bed and room look nice and tidy. Sometimes Mildred says that she will try to kill herself, using a razor blade or a pair of scissors. Rebecca finds it difficult to know how to respond at such moments.

> Well, sometimes you don't give a very wise answer, I guess. It's more like "Think of your children, do you really want them to remember you like that?" and then she goes "Well, no, I don't."

Hence, dying and death *is* a recurring topic of conversation between Mildred and Rebecca. Perhaps that is why Rebecca, in the situation described above, does not try to elaborate, but instead attempts to distract Mildred by talking about her great-grandchildren. Mildred may be perceived as dwelling upon death without getting closer to being prepared for it with a peaceful mind, and distraction is found to be the best solution to manage this.

5.2.3. Comforting

Close to the distracting strategy is the strategy of comforting. The ANs are expected to give comfort to the residents and improve their well-being in whatever way they can. It is a natural part of their work, which is illustrated in the following strategy.

Alice, a resident known to have severe anxiety and suffer from panic attacks, is seated by her kitchen table at the window. She looks sad and worried. "I'm sitting here, waiting for the end," she says. She explains that she has trouble breathing, and she is taking short, quick breaths. Barbara sits down calmly beside her and asks in a gentle tone if Alice wants some water. Alice does not answer, but continues to say that she is near the end now. Barbara says "Oh, no" with a comforting voice and squeezes Alice's hand. She reminds Alice that she has had this feeling several times before, and it will pass. Barbara soothingly pats Alice's back and tries to ease her by talking about the coming musical entertainment this afternoon and says that Alice may be feeling better by then. Alice says that she would feel better if she could get some medication. Barbara takes her request seriously and unlocks the medication locker in the kitchen and checks the medication signing list. Alice received a mild sedative earlier in the morning, and Barbara asks Alice if she could take aspirin instead. Alice says she prefers something stronger. Barbara notes that she has to phone the nurse in that case, and she takes her phone from her pocket. Talking to the nurse, Barbara explains that she wants to give Alice an aspirin, and the nurse asks if Alice is in pain. "No, she's worried and she's not feeling well," Barbara says. The nurse and Barbara agree to give Alice two aspirin, saving the second daily dose of the sedative for the evening. Alice seems to be more relaxed now and content with the solution, and she takes the two aspirin Barbara gives her. Barbara gives Alice an encouraging smile and tells her she will be back later, in time for lunch, to check how she is feeling.

Alice's anxiety has consequences for the way she is treated. When Alice says that she is sitting there and waiting for the end, it is not regarded as an opening to a conversation about death. Instead, it is interpreted as an illness that needs to be treated. Barbara manages the situation by listening to Alice and trying to comfort her, but she does not ask any questions about Alice´s thoughts about death and dying.

5.2.4. Disregarding

Disregarding is a strategy to avoid listening or talking about death and dying. This may occur when the AN perceive risks with conversations about death and dying, as in the next example. Jean, a resident who suffers from mild dementia, is sitting in the corridor on her walker. When I (the first author) walk by, she turns to me and says that there is no point anymore. "I feel so alone," she tells me, and looks sad. "I don't know what to do," she says. One of the ANs, Pamela, arrives, and she seems to be in a hurry. She does not answer Jean, but suggests that Jean could water the flower pots in the windows, saying, "You can also take away the petals that have wilted, you like to do that." Jean replies that she does not want to water any flowers, but Pamela ignores her and goes to get the watering can in the next room.

A little later, we bump into Jean again. She is standing by her walker in the corridor and is still looking sad. She tells Pamela that she is going to hang herself. "Why, no," Pamela responds dismissively. Jean insists that she is going to kill herself, and Pamela gives her an absentminded pat on the cheek, saying that she could not manage without Jean, and then we continue down the corridor.

In a later discussion with Pamela, she notes that Jean is getting worse, with more anxiety and perhaps depression. She believes it could be a great risk talking about death and dying with someone like Jean, who has suicidal thoughts. Such a conversation would only make Jean feel worse. Pamela explains that as an assistant nurse, she always has to consider the possible consequences of conversations about death and dying. The fear is also that older people with dementia may be upset with the topic. In order to manage this, any conversations about death and dying should be avoided.

6. Discussion

This study illustrates perceived barriers to and strategies for managing conversations about death and dying between ANs and nursing home residents. The results should be considered within a context of an overarching ideal of dying well, where health care staff are expected to help dying individuals prepare for a good and dignified death [1,13]. As the ANs were part of KUPA, an implementation project concerning palliative care [33], they also described having gained tools and knowledge for how to talk about death and dying with residents. However, the results from the 110 hours of observations of conversations between residents and ANs show that ANs used strategies to circumvent issues of death and dying raised by the residents. These issues were not understood as a need by the residents to prepare for their own death, but as a sign of illness. The results point toward the complex needs of these frail residents and the importance of multi-professional team support and supervision for the ANs to enable differentiation between healthy and unhealthy talk of death. Also, being halfway through the implementation project appears to be insufficient to support ANs in the observed conversations about death and dying with residents.

ANs need more training and supervision to ease the experienced emotional strain and communicate with different residents in a time-stressed work context. Other studies [20,22] show that nursing home staff members feel that it is difficult to find time for nonscheduled tasks such as conversations or just being by an older person's side. Åhsberg and Carlsson [20] state that a conflict exists between what nursing assistants would like to do and what they are able to do for a dying person given the resources at hand. In our study, lack of time was perceived as an obstacle, but the overall opinion was that such difficulties must be solved, and the ANs generally seem to depend on individual strategies to find enough time.

Another barrier found in our study was the experience of emotional strain. This finding aligns with previous studies reporting that ANs find talking about existential questions to be a difficult and emotionally demanding task for which they lack competence [17,37,38]. Sundler et al. [39] also described ANs' experience of unexpected turns in conversations when caring for older people and difficulties in detecting their needs. These situations challenged their competence, and they felt unprepared. Similar feelings of distress and powerlessness when caring for people at the end of life have been discussed by Young et al. [40]. However, the implementation project seems to have empowered the ANs with tools, to a certain degree.

We found that the ANs used different strategies when managing conversations about death and dying. The disregarding strategy seemed to arise when the older person's contemplations about death and dying were understood as signs of disorder, disease, and diagnosis. The AN's reflections in this situation were concerned with health conditions of the older person and was not perceived as part of a dying process. Costello [41] calls this a curative ideology that values treatment and cures rather than death and terminal care, which, together with society's expectations for optimal health, may contribute to how care work is performed [41,42]. Conditions such as anxiety and dementia also prompted the opinion that the risk is too great, since conversations about death and dying will intensify anxiety and perhaps increase suicidal thoughts. Therefore, a diagnosis such as anxiety, depression, or dementia, or a suspicion of this kind of condition, might be a hindrance to having conversations about death and dying. Saini et al. [43] discuss how nursing home staff attribute any symptoms to dementia and similar diseases and fail to see other possible underlying causes of symptoms and behaviors; however, multiprofessional team support and supervision are paramount in understanding these symptoms and behaviors.

In another example, the older person is rehashing the subject of death and dying without achieving a sense of closure and readiness for the end of life. This differs from the ideal of the good dying process [7,44] grounded in palliative care and the idea of providing a good death, drawing upon a culturally established framework of how dying should occur and be experienced. Equally, in our study, when the ANs experience behavior and communication from the residents that is not in accordance with an assumed good dying process, they may respond with distraction. The notion of dying well may provide knowledge of how to proceed and what to achieve, but it also frames and decides the "right" way of dying. As Costello [41] formulates it, beliefs and ideologies about death and dying significantly shape the experiences of older dying patients and, as we have seen here, of the ANs.

A critical question, then, is how the principles of palliative care, including existential issues, can be implemented in nursing homes [8]. According to the Advance Care Planning (ACP) recommendations from the European Association for Palliative Care [45], planning and delivering palliative care should take into account the patient's preferences, resources, and best medical advice. However, Mignani et al. [26] point out that even when applying ACP, there seems to be a lack of communication between older people and their relatives and health care professionals about their wishes. The authors conclude that choosing the right moment and appropriate wording could have a profound impact on the value and effect of the communication, and that staff members who know the older person well are considered the ideal group to initiate an ACP discussion [26]. In Sweden, ACP is not yet standard and occurs infrequently in older people's nursing homes. The implementation context of this study, connected to an educational intervention based on knowledge-based palliative care principles, is in line with previous findings mentioned above, and it also illustrates the complexity of these conversations that need to be addressed.

In this study, doing participant observations facilitated an understanding of what people do and how their actions change in response to different situations and contexts [46,47]. "Thick descriptions" [46] were made, where meaningful and extensive details were recorded to illustrate the element of presence and trustworthiness, thus strengthening descriptive validity [48,49]. During the observations, the first author reflected upon how her presence might affect the situations and critically reflected upon what caught her attention in each situation and why. The data analysis process was done in collaboration with the first, second, and last author, which increased the credibility.

7. Conclusions

This study shows that conducting conversations about death and dying can have obstacles in practice. The ANs in this study experienced increased security in conducting these conversations halfway into the seminars of a project on implementing knowledge-based palliative care (KUPA);

however, barriers such as limited time and emotional stress were said to hinder the conversations from taking place. Apart from gaining tools to manage conversations, the ANs also used the strategies of distracting, comforting, and disregarding when they perceived the residents' reflections on death and dying either as part of their illness and disease or when there was a lack of alignment between their contemplations and the ideal good dying process. The expressed ambivalence and ambiguity around conversations about death and dying should be taken into consideration in future training, with the aim of developing and supporting ANs' communicative skills in practice. The knowledge from this study will be used and translated into guidelines for continued implementation in new nursing homes after the KUPA project is finalized.

8. Data Availability

The data generated and analyzed during the current study are not publicly available due to the sensitive information with respect to a vulnerable group, older persons living in nursing homes. Therefore, before approving the study, the Regional Ethics Review Board in Lund set restrictions regarding accessibility of the data. However, after the principal researcher (GA) of the KUPA project consults with the review board, data may be available upon reasonable request.

Author Contributions: Å.A. designed the study in collaboration with G.A. (PI of the KUPA project). Å.A. collected data in the fieldwork. The qualitative analysis was performed by Å.A., B.H.R. and G.A. And Å.A. wrote the first draft of the manuscript, together with B.H.R. and G.A. Comments on the results of the categorization and improvement of the draft were made by B.H.R., G.A., A.S., L.B., E.B., B.W. and P.N. All authors approved the final version of the manuscript.

Funding: This study is part of the KUPA project and supported by the Swedish Research Council (grant number 2014-2759); the Vårdal Foundation (grant number 2014-0071); the Medical Faculty of Lund University; the Kamprad Family Foundation; the Faculty of Health and Life Sciences, Linnaeus University; the City of Lund; the Institute for Palliative Care, Region Skane and Lund University; the Greta and Johan Kocks Foundation; and the Ribbingska Memorial Fund. A grant to cover the cost of publishing in Open Access was received from the Swedish Research Council.

Acknowledgments: We are grateful to the assistant nurses who took part in this research, and we would like to thank the nursing home manager, who helped with recruitment.

References

1.   Kellehear, A. *A Social History of Dying*; Cambridge University Press: Cambridge, UK; New York, NY, USA, 2007.

2.   Walter, T. *The Revival of Death*; Routledge: London, UK; New York, NY, USA, 1994.

3.   Werkander Harstade, C.; Sandgren, A. Confronting the forthcoming death: A classic grounded theory. *J. Palliat. Care Med.* **2016**, *6*, 289. [CrossRef]

4.   Hall, S.; Petkova, H.; Tsouros, A.; Constantini, M.; Higginson, I. *Palliative Care for Older People: Better Practices*; World Health Organization, Regional Office for Europe: Copenhagen, Denmark, 2011.

5.   Chan, H.Y.; Pang, S.M. Quality of life concerns and end-of-life care preferences of aged persons in long-term care facilities. *J. Clin. Nurs.* **2007**, *16*, 2158–2166. [CrossRef] [PubMed]

6.   WHO Definition of Palliative Care. Available online: http://www.who.int/cancer/palliative/definition/en/ (accessed on 7 May 2018).

7.   Howarth, G. *Death and Dying: A Sociological Introduction*; Polity Press: Cambridge, UK, 2007.

8.   Froggatt, K.; Payne, S.; Morbey, H.; Edwards, M.; Finne-Soveri, H.; Gambassi, G.; Pasman, H.R.; Szczerbinska, K.; Van den Block, L.; PACE. Palliative care development in European care homes and nursing homes: Application of a typology of implementation. *J. Am. Med. Dir. Assoc.* **2017**, *18*, 550.e7–550.e14. [CrossRef] [PubMed]

9.   Broad, J.B.; Gott, M.; Kim, H.; Boyd, M.; Chen, H.; Connolly, M.J. Where do people die? An international comparison of the percentage of deaths occurring in hospital and residential aged care settings in 45 populations, using published and available statistics. *Int. J. Public Health* **2013**, *58*, 257–267. [CrossRef] [PubMed]

10. Hakanson, C.; Ohlen, J.; Morin, L.; Cohen, J. A population-level study of place of death and associated factors in Sweden. *Scand. J. Public Health* **2015**, *43*, 744–751. [CrossRef] [PubMed]

11. Elderly Care in Sweden. Available online: https://sweden.se/society/elderly-care-in-sweden/ (accessed on 11 April 2018).

12. Tornquist, A.; Andersson, M.; Edberg, A.-K. In search of legitimacy–registered nurses' experience of providing palliative care in a municipal context. *Scand. J. Caring Sci.* **2013**, *27*, 651–658. [CrossRef] [PubMed]

13. Hviid Jacobsen, M. *Deconstructing Death: Changing Cultures of Death, Dying, Bereavement and Care in the Nordic Countries*; University Press of Southern Denmark: Odense, Denmark, 2013.

14. Davies, E.; Higginson, I.J. *Better Palliative Care for Older People*; WHO Regional Office for Europe: Copenhagen, Denmark, 2004.

15. Gott, M.; Ingleton, C. *Living with Ageing and Dying: Palliative and End of Life Care for Older People*; Oxford University Press: Oxford, UK; New York, NY, USA, 2011.

16. Jenull, B.; Brunner, E. Death and dying in nursing homes: A burden for the staff? *J. Appl. Gerontol.* **2008**, *27*, 166–180. [CrossRef]

17. Beck, I.; Tornquist, A.; Brostrom, L.; Edberg, A.-K. Having to focus on doing rather than being-nurse assistants' experience of palliative care in municipal residential care settings. *Int. J. Nurs. Stud.* **2012**, *49*, 455–464. [CrossRef] [PubMed]

18. Froggatt, K.; Parker, D. Guest editorial: Development of palliative care in long term-care facilities: A new evidence base. *Int. J. Older People Nurs.* **2014**, *9*, 91–92. [CrossRef] [PubMed]

19. Tornoe, K.; Danbolt, L.J.; Kvigne, K.; Sorlie, V. A mobile hospice nurse teaching team's experience: Training care workers in spiritual and existential care for the dying—A qualitative study. *BMC Palliat. Care* **2015**, *14*, 43. [CrossRef] [PubMed]

20. Ahsberg, E.; Carlsson, M. Practical care work and existential issues in palliative care: Experiences of nursing assistants. *Int. J. Older People Nurs.* **2014**, *9*, 298–305. [CrossRef] [PubMed]

21. Adams, J. Life and death in English nursing homes: Sequestration or transition? *Nurs. Older People* **2001**, *13*, 8. [CrossRef] [PubMed]

22. Dwyer, L.-L.; Hansebo, G.; Andershed, B.; Ternestedt, B.-M. Nursing home residents' views on dying and death: Nursing home employee's perspective. *Int. J. Older People Nurs.* **2011**, *6*, 251–260. [CrossRef] [PubMed]

23. Osterlind, J.; Hansebo, G.; Andersson, J.; Ternestedt, B.M.; Hellstrom, I. A discourse of silence: Professional carers reasoning about death and dying in nursing homes. *Ageing Soc.* **2011**, *31*, 529–544. [CrossRef]

24. Handley, M.; Goodman, C.; Froggatt, K.; Mathie, E.; Gage, H.; Manthorpe, J.; Barclay, S.; Crang, C.; Iliffe, S. Living and dying: Responsibility for end-of-life care in care homes without on-site nursing provision—A prospective study. *Health Soc. Care Community* **2014**, *22*, 22–29. [CrossRef] [PubMed]

25. Cronfalk, B.S.; Ternestedt, B.-M.; Larsson, L.-L.F.; Henriksen, E.; Norberg, A.; Osterlind, J. Utilization of palliative care principles in nursing home care: Educational interventions. *Palliat. Support. Care* **2015**, *13*, 1745–1753. [CrossRef] [PubMed]

26. Mignani, V.; Ingravallo, F.; Mariani, E.; Chattat, R. Perspectives of older people living in long-term care facilities and of their family members toward advance care planning discussions: A systematic review and thematic synthesis. *Clin. Interv. Aging* **2017**, *12*, 475–484. [CrossRef] [PubMed]

27. Stone, L.; Kinley, J.; Hockley, J. Advance care planning in care homes: The experience of staff, residents, and family members. *Int. J. Palliat. Nurs.* **2013**, *19*, 550–557. [CrossRef] [PubMed]

28. Hockley, J.M. *Developing High Quality End-of-Life Care in Nursing Homes*; University of Edinburgh: Edinburgh, UK, 2006.

29. National Board of Health and Welfare. *The National Knowledge Support Document for Good Palliative Care at the End of Life*; National Board of Health and Welfare: Stockholm, Sweden, 2013. (In Swedish)

30. Regional Co-Operative Cancer Centers. *The National Care Program for Palliative Care 2012–2014*; Regional Co-Operative Cancer Centers (Regionala Cancercentrum i Samverkan): Stockholm, Sweden, 2012. (In Swedish)

31. Smedback, J.; Ohlen, J.; Arestedt, K.; Alvariza, A.; Furst, C.J.; Hakanson, C. Palliative care during the final week of life of older people in nursing homes: A register-based study. *Palliat. Support. Care* **2017**, *15*, 417–424. [CrossRef] [PubMed]

32. National Board of Health and Welfare. The Eldery Guide 2017 (In Swedish: Äldreguiden 2017). Available online: http://oppnajamforelser.socialstyrelsen.se/aldreguiden/Sidor/default.aspx (accessed on 6 June 2018).

33. Ahlstrom, G.; Nilsen, P.; Benzein, E.; Behm, L.; Wallerstedt, B.; Persson, M.; Sandgren, A. Implementation of knowledge-based palliative care in nursing homes and pre-post post evaluation by cross-over design: A study protocol. *BMC Palliat. Care* **2018**, *17*, 52. [CrossRef] [PubMed]

34. Nilsen, P.; Wallerstedt, B.; Behm, L.; Ahlstrom, G. Towards evidence-based palliative care in nursing homes in Sweden: A qualitative study informed by the organizational readiness to change theory. *Implement. Sci.* **2018**, *13*, 1. [CrossRef] [PubMed]

35. Gray, A. *Research Practice for Cultural Studies: Ethnographic Methods and Lived Cultures*; SAGE: London, UK; Thousand Oaks, CA, USA, 2003.

36. Riessman, C.K. *Narrative Methods for the Human Sciences*; Sage Publications: Los Angeles, CA, USA, 2008.

37. Albinsson, L.; Strang, P. A palliative approach to existential issues and death in end-stage dementia care. *J. Palliat. Care* **2002**, *18*, 168–174. [PubMed]

38. Casey, D.; Murphy, K.; Ni Leime, A.; Larkin, P.; Payne, S.; Froggatt, K.A.; O'Shea, E. Dying well: Factors that influence the provision of good end-of-life care for older people in acute and long-stay care settings in ireland. *J. Clin. Nurs.* **2011**, *20*, 1824–1833. [CrossRef] [PubMed]

39. Sundler, A.J.; Eide, H.; van Dulmen, S.; Holmstrom, I.K. Communicative challenges in the home care of older persons—A qualitative exploration. *J. Adv. Nurs.* **2016**, *72*, 2435–2444. [CrossRef] [PubMed]

40. Young, A.; Froggatt, K.; Brearley, S.G. 'Powerlessness' or 'doing the right thing'—Moral distress among nursing home staff caring for residents at the end of life: An interpretive descriptive study. *Palliat. Med.* **2017**, *31*, 853–860. [CrossRef] [PubMed]

41. Costello, J. Nursing older dying patients: Findings from an ethnographic study of death and dying in elderly care wards. *J. Adv. Nurs.* **2001**, *35*, 59–68. [CrossRef] [PubMed]

42. Kellehear, A. Health-promoting palliative care: Developing a social model for practice. *Mortality* **1999**, *4*, 75–82. [CrossRef]

43. Saini, G.; Sampson, E.L.; Davis, S.; Kupeli, N.; Harrington, J.; Leavey, G.; Nazareth, I.; Jones, L.; Moore, K.J. An ethnographic study of strategies to support discussions with family members on end-of-life care for people with advanced dementia in nursing homes. *BMC Palliat. Care* **2016**, *15*, 55. [CrossRef] [PubMed]

44. Wright, D.K.; Brajtman, S.; Cragg, B.; Macdonald, M.E. Delirium as letting go: An ethnographic analysis of hospice care and family moral experience. *Palliat. Med.* **2015**, *29*, 959–966. [CrossRef] [PubMed]

45. Radbruch, L.; Payne, S. White paper on standards and norms for hospice and palliative care in Europe: Part 2. *Eur. J. Palliat. Care* **2010**, *17*, 22–33.

46. Geertz, C. *The Interpretation of Cultures: Selected Essays*; Basic Books: New York, NY, USA, 1973.

47. Walshe, C.; Ewing, G.; Griffiths, J. Using observation as a data collection method to help understand patient and professional roles and actions in palliative care settings. *Palliat. Med.* **2012**, *26*, 1048–1054. [CrossRef] [PubMed]

48. Draper, J. Ethnography: Principles, practice and potential. *Nurs. Stand.* **2015**, *29*, 36–41. [CrossRef] [PubMed]

49. Maxwell, J.A. Understanding and validity in qualitative research. *Harvard Educ. Rev.* **1992**, *62*, 279–300. [CrossRef]

7

Systematic Approach to the Diagnosis and Treatment of Lyme Carditis and High-Degree Atrioventricular Block

Cynthia Yeung⑩ and Adrian Baranchuk *

Department of Medicine, Queen's University, Kingston, ON K7L 3N6, Canada; cyeung@qmed.ca
* Correspondence: Adrian.Baranchuk@kingstonhsc.ca

Abstract: Lyme carditis (LC) is a manifestation of the early disseminated stage of Lyme disease and often presents as high-degree atrioventricular (AV) block. High-degree AV block in LC can be treated with antibiotics, usually resolving with a highly favorable prognosis, thus preventing the unnecessary implantation of permanent pacemakers. We present a systematic approach to the diagnosis and management of LC that implements the Suspicious Index in Lyme Carditis (SILC) risk stratification score.

Keywords: Lyme disease; Lyme carditis; atrioventricular block

1. Introduction

Lyme disease is an infection that can manifest in a multi-system nature, usually transmitted by the tick *Ixodes scapularis* and caused by a Gram-negative spirochete bacteria, *Borrelia burgdorferi*. The most commonly reported vector-borne disease in North America [1], Lyme disease presents mainly between March and October, with over 60% of reported cases in June and July [2].

Lyme carditis (LC) was first described in 1980 by Steere, et al. and is an early manifestation of Lyme disease, appearing within one to two months (range < 1 to 28 weeks) after the onset of infection [3,4]. The incidence of cardiac involvement in Lyme disease is estimated to be 0.3% to 4% [5]. Compared to the relatively equal prevalence of Lyme disease by sex, LC has a strong male predominance of approximately 3:1 [2]. Although other asymptomatic conduction disorders are possible—including sinus node disease, intraatrial block, abnormal nodal recovery time, and interventricular delay [5–9]—high-degree atrioventricular (AV) block is the most common, in approximately 90% of LC, and requires cardiac monitoring [3,7].

The transmural inflammation in LC is predominantly comprised of macrophages and lymphocytes [10], and is concentrated at the base of the heart, the basal interventricular septum, and the perivascular regions [10,11]. The pathophysiology of AV node involvement in LC may be explained by its anatomical location, histology, and metabolic mechanisms [12]. The block is often above the bundle of His at the AV node level [4]. Patients with a PR interval > 300 milliseconds are at the highest risk for progression to complete AV block [4]. Progression to complete heart block can be rapid, and if untreated, potentially fatal [13–15].

In general, the treatment for a high-degree AV block is pacing. However, the AV block in LC may revert back to normal conduction, and usually resolves within the first 10 days of antibiotic administration [12,16,17]. If the AV block in LC is indeed transient, then a permanent pacemaker is not indicated [16]. Therefore, the identification of LC in patients with a high-degree AV block is imperative to prevent the inherent risks of pacemaker implantation, such as periprocedural infections, lead dislodgement, and erosions [18]. Furthermore, given the young demographic of patients with

LC, unnecessary pacemaker implantation would result in the subsequent lifetime of multiple pulse generator changes and burden of associated cumulative health care costs [19].

2. Systematic Approach to the Diagnosis and Management of Lyme Carditis

Case series have demonstrated that patients often present several times before the LC is suspected [19]. Many patients with LC do not recall a clear history of a tick bite. Although erythema migrans is present in 70–80% of Lyme disease cases [6,20], the pathognomonic rash is less common (40%) in LC [5]. Prompt treatment of LC shortens the duration of the cardiac manifestations and prevents later complications of Lyme disease [5,21]. Failure to recognize and treat Lyme disease aggressively in its early stages may increase the need for temporary or permanent pacing [17].

2.1. The Suspicious Index in Lyme Carditis (SILC) Risk Score

In order to evaluate the likelihood that a patient's high-degree heart block is caused by LC, we proposed the Suspicious Index in Lyme Carditis (SILC) score (Table 1) [22]. This novel risk score assigns weights to several risk factors: age < 50 [5,6,19]; male sex [2]; outdoor activity or endemic area [2,23]; constitutional symptoms of Lyme disease, including fever, malaise, arthralgia, dyspnea, pre-syncope, and syncope [4,24]; history of a tick bite [19]; and erythema migrans [6]. A preliminary validation study in which the SILC risk stratification tool was retrospectively applied to 88 cases of LC (83 from a systematic review of all published cases of LC with high degree AV block and five from our own experience) demonstrated a sensitivity of 93.2% (if a variable was not available, it was conservatively assigned a zero). The sensitivity increased to 100% when the SILC score was applied to cases that reported on all SILC variables ($n = 32$) [22].

Table 1. The Suspicious Index in Lyme Carditis (SILC) score evaluates the likelihood that a patient's high-degree heart block is caused by Lyme carditis. The total summed score indicates low (0–2), intermediate (3–6), or high (7–12) suspicion of Lyme carditis.

Variable	Value
Age < 50 years	1
Male	1
Outdoor activity/endemic area	1
Constitutional symptoms [1]	2
Tick bite	3
Erythema migrans	4

[1] Fever, malaise, arthralgia, dyspnea, pre-syncope, and syncope.

2.2. Algorithm for the Diagnosis and Management of Lyme Carditis

A flowchart summarizing our algorithm for the systematic approach to the diagnosis and management of LC is presented in Figure 1. The SILC score should be calculated for the patient presenting with a high-degree AV block. If the summed SILC score is 0–2 (low risk), then standard treatment for a high-degree AV block should be followed. If the summed SILC score is 3–6 (intermediate risk) or 7–12 (high risk), serological tests for Lyme disease (positive enzyme-linked immunosorbent assay (ELISA) and Western blot) should be ordered to confirm the infection [25–27].

Blood serologies can be falsely negative due to the delayed immune response, and consequently, negative serology does not always rule out early Lyme infection. However, since LC is a manifestation of the disseminated stage of Lyme disease, the vast majority of patients with LC have positive serologic responses with either IgM and/or IgG antibodies [28]. Notably, serum IgG antibodies may be present long after recovery from Lyme disease, and thus, seropositivity may not translate to a recent *B. burgdorferi* infection being the cause of a cardiac presentation.

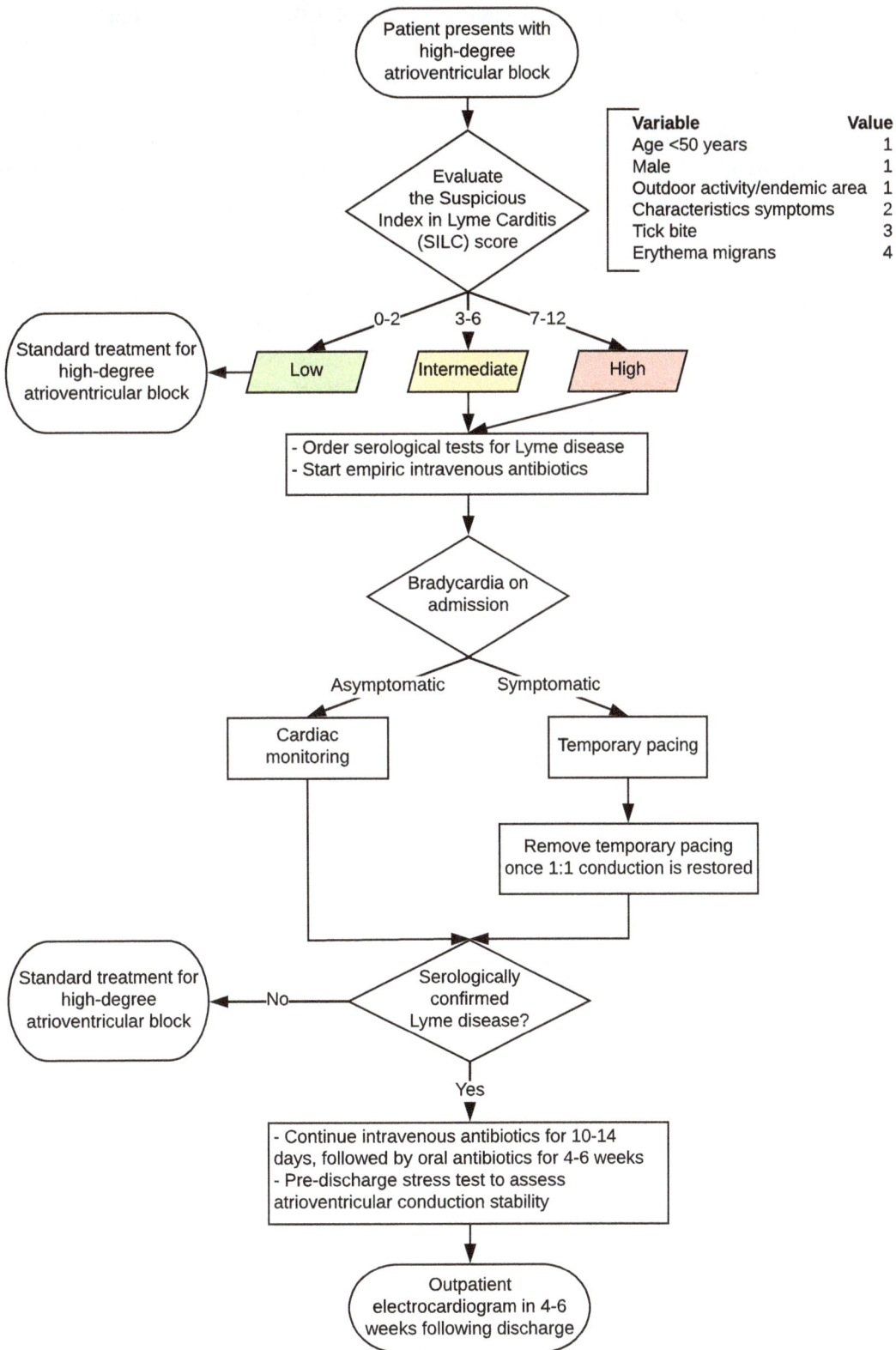

Figure 1. Systematic approach to the diagnosis and management of Lyme carditis and high-degree atrioventricular block.

While the results of the Lyme serology are being processed, empiric intravenous (IV) antibiotics should be started [21]. Despite the lack of comparative trials on the optimal antibiotic regimen or route for LC, expert opinion and supportive data from case reports indicate that ceftriaxone (2 g IV once daily in adults; 50–75 mg/kg IV once daily in children) is first-line therapy, but appropriate alternatives include IV cefotaxime or penicillin G.

Management for bradycardia on admission is dependent on whether it is symptomatic. Asymptomatic bradycardia should be followed with cardiac monitoring, because patients with LC can progress from a prolonged PR interval to complete block and asystole, and the degree of AV block can fluctuate rapidly [29,30]. Symptomatic bradycardia should be managed with temporary pacing (standard or temporary-permanent pacemaker). Approximately one-third of patients with LC require temporary pacing [3,16,19].

If Lyme disease is serologically confirmed, IV antibiotics should be continued for 10–14 days, followed by a four to six weeks oral antibiotic regimen. Appropriate oral antibiotics include doxycycline, amoxicillin, and cefuroxime axetil (doxycycline should not be used in pregnant women or children <8 years). A pre-discharge stress test should be ordered to assess the stability of atrioventricular conduction. An outpatient electrocardiogram arranged for four to six weeks post-discharge is appropriate to confirm a normal PR interval and the lack of any other rhythm or conduction abnormalities.

3. Conclusions

The SILC risk score may help identify LC in patients presenting with high-degree AV block. High-degree AV block in LC can be treated with antibiotics, often resolving with a highly favorable prognosis, thus preventing the unnecessary implantation of permanent pacemakers.

Author Contributions: The authors contributed equally to this work.

Funding: This research received no external funding.

References

1. Mead, P.S. Epidemiology of Lyme disease. *Infect. Dis. Clin. N. Am.* **2015**, *29*, 187–210. [CrossRef] [PubMed]
2. Bacon, R.M.; Kugeler, K.J.; Mead, P.S.; Centers for Disease Control and Prevention. Surveillance for Lyme disease—United States, 1992–2006. *MMWR Surveill Summ.* **2008**, *57*, 1–9. [PubMed]
3. McAlister, H.F.; Klementowicz, P.T.; Andrews, C.; Fisher, J.D.; Feld, M.; Furman, S. Lyme carditis: An important cause of reversible heart block. *Ann. Intern. Med.* **1989**, *110*, 339–345. [CrossRef] [PubMed]
4. Steere, A.C.; Batsford, W.P.; Weinberg, M.; Alexander, J.; Berger, H.J.; Wolfson, S.; Malawista, S.E. Lyme carditis: Cardiac abnormalities of Lyme disease. *Ann. Intern. Med.* **1980**, *93*, 8–16. [CrossRef] [PubMed]
5. Krause, P.J.; Bockenstedt, L.K. Cardiology patient pages. Lyme disease and the heart. *Circulation* **2013**, *127*, e451–e454. [CrossRef] [PubMed]
6. Nagi, K.S.; Joshi, R.; Thakur, R.K. Cardiac manifestations of Lyme disease: A review. *Can. J. Cardiol.* **1996**, *12*, 503–506. [PubMed]
7. Van der Linde, M.R. Lyme carditis: Clinical characteristics of 105 cases. *Scand. J. Infect. Dis. Suppl.* **1991**, *77*, 81–84. [PubMed]
8. Reznick, J.W.; Braunstein, D.B.; Walsh, R.L.; Smith, C.R.; Wolfson, P.M.; Gierke, L.W.; Gorelkin, L.; Chandler, F.W. Lyme carditis. Electrophysiologic and histopathologic study. *Am. J. Med.* **1986**, *81*, 923–927. [CrossRef]
9. Van der Linde, M.R.; Crijns, H.J.; De Koning, J.; Hoogkamp-Korstanje, J.A.; De Graaf, J.J.; Piers, D.A.; Van der Galien, A.; Lie, K.I. Range of atrioventricular conduction disturbances in Lyme borreliosis: A report of four cases and review of other published reports. *Br. Heart J.* **1990**, *63*, 162–168. [CrossRef] [PubMed]
10. Cadavid, D.; Bai, Y.; Hodzic, E.; Narayan, K.; Barthold, S.W.; Pachner, A.R. Cardiac involvement in non-human primates infected with the lyme disease spirochete borrelia burgdorferi. *Lab. Investig.* **2004**, *84*, 1439–1450. [CrossRef] [PubMed]
11. Armstrong, A.L.; Barthold, S.W.; Persing, D.H.; Beck, D.S. Carditis in Lyme disease susceptible and resistant strains of laboratory mice infected with borrelia burgdorferi. *Am. J. Trop. Med. Hyg* **1992**, *47*, 249–258. [CrossRef] [PubMed]

12. Sharma, A.K.; Almaddah, N.; Chaudhry, K.; Ganatra, S.; Chaudhry, G.M.; Silver, J. Without further delay: Lyme carditis. *Am. J. Med.* **2018**, *131*, 384–386. [CrossRef] [PubMed]

13. Centers for Disease Control and Prevention. Three sudden cardiac deaths associated with Lyme carditis—United States, November 2012–July 2013. *MMWR Morb. Mortal. Wkly. Rep.* **2013**, *62*, 993–996.

14. Forrester, J.D.; Meiman, J.; Mullins, J.; Nelson, R.; Ertel, S.H.; Cartter, M.; Brown, C.M.; Lijewski, V.; Schiffman, E.; Neitzel, D.; et al. Notes from the field: Update on Lyme carditis, groups at high risk, and frequency of associated sudden cardiac death—United States. *MMWR Morb. Mortal. Wkly. Rep.* **2014**, *63*, 982–983. [PubMed]

15. Muehlenbachs, A.; Bollweg, B.C.; Schulz, T.J.; Forrester, J.D.; DeLeon Carnes, M.; Molins, C.; Ray, G.S.; Cummings, P.M.; Ritter, J.M.; Blau, D.M.; et al. Cardiac tropism of borrelia burgdorferi: An autopsy study of sudden cardiac death associated with Lyme carditis. *Am. J. Pathol.* **2016**, *186*, 1195–1205. [CrossRef] [PubMed]

16. Fuster, L.S.; Gul, E.E.; Baranchuk, A. Electrocardiographic progression of acute Lyme disease. *Am. J. Emerg Med.* **2017**, *35*, 1040.e5–1040.e6. [CrossRef] [PubMed]

17. Fu Md, J.; Bhatta, L. Lyme carditis: Early occurrence and prolonged recovery. *J. Electrocardiol.* **2018**, *51*, 516–518. [CrossRef] [PubMed]

18. Wan, D.; Baranchuk, A. Lyme carditis and atrioventricular block. *CMAJ* **2018**, *190*, E622. [CrossRef] [PubMed]

19. Wan, D.; Blakely, C.; Branscombe, P.; Suarez-Fuster, L.; Glover, B.; Baranchuk, A. Lyme carditis and high-degree atrioventricular block. *Am. J. Cardiol.* **2018**, *121*, 1102–1104. [CrossRef] [PubMed]

20. Ogden, N.H.; Lindsay, L.R.; Morshed, M.; Sockett, P.N.; Artsob, H. The emergence of Lyme disease in Canada. *CMAJ* **2009**, *180*, 1221–1224. [CrossRef] [PubMed]

21. Wormser, G.P.; Dattwyler, R.J.; Shapiro, E.D.; Halperin, J.J.; Steere, A.C.; Klempner, M.S.; Krause, P.J.; Bakken, J.S.; Strle, F.; Stanek, G.; et al. The clinical assessment, treatment, and prevention of Lyme disease, human granulocytic anaplasmosis, and babesiosis: Clinical practice guidelines by the infectious diseases society of America. *Clin. Infect. Dis.* **2006**, *43*, 1089–1134. [CrossRef] [PubMed]

22. Besant, G.; Wan, D.; Blakely, C.; Branscombe, P.; Suarez-Fuster, L.; Redfearn, D.; Simpson, C.; Abdollah, H.; Glover, B.; Baranchuk, A. Lyme carditis presenting with high-degree atrioventricular block: A systematic review. *J. Electrocardiol.* **2018**, in press.

23. Schwartz, B.S.; Goldstein, M.D. Lyme disease in outdoor workers: Risk factors, preventive measures, and tick removal methods. *Am. J. Epidemiol.* **1990**, *131*, 877–885. [CrossRef] [PubMed]

24. Applegren, N.D.; Kraus, C.K. Lyme disease: Emergency department considerations. *J. Emerg. Med.* **2017**, *52*, 815–824. [CrossRef] [PubMed]

25. Russell, H.; Sampson, J.S.; Schmid, G.P.; Wilkinson, H.W.; Plikaytis, B. Enzyme-linked immunosorbent assay and indirect immunofluorescence assay for Lyme disease. *J. Infect. Dis.* **1984**, *149*, 465–470. [CrossRef] [PubMed]

26. Engstrom, S.M.; Shoop, E.; Johnson, R.C. Immunoblot interpretation criteria for serodiagnosis of early Lyme disease. *J. Clin. Microbiol.* **1995**, *33*, 419–427. [PubMed]

27. Dressler, F.; Whalen, J.A.; Reinhardt, B.N.; Steere, A.C. Western blotting in the serodiagnosis of Lyme disease. *J. Infect. Dis.* **1993**, *167*, 392–400. [CrossRef] [PubMed]

28. Steere, A.C.; McHugh, G.; Damle, N.; Sikand, V.K. Prospective study of serologic tests for lyme disease. *Clin. Infect. Dis.* **2008**, *47*, 188–195. [CrossRef] [PubMed]

29. Steere, A.C. Lyme disease. *N. Engl. J. Med.* **2001**, *345*, 115–125. [CrossRef] [PubMed]

30. Pinto, D.S. Cardiac manifestations of Lyme disease. *Med. Clin. N. Am.* **2002**, *86*, 285–296. [CrossRef]

8

An Evaluation of Alternatives for Providing Care to Veterans

Lawrence V. Fulton *[ID] and Matthew S. Brooks

Department of Health Administration, Texas State University, HPB 250, 601 University Drive, San Marcos, TX 78666, USA; mbrooks@txstate.edu
* Correspondence: Lf25@txstate.edu

Abstract: In 2014, a whistleblower reported that many U.S. veterans died while waiting for care at the Phoenix VHA. Problems with veteran's care through 2018 reveal ongoing and systematic problem. In March 2018, the VA Inspector General identified critical deficiencies at the Washington, DC VA Medical Center including failures to track patient safety events accurately, ineffective sterile processing and more than 10 thousand open or pending prosthetic/sensory aid consults. The VHA clearly has problems with access and quality in a budget-constrained environment. In this policy analysis, four separate interventions that address the gap between the magnitude as well as the use of the VHA's fixed budget versus access and cost expectations are explored. These policy interventions include maintaining the status quo, returning to a "VHA-only" option, transitioning to a CMS central payer system and consolidating care under the DoD TRICARE insurance plans. An objective evaluation suggests that extending TRICARE to veterans during the phasing out the VHA's care responsibilities, while politically unpalatable, would likely provide the best of four possible solutions under various criterion weighting schemes. A central payer solution under the CMS would also be a viable consideration. Results suggest that TRICARE patient perceptions of quality are superior to VHA and non-VHA/non-DoD, that access provided by the TRICARE program is ranked second in terms of venue acceptance only to the CMS solution set based on primary provider acceptance and that the cost per beneficiary of a TRICARE solution ($6.5 K/beneficiary) is far better than a VHA-only solution ($14.0 K/beneficiary), the CMS central payer solution ($12.2 K/beneficiary), or the status quo (between $12.2 K and $14.0 K/beneficiary). The intent of this paper is to provoke thoughtful consideration of solutions for providing access to high-quality healthcare for veterans within or outside of the VHA.

Keywords: health policy; VHA; VA; CMS TRICARE; scandal

1. Introduction

The United States Veteran's Health Administration (VHA) is the "largest integrated healthcare system, providing care at 1240 facilities, including 170 medical centers and 1061 outpatient sites of care of varying complexity (VHA outpatient clinics), serving 9 million enrolled veterans each year" [1]. For FY2019, the VHA will maintain more than 315,000 full-time equivalents and a budget (both mandatory and discretionary with stepped down administrative costs) estimated to be nearly $98 billion [2]. The organization's mission is to "Honor America's Veterans by providing exceptional health care that improves their health and well-being" [3]. Unfortunately, the VHA's recent and historical problems with mismanagement, reporting falsification and preventable deaths have made it "exceptional" in unfortunate ways. This problem has been characterized as "system-wide" by Concerned Veterans of America [4]. These recent problems provide the United States an opportunity to evaluate alternatives that provide veterans cost-effective and quality-centered health services.

This policy analysis paper identifies the VHA system problems and ongoing policy interventions, evaluates possible additional policy interventions by drawing from other systems external and internal to the US, analyzes these possible interventions against developed criterion and leverages utility matrices to evaluate them.

1.1. Problem Background

In 2014, a whistleblower reported that "at least 40" U.S. veterans died while waiting for care at the Phoenix VHA. More than 1400 of these veterans were placed on a "secret" waiting list in an apparent effort to hide the actual treatment delays [5]. The VA Office of the Inspector General's (IG's) investigation confirmed the existence of an "off-book" waiting list and further identified 28 cases of clinically significant delays with 6 associated deaths. By August of 2014, the VA IG was investigating 93 VHA facilities for manipulating wait times but had confirmed manipulations of wait time were prevalent. One of the conclusions of the IG was that emphasis on goals (linked to financial incentives) provided a "misleading portrayal" of veterans' access and that the reported outcomes were both inaccurate and unsupported [6]. The demand from high-need returning veterans likely outstripped the supply and the VHA handled it poorly [7].

Similar misconduct occurred in the United Kingdom. Between January 2005 and March 2009, Britain's National Health Service (NHS) experienced a scandal, which was discovered when mortality rates were increasing [8]. The UK government was incentivizing frugality by offering autonomy and a share of savings for those facilities attaining "Foundation" status [9]. The focus on performance targets was associated with an unexpected increase in deaths during this period (estimated to be as many as 1200). In another example from 2001, the National Audit Office identified nine trusts that were inappropriately manipulating waiting lists, identical to the problem of the VHA. Some of the problems identified in the report include altering of patient records, deletions from waiting lists and non-reporting of patients waiting 18 months or more. The report found that some managers simply sought to meet performance benchmarks [10].

In both government-run and government-funded organizations (the VHA and NHS), management's focus appeared to be on performance targets rather than patients and incentives for fraud existed. In the case of the VHA, the problems continue today. A recent report from the VA IG confirmed that the VHA's Eastern Colorado Health Care System was using "off-book" patient scheduling which under-reported treatment delays [11]. Waiting time manipulation since 2014 has occurred in at least seven states [12]. In 2016, the Phoenix VHA again became the subject of investigation, as VA IG inspectors identified 215 deceased patients who were awaiting specialist consultations on the date of death. Staff were still not managing or scheduling consults according to VHA policy [13].

1.2. Problem and Significance

The problem for the VHA and under consideration here is the identification of possible policy solutions that improve on status quo performance and address the gap between the magnitude as well as the use of the VHA's annual and performance expectations for quality and access [8]. The significance of this problem may be measured in mortality and morbidity. The true scope of the problem is unknown, as metrics are only available for those who successfully accessed the system. Those veterans discouraged with access issues may not seek care and are of unknown quantity.

Like the NHS, the VHA operates with an annual budget and has certain benchmarks for quality and access. This budget versus benchmark relationship may be irreconcilable at the current operating efficiency level. Policy efforts have attempted to fill the budget versus benchmark gap by increasing funding and access; however, the success of these interventions has been mixed. The purpose of this policy analysis is to assess current and future policy interventions that might address the requirement to provide veterans access to high-quality, cost-effective healthcare.

1.3. Previous Policy Interventions

As a direct response to the 2014 VHA scandal, President Obama signed the Veterans Access, Choice and Accountability Act of 2014 (PL 113-146). This law approved $10 billion for the Veterans Choice plan, authorizing civilian care opportunities to veterans who live more than 40 miles from a VA facility or who wait for more than 30 days for healthcare. Further, it offered another $5 billion to the VHA for personnel and facilities, prevented bonus payments from being tied to wait-time goals, implemented additional oversight of facilities and provided the VA Secretary expanded authority to fire poorly performing managers. Initial funding for Veterans Choice ended on 31 May 2018 [14]. A 2017 NPR investigation, however, revealed that the VA hired no more providers than it would have without the funding, that the new hires were not sent to the hospitals with the longest waiting times and that the facilities which received the new hires were not more likely to see improved waiting times [15].

On 6 June 2018, President Trump signed the VA Maintaining Systems and Strengthening Integrated Outside Networks Act (VA Mission Act of 2018). This act (among other things) provided a community health program for veterans and extended Veterans Choice coverage until the Mission Act is implemented. Under the new law, veterans are entitled access to community care if the VHA does not offer the care or services required, it does not operate a full-service medical facility in the veteran's state, the veteran lives more than 40 miles from a VHA facility, the VHA is not able to meet the designated access standards it establishes, or the veteran and clinician agree that community care would be in the veteran's best interest [16]. The Congressional Budget Office (CBO) estimates the VA Mission Act will cost $55.2 billion over 5 years with $5.2 billion extending the Veterans Choice program, $4.5 billion extending certain Medicaid-eligible veteran pension benefits and $46.5 billion for the community healthcare program [17].For FY2019, $14.2 billion is provided for community care [2].

Coupled with this $14.2 billion is the VHA FY2019 requested budget of $76.5 billion for medical care, $1.2 billion for an electronic health record (EHR) system, $0.7 billion for research and $1.5 billion for construction for a total of $79.9 billion [2].Assigning 80% of the requested $4.2 billion for informational technology, $0.4 for general administration and $0.2 for IG functions to the VHA (due to its sheer size relative to the other organizations within the VA) results in an adjusted VHA estimated budget of $83.8 billion. While the organization reports on its website that there are 9 million enrolled veterans, its budget request is for 7.0 million treated veterans [2]. NOTE: A veteran "enrolled" in the VHA may never use the system, as he or she may have secondary insurance such as TRICARE (e.g., military retirees) or through other employment, so the "treated veterans" is likely the better estimate of actual beneficiaries. This dual eligibility provides some complication when accounting for the number of true beneficiary users, particularly if users split care between systems. With the $14.2 billion for community care, the total cost for veteran care becomes an estimated $98 billion or $14.0 K per veteran per year. Understanding this baseline becomes important when considering additional policy alternatives.

1.4. Why Are Policies Shifting towards External Care for Veterans?

Veterans Choice and the VA Mission Act pave an avenue to civilian care for veterans, which is a shift in policy. The question becomes "why?" The VA indicates that "there is no effort underway to privatize [6] VA and to suggest otherwise is completely false and a red herring designed to distract and avoid honest debate on the real issues surrounding Veterans' health care" [18]. In this statement, the VA points to increases in budget, employees and facilities over two decades. President Trump has indicated a shift in policy towards joint community and VHA care, by stating, "We're allowing our veterans to get access to the best medical care available, whether it is at the VA or at a private provider" [19]. Further, the VA Mission Act also established a commission charged with reviewing the VA infrastructure assets for closure (i.e., the 1240 facilities), a commission that will not have any VA representation [20]. It is possible that there will be a blended VA system for quite some time; however, it is fathomable that the incorporation of external healthcare providers may be logical incrementalism [21], a slow move away from the VHA's NHS-like structure in favor of a single payer system for veterans. From a broader perspective, it is also possible that the VHA may see transformational change through additional policy.

1.5. Some Major Stakeholders

Some of the major actors in the veterans' healthcare crisis problem are the veterans themselves, veterans' groups, the public, the VHA, the Congressional Democrats, the Congressional Republicans, the Executive Branch and the media. Each of these stakeholders has evidence-based positions on policy.

1.5.1. Veterans, Veterans' Groups and the Public

A somewhat-dated poll (2015) indicates that 64% of veterans oppose "privatization" of the VHA system, although that definition is not well defined [22]. Veterans' groups such as the Concerned Veterans for America have emerged as powerful players in this administration [23]. The public itself is influential and there is highest level of grass-roots support for increased spending on veterans in two decades [24].

1.5.2. The VHA

The VHA opposes any policy that results in further dilution of organic management and treatment [18]. But the VHA may have little power in the process as evidence by the fact that the VA Mission Act excludes them from even having a representative on the committee that will evaluate infrastructure for elimination [20].

1.5.3. Congress and the President

Democrats and Republicans demonstrated significant bi-partisanship when passing the VA Mission Act, with the Senate voting 92% in favor and the House voting 81% in favor. Both parties officially oppose "privatization," an ill-defined buzzword which may trigger emotional responses in constituencies [25]. Republicans are characteristically more supportive of small government [26] relative to Democrats, so one might assume their support for a smaller VHA. As a former business leader, the President favors business solutions [27]. By extending community care for veterans further and by approving plans for infrastructure assessment, he may be sending a message that the VHA is inefficient.

1.5.4. The Media

The media is likely to report incremental changes to the veteran's healthcare system which result in negative outcomes are likely to be reported widely. As in the initial scandal, the media can make a difference [28].

1.6. The Political Environment

Given the current political environment, additional major changes in veterans' healthcare may not be supported. Without bi-partisan support for additional interventions, policy changes would require executive orders and the rule-making process. It is here where the courts may have a significant role.

1.7. Synopsis

As the VHA continues to struggle with executing its mission, Congress and the President have stepped in with money and programs to attempt to fill the void. Despite the lackluster performance of the Veterans Choice program, there may be reasonable hope that the VA Mission Act will improve veterans care. The question then becomes what other policy interventions are available.

2. Materials & Methods

For this policy analysis, the framework of MacRae and Wilde is loosely followed [29]. The use of utility (decision or performance) matrices in decision-making has been promulgated for health interventions [30] and that is the approach used here. A utility matrix evaluates health policy interventions against policy goals. Assume that three policies, {A, B, C}, are being evaluated against three operationalized criteria, {X, Y, Z}. Qualitative or quantitative analysis of each potential policy against each criterion is made based on the definitions provided for the criteria. Once all assessments are completed for all criteria and all policies, the assessments for each criterion across all policies are converted to ranks. For this policy analysis, lower values reflect better rankings. Decision makers often weight criteria based on relative importance or political consequences and these weights are applied to each ranking within that criterion. If the weights across all criterion sum to the number of criterion (e.g., the sum of the weights equals 3 in this case), then the sum of the values in the weighted table will be identical to the sum of values in the unweighted table. Sensitivity analysis is often conducted by manipulating the weights to identify under what weighting conditions other policy interventions might emerge. Table 1 discusses the use of a decision matrix for this example.

Table 1. This table illustrates a typical weighted utility matrix. The left-hand column contains the policies under consideration, {A, B, C}. The top row contains the criteria for evaluating the policies, {X, Y, Z}. The assessed values for each criterion across all policies sum to 6, 1 + 2 + 3. Ties receive an average of the occupied position as illustrated under criterion Z where 2 values of 2.5 exist representing a tie for positions 2 and 3 for policies A and C, (2 + 3)/2 = 2.5. Since lower values indicate a higher assessment, the unweighted decision would be policy A, as its sum is 5.5 compared to 6.0 and 6.5. Weights are assigned to each criterion such that the sum of those weights (0.5 + 0.5 + 2.0) equals the number of criteria (3) to keep the magnitude of the unweighted and weighted decisions the same. (Both the unweighted and weighted solution values sum to 18). The weighted decision values are calculated by applying the weights to the assessed values for each policy. For example, policy A's weighted solution is calculated as follows: $0.5 \times 1.0 + 0.5 \times 2.0 + 2.0 \times 2.5 = 6.5$. In this example, the weighted decision would be policy B versus policy A. The weights are often adjusted to provide sensitivity analysis.

	Criteria			Decision	
Policy	X	Y	Z	Unweighted	Weighted
A	1.0	2.0	2.5	5.5	6.5
B	2.0	3.0	1.0	6.0	4.5
C	3.0	1.0	2.5	6.5	7.0
Sum	6.0	6.0	6.0	18.0	18.0
Weights	0.5	0.5	2.0	Lower is better.	

2.1. Goals and Objectives of Public Policy for the VHA Problem

The U.S. government and public in general expect veterans to receive timely access to quality, cost-effective care. These principles reflect the "Iron Triangle of Healthcare" promulgated by William Kissick and form three of the evaluation criteria: cost, quality and access [31]. Further, any evaluation of policies should consider analysis of political feasibility [32], as well as administrative feasibility (ability to obtain resources and administer the policy). Operational definitions for each selected criterion are then required.

Healthcare costs are difficult to assess even with assembled panels of experts. In the case of this analysis, annual cost per beneficiary is the primary measure when available. If this metric cannot be estimated (as in the case of one policy intervention), then comparative analysis of fixed and variable costs using the status quo is used. Cost is measured in dollars with lower costs indicating a better solution for this criterion.

Measuring quality associated with a policy intervention is difficult, particularly when fraudulent or inaccurate reporting of metrics may exist by all parties involved. For example, a GAO audit recently identified that the VHA does not capture data from all providers including contract providers as well as advanced practice providers, so the reported quality metrics are a non-random subsample. Further, the audit indicated that the VHA does not oversee its medical centers' monitoring efforts, which is inconsistent with federal controls [33]. Also problematic is that the VHA has been violating federal law for at least 15 years by hiring clinicians whose licenses have been revoked in other states. For example, a neurosurgeon whose license was revoked was hired by the Iowa City VA based on VA's national guidance [34]. Given the VHA's recent scandals, confidence in their self-reported quality metrics should be low. In this study, quality will be measured by the patient experience metrics in the most recent Hospital Compare dataset [35]. The Medicare Hospital Compare dataset provides standardized information for all hospital facilities which receive Medicare reimbursement including patient satisfaction scores. Because the VHA quality outcome data are flawed, comparing VHA versus non-VHA facilities must be done on identically gathered and reported reliable data. The data that best meet this criterion are the Hospital Consumer Assessment of Healthcare Providers and Systems (HCAHPS) patient satisfaction data gathered by Hospital Compare and the VHA equivalent, the Survey of Healthcare Experiences of Patients (SHEPS). Both instruments contain 11 identical HCAHPS questions, which may be quantitatively used to assess quality. These surveys provide reasonable comparisons of quality across systems [36]. One should note that some studies have shown that VHA facilities provide at least the same quality as non-VHA facilities using the VHA's non-random subsample (and flawed reporting), while satisfaction may be lower [37,38].

Access is a difficult variable to define, as most associated metrics fail to consider individuals who wanted access and were not provided it. VHA reports patient access data on its website [39]; however, there is no analogous report for civilian facilities and some of the VHA reporting appears to contain errors. Examples of the problem were seen when evaluating bi-monthly access reports from January through June 2017 ($N = 11$ reports). Of specific interest was the variability of the visit counts and the variability of the proportion of appointments made within 30 days. For facilities with an average appointment count between 10,000 and 12,000 during the survey time ($n = 30$), one facility's standard deviation for appointment counts was 82.4 over this 6-month period versus 751.9 for all others, a statistical outlier with $F_{(319,11)} = 83.2$, $p < 0.001$. This same facility's variation in the proportion of 30-day appointments provided averaged 99.3% (with no reports of 100%) and the standard deviation was 0.0006% compared to 0.1245% for all other facilities (none of which had reports of 100% availability), $F_{(319,11)} = 214.9$, $p < 0.001$. As another example, the coefficient of variation for appointment counts (CV = $s/\mu \times 100$), a measure of standardized variability, was less than one (CV = 0.694) for a facility with on-average 5622 patient appointments per month. That same facility had 3 out of 11 reports with identical proportion of appointments within 30 days (99.37%). While these examples might reflect true outliers, they and other statistics are somewhat suggestive of reporting errors. There is also evidence from late 2017 that VHA access metrics are problematic [11]. Given that access metrics for non-VHA facilities are not available and that VHA access metrics may reflect actual waiting time, access will be measured as the number healthcare venue options veterans are provided. If a veteran has access to only one system, this would be worse than having access to two or more systems. While this is an imperfect measure, it allows for policy comparison at least at the macro level.

Both political and administrative feasibility are assessed qualitatively. Political feasibility is assessed via ranking of policy alternatives based on known or inferred positions of actors, an evaluation of the current environment and an assessment of events that would either favor or not favor a particular policy. Policies assessed to be more politically palatable are deemed better than others. Administrative feasibility is a ranking assessment of ease in which a plan might be implemented based on required resources and overhead. Some of these resources include facilities as well as personnel. Where possible, evidence of administrative complexity from the baseline status quo is provided.

2.2. Weighting

Weighting of decision matrices is subjective and should be coupled with sensitivity analysis. To assign weights, Table 2 is used to depict importance values which are converted to weights. The sum of the importance assessment by criterion is {8, 10, 10, 7, 6} for {cost, quality, access, political feasibility, administrative feasibility}, respectively. Converting these to weights (dividing each value by the sum of the criteria importance and multiplying by the number of criteria) results in starting weights of {0.98, 1.22, 1.22, 0.85, 0.73} for each of the respective criteria.

Table 2. Patient satisfaction scores for 1 April 2016 through 31 March 2017 for the VHA, non-VHA and DoD.

	Item: Patients Who	VHA	Other Facilities	DoD
1.	"Strongly Agree" they understood their care when they left the hospital	0.554	0.521	0.605
2.	gave their hospital a rating of 9 or 10 on a scale from 0 (lowest) to 10 (highest)	0.684	0.727	0.716
3.	reported that staff "Always" explained about medicines before giving it to them	0.663	0.651	0.752
4.	reported that the area around their room was "Always" quiet at night	0.566	0.622	0.681
5.	reported that their doctors "Always" communicated well	0.779	0.818	0.868
6.	reported that their nurses "Always" communicated well	0.763	0.802	0.857
7.	reported that their pain was "Always" well controlled	0.640	0.710	0.735
8.	reported that their room and bathroom were "Always" clean	0.733	0.742	0.766
9.	reported that they "Always" received help as soon as they wanted	0.649	0.682	0.785
10.	reported that YES, they were given information about what to do during their recovery at home	0.871	0.873	0.907
11.	reported YES, they would definitely recommend the hospital	0.695	0.720	0.727

2.3. Policy Options

With the operational definitions of the criteria complete, an analysis of reasonable policy options is necessary. Here, we explore four possible policy interventions: expansion of the VHA system to provide all required veteran care, phased elimination of the VHA in favor of central payment system at the Centers for Medicare and Medicaid (CMS), expansion of military retiree subsidized insurance plan to include all veterans regardless of retirement status (private insurance), retention of the status quo. All interventions except for the status quo would require legislative action. Each of these policy options might achieve the goals of providing cost-effective, quality care for veterans.

The first option (short title: VHA only) expands the VHA sufficiently to address the unmet demand of veterans. This would return the treatment currently outsourced to the VHA. To do so would require an understanding of where that demand exists and in what quantity.

The second option (short title: CMS) is a long-term, phased elimination of the VHA in favor of a central payment system. This plan would leverage facility closings or acquisitions to divest VHA assets while simultaneously expanding the VA Mission Act so that all veterans would receive care in private facilities. Funding control and program rules would logically move to the Centers for Medicare and Medicaid (CMS). Entitled veterans would receive this care without additional payment.

A third option (short title: PI) would expand the current, subsidized Department of Defense insurance program (TRICARE Prime managed care plan, TRICARE Select fee for service plan and TRICARE for Life Medicare wraparound coverage) to the entitled veteran population. For TRICARE Prime, veterans would be required annual payments, which are currently a fraction of the actual cost of care. (Annual plan rates for 2018 are $289.08 with no deductible and nominal co-pays.) For TRICARE Select, the veteran would need to cover an annual deductible (currently $150 for an individual), co-pays, an annual enrollment (currently $450 for retirees) and out of network charges if appropriate. Some or all of these costs might be waived. For TRICARE for Life, veterans would only pay the Medicare Part B premiums [40].These insurance plans would need to be negotiated among regional providers, the Department of Defense and the Department of Veterans Affairs. A logical incrementalism approach would eventually merge the VHA functions with the DoD, phasing out VHA's direct treatment responsibilities.

The status quo option (short title: SQ) retains the current VHA Mission Act components. This Act effectively mixes an NHS-style system (the VHA) with an NIH-component (centralized payment to non-government run facilities). Some of the details of the plan as well as long-term funding have yet to be established; however, the intent is to provide all required care by allowing eligible veterans to receive treatment in the VHA system or in non-VHA facilities under certain circumstances.

3. Results

The policies presented each have secondary and tertiary effects. These will be explicated here by evaluating cost, quality, access, political feasibility (including public expectations) and administrative feasibility. For those unfamiliar with decision matrices, a review of Table 1 up-front might be helpful prior to reading the alternative assessments.

3.1. Option 1: VHA-Only Assessment

Cost. The VHA-only option would require expansion in facilities and resources to handle unmet demand. If the magnitude of unmet demand is calculated as a proportion of annual community care payments ($14.2 billion) over all annual costs ($98.0 billion), then the unmet demand would be nearly 14% of total workload. However, the $98.0 billion reflects many VHA fixed costs rather than variable costs of care, so the 14% estimate may be low, even if the variable costs of the VHA are cheaper. To accommodate a 14% increase in the VHA system, facility and materiel acquisitions as well as faculty and staff would be required at some level and those costs are dependent on the way the VHA expands [41]. Further, "VA faces challenges regarding the reliability, transparency and consistency of its budget estimates for medical services, as well as weaknesses in tracking obligations for medical services and estimating budgetary needs for future years" [42]. A VHA-only option is assessed to be more expensive than the status quo ($14.0 K/beneficiary) at least in the short term due to the increase in construction with associated fixed costs.

Quality. An analysis of the SHEP items for patient satisfaction (1 April 2016 through 31 March 2017) against the identical HCAHPS items for all other facilities revealed lower satisfaction on 9 of 11 of the identical metrics (Table 2). Under the binomial assumption of equal likelihood, the probability that 9 or more of the 11 identical measures would be higher for "other facilities" is small (0.032); however, the size of the proportional distances is small except for the pain control measure. Quality based on patient experience metrics is assessed to be lower in the VHA.

While hospital outcome analysis is not accurate due to reporting issues in the VHA, a newly-released report suggests that VHA nursing homes performed poorly on quality compared to their community counterparts during the 2017 calendar year. Table 2 illustrates data acquired by USA Today and the Boston Globe [43]. One metric that seems particularly problematic in Table 3 is that 8.51% of VHA residents at high-risk experienced decubitus ulcers during this reporting period. These are "never happen" events. Given these metrics, it would be hard to justify an assessment that the VHA delivers higher quality healthcare than its civilian counterparts.

Access. Veteran access under an expanded VHA system should improve under this proposal. However, a National Public Radio (NPR) study demonstrated the VHA struggled to execute expanded care when provided additional funds [15]. Further, the unmet demand may be more significant than anticipated and adding facilities may just remove backlog associated with on and off-the-books waiting lists. Evidence of this backlog includes a March 2018 report from the VA Inspector General which identified critical deficiencies at the Washington, DC VA Medical Center, including more than

10 thousand open and pending prosthetic and sensory aid consults [44]. Further, availability for care in only one system is defined as reduced access, as veterans' options are limited.

Table 3. The 2017 quality care comparison for nursing homes does not reflect case complexity; however, certain measures such as the administration of anti-psychotics, catheter mistakes and decubitus ulcers are problematic.

Measure	VHA	Non-VHA
• Reported Pain within the Past Five Days	32.64%	5.59%
• Received Anti-Psychotic Medication, which the FDA has Associated with an Increased Risk of Deaths in Elderly Dementia Patients	20.89%	15.48%
• Experienced Marked Decrease in Abilities to Perform Acts of Daily Living	16.70%	14.99%
• Had a Catheter Left in Their Bladder, which can lead to Urinary or Blood Infections and Other Complications	11.96%	1.83%
• High-risk Residents with Serious Bed Sores, which may be Prevented by Repositioning/Cushioning	8.51%	5.57%

Political Feasibility. Given the predilection of the current and previous administrations to provide outsourced community care to support the veterans and the multitude of ongoing oversight actions, it is unlikely that a return to a VHA-only system would be palatable at this point. The leadership changes over the past several years suggest a lack of confidence in the VA in general. Since veterans group generally support the VHA [25], this option is likely to achieve significant levels of public support.

Administrative Feasibility. Administering a VHA-only policy would certainly be more problematic and likely more expensive than the status quo solution. This policy would be a multi-year transition during construction and hiring and during that time, access would continue to be a problem without the continued use of community care options. While the VA Mission Act would provide the community care option, the VHA would have to implement real systems capable of supporting that access during the transition. The VHA's history in supporting payments to third parties under legislative directive is suspect as evidence by its failures under the Veterans Choice Act [45].

3.2. Option 2: CMS Assessment

Cost. For this policy option, CMS gradually takes over funding of all veteran healthcare through its existing Medicare processes. The fixed costs associated with the VHA-operated facilities (roughly $6.2 billion in FY2019) would phase out over time and facilities as well as equipment would be divested. While the fixed costs of care would disappear, the variable costs would likely but not necessarily rise. As indicated by the CBO, the VHA's actual knowledge of current costs is poor [41]. While dated studies relying on data from 1999 or earlier indicated that the VHA care was less expensive than private-sector care, the cost comparisons may not be relevant now due to changes in patient mix, demand and so forth. Further, the cost-effectiveness of that care is unknown and "comparing health care costs in the VHA system and the private sector is difficult partly because the Department of Veterans Affairs [6], which runs VHA, has provided limited data to the Congress and the public about its costs and operational performance" [41]. The most recent study (VA sponsored and dated) from Nugent et al. in 2004 evaluated six non-randomly selected facilities to estimate cost-savings over Medicare between 17–20% [46]. That study is not relevant today. First, 49% of the estimated "cost offsets" based on an inflated workload estimate were associated with the VA's ability to negotiate pharmaceutical prices ($81, 946/$167, 383). Fourteen years ago, that estimate might have been reasonable. With Medicare Part D, CMS has demonstrated the bargaining power to reduce pharmaceutical costs by 55% [47]. Second, adjustments of 3.3% for corporate overhead, interest on capital assets and torts were included in the authors' study; however, legal settlements in the VA more than tripled from 2011 to 2015 going from $98 million to $338 million [48].

Aside from the Nugent's study cost analysis, one can compare the estimate of $14.0 K per enrolled veteran per year with the Medicare spending provided by the Henry J. Kaiser Foundation and derived from CMS and Census Bureau data. The per enrollee Medicare spending in 2014 was $10,986 [49]. Inflating these values using the Bureau of Labor Statistics inflation rates from May 2015 through May 2018, {2.8%, 3.1%, 2.7%, 2.4%} [50], results in a revised estimate of $12.2 K per beneficiary. This would imply that Medicare expenditures per patient with access may be less than the VHA.

Quality. CMS relies on Medicare approved facilities for providing care. As national insurance for the elderly, it demands and incentivizes quality through a variety of mechanisms such as Accountable Care Organizations (ACOs), accreditation and Quality Improvement Organizations. Thus, shifting care from VHA facilities to private facilities which accept Medicare should result in quality at least as good as the VHA. From a patient experience view, non-VHA facilities scored better than VHA facilities on 9 of 11 common satisfaction survey items as discussed earlier. Table 2 contains the DoD satisfaction results. A Friedman's non-parametric repeated measures test for satisfaction scores indicated differences among the three groups ($\chi_2^2 = 16.545$, $p = 0.0002$). Wilcoxon Rank Sum post-hoc tests found differences between non-VHA and VHA ($V = 57.5$, $p = 0.033$), between VHA and DoD ($V = 66$, $p = 0.004$) and between DoD and non-VHA ($V = 64$, $p = 0.003$). All tests were performed in R Statistical Software [51].

Access. With a logical incrementalism approach and the opportunity for large systems to acquire VHA facilities built into this option, access to care should be better than the VHA only system, as veterans would have access to all Medicare-accepting organizations. This option expands choice and would therefore be preferred over the VHA-only option.

Political Feasibility. Members on both sides of the aisle as well as some veterans' groups (i.e., the Veterans of Foreign Wars) have indicated they are not in favor of VHA "privatization" [25]. The word "privatization" is politically charged; therefore, many who actually are in favor moving towards a single payer system avoid it [25]. Still, open discussion of a CMS option would be politically charged and the public would likely take their cues from both the veterans groups and media. Implementation of a plan such as this would require strong leadership and face many challenges. Arguably, the simplest method to implement this plan would be incrementally without discussion.

Administrative Feasibility. While the CMS already manages Medicare, the inclusion of payments on behalf of veterans would be a new mission and difficult to execute. Further, the sale and extraction of residual from the existing VHA properties would require significant planning. Administratively, this plan would likely be more difficult to implement than the VHA only option.

3.3. Option 3: PI

Cost. Option 3 expands TRICARE subsidized insurance to veterans. In 2012, the Department of Defense spent $52 billion on TRICARE to cover 9.5 million beneficiaries, an average of $5.5 K per covered individual [46]. Inflating this to 2018 dollar using the BLS medical inflation rates for May 2013 through May 2018 [52] results in a revised estimate of $6.5 K per beneficiary. While some might suggest that the lower cost per beneficiary user is due to case mix, this may or may not be true. Post-traumatic stress disorder, polytrauma combat veterans, burn victims and so forth are part of the DoD as well as the VA. Further, dual eligible veterans (those who are entitled to care from the VHA) also seek care from TRICARE. The cost structure of TRICARE appears to be better than either a VHA only option or the CMS option.

Quality. TRICARE is an insurance-based program. Outcomes are likely to be similar to the other two options. When comparing the most recent patient experience metrics for the DoD (a proxy for TRICARE) [53] versus all other facilities and the VHA using the Hospital Compare data, the DoD metrics are superior to the VHA for all 11 questions and are superior in 10 of 11 categories to all other facilities. In both cases, the results are unlikely due to chance alone ($p < 0.001$, $p < 0.006$ respectively using binomial models). In terms of patient experiences, this option is preferred over VHA-only and CMS.

Access. TRICARE Prime provides access through participating providers both within and outside of the military healthcare system. Because TRICARE includes both a managed care and indemnity insurance option, the access to care is better than a VHA-only system and similar to that of the status quo. The CMS option arguably provides more options for access, as the acceptance rate for new patients in 2015 was 72% for Medicare versus 67% for TRICARE in 2012 [54].

Political Feasibility. While the consolidation of veterans' care with DoD beneficiary care may make sense from the aspects of cost, quality and access, the political feasibility would be problematic. Transitioning to DoD insurance plans might (1) be a non-clandestine threat to the existence of the VHA; (2) require contributions from veterans unless waived, which would be highly unpopular and (3) be opposed by many in Congress whose constituencies include many veterans. From a feasibility perspective, this option probably ranks below VHA-only and incremental transition to the CMS.

Administrative Feasibility. From an administrative viewpoint, this option is feasible. The VHA already uses one of the major TRICARE contractors (Health Net Federal Services) to support the existing Veterans Choice program [55,56]. Combining TRICARE and (in the future) VA Mission Act contracts would be feasible, arguably more feasible than expanding the VHA-only option.

3.4. Option 4: SQ

Cost. The status quo option costs are currently estimated to be $14.0 K per treated veteran per year. Based on the previous cost analyses, this option is probably only superior to the VHA-only option and inferior to all others.

Quality. Under the status quo, outcome quality should be at least as good as all other plans; however, experience of care (satisfaction) metrics should be a mix of the VHA current scores and the other facility scores in Table 3. Using this logic, the status quo is superior to VHA-only but inferior to all other options on this criterion.

Access. With access to the VHA and contracted facilities, veterans should have more choice than the VHA only option but less choice than PI or CMS. PI and CMS provide a wider array of options.

Political Feasibility. Since this is the status quo solution, it has proven to be palatable. In fact, the expansion of community care indicates that support for expanding such action exists. This intervention ranks first in political feasibility.

Administrative Feasibility. This criterion might be an issue despite the VA Mission Act having been enacted already. The responsibility for coordinating the outside care for veterans lies within the VHA. The question remains whether the VHA be able to improve upon its demonstrated performance with the Veterans Choice Act. Still, there is some experience in contracting care within the VHA, so it probably ranks first in administrative feasibility.

3.5. Comparisons

The use of the evaluation criteria provides a mechanism for building a combined evaluation and comparison matrix, both weighted and unweighted (Table 4). The unweighted and weighted solutions both favor PI, the TRICARE insurance option. This option was ranked first or second in all but one category, political feasibility. In the unweighted matrix, both CMS and SQ solutions tied for second, while CMS took second position by itself under weighting. The VHA only solution was assessed to be the worst solution weighted and unweighted, primarily because of quality metrics and access metrics.

For the CMS policy intervention to be selected as the weighted choice, the weight for access would have to increase to nearly 2.0 with all other criterion being held constant. Alternatively, the weight for political feasibility would have to increase above 1.22. For SQ to be selected, the weight for either political feasibility or for administrative feasibility would need to be increased above 2.4 with all other weights held constant. VHA-only is a dominated solution that is never selected under any weighting scheme. Given this analysis, the PI or CMS solutions are better options than the status quo or VHA only; however, the PI is preferred due to the better cost and quality metrics.

Table 4. Evaluation and comparison of possible policy interventions is depicted. The unweighted and weighted recommendations are initially identical without sensitivity analysis and in favor of the TRICARE option.

Policy	Cost	Quality	Access	Political	Admin.	Unweighted	Weighted
		Criteria				**Decision**	
VHA Only	4.0	4.0	4.0	3.0	3.0	18.0	18.4
CMS	2.0	2.0	1.0	2.0	4.0	11.0	10.2
PI	1.0	1.0	2.0	4.0	2.0	10.0	9.5
SQ	3.0	3.0	3.0	1.0	1.0	11.0	11.8
Sum	10.0	10.0	10.0	10.0	10.0	50.0	50.0
Weights	0.98	1.22	1.22	0.85	0.73	Lower is better.	

4. Discussion

The United States has a long-standing obligation to provide veterans access to high quality care. Failures in the system have resulted in unnecessary morbidity and mortality. The country has an obligation to provide a lasting solution to wicked problem that balances the components of the "Iron Triangle".

The policy analysis suggests that PI is probably the best solution and it is certainly worth exploring. This solution, however, might not be politically viable. The CMS solution, on the other hand, may be implemented through incremental steps such as the expansion of the VA Mission Act and appears to be reasonably implementable. The current status quo provides an access relief valve but fewer choices and additional costs, particularly when compared to the PI solution; however, expanding the VA Mission Act incrementally might achieve a permanent solution to the problem.

Any policy analysis always has major limitations. While care is taken in the selection of criteria, there is no perfect method for doing so. An infinite number of policy interventions are available and subsets of these might be evaluated differently. Weighting selection for criteria are subject to debate. Analysis of rankings on selected criteria may be second-guessed. But the objective analysis of potential policies serves one purpose well: it invokes debate.

The VHA has been involved in repeated scandals since 2014 and yet it is the veterans who suffer. Leadership at all levels of the Government have an obligation to fix these problems. The VA Mission Act passed by the Congress and signed by President Trump may be a good start but it relies on the VHA for implementation. Should the public place its confidence yet again in this organization? More importantly, should our veterans?

Author Contributions: L.V.F. and M.S.B. contributed to the writing and research of this article.

Funding: This research was not funded.

References

1.   VA. Veterans Health Administration. 2018. Available online: www.va.gov/health (accessed on 21 June 2018).
2.   VA. Office of Budget. 2018. Available online: https://www.va.gov/budget/products.asp (accessed on 21 June 2018).
3.   VA. About VHA. 2018. Available online: www.va.gov/health/aboutvha.asp (accessed on 21 June 2018).
4.   Landon, R. Pattern of Problems with Veterans Affairs Healthcare System. *Modern Healthcare*, 7 May 2014.
5.   Bronstein, S.; Griffin, D. *A Fatal Wait: Veterans Languish and Die on a VA Hospital's Secret List*; Cable News Network: Atlanta, GA, USA, 2014.
6.   VA Office of the Inspector General. *Veterans Health Administration Review of Alleged Patient Deaths, Patient Wait Times, and Scheduling Practices at the Phoenix VA Health Care System*; VA Office of the Inspector General: Washington, DC, USA, 2014.
7.   Hayward, R.A. Lessons from the Rise-and Fall?-of VA Healthcare. *J. Gen. Int. Med.* **2017**, *32*, 11–13. [CrossRef] [PubMed]

8. Bloche, M.G. Scandal as a Sentinel Event–Recognizing Hidden Cost-Quality Trade-offs. *N. Eng. J. Med.* **2016**, *374*, 1001–1003. [CrossRef] [PubMed]

9. Telegraph Reporters. Mid Staffordshire Trust Inquiry: How the Care Scandal Unfolded. *The Telegraph*, 6 February 2013.

10. National Audit Office. *Inappropriate Adjustments to NHS Waiting Lists*; National Audit Office: London, UK, 2001.

11. VA Office of the Inspector General. *Review of Alleged Use of Inappropriate Wait Lists for Group Therapy and Post-Traumatic Stress Disorder Clinic Team, Eastern Colorado Health Care System*; VA Office of the Inspector General: Washington, DC, USA, 2017.

12. Slack, D. VA Bosses in 7 States Falsified Vets' Wait Times for Care. *USA Today*, 11 April 2016.

13. VA Office of the Inspector General. *Review of Alleged Consult Mismanagement at the Phoenix VA Health Care System*; VA Office of the Inspector General: Washington, DC, USA, 2017.

14. VA Office of the Inspector General. *Veterans Access, Choice, and Accountability Act of 2014*; VA Office of the Inspector General: Washington, DC, USA, 2014.

15. Elosua, J. *VA Hospitals Still Struggling with Adding Staff Despite Billions from Choice Act*; NPR: Washington, DC, USA, 2017.

16. VA Office of the Inspector General. *VA Maintaining Internal Systems and Strengthening Integrated Outside Networks Act of 2018, PL 115-182*; VA Office of the Inspector General: Washington, DC, USA, 2018.

17. CBO. H.R. 5674, VA Maintaining Internal Systems and Strengthening Integrated Outside Networks Act of 2018. 2018. Available online: https://www.cbo.gov/publication/53871 (accessed on 21 June 2018).

18. VA. Debunking the VA Privatization Myth. 2018. Available online: https://www.va.gov/opa/pressrel/pressrelease.cfm?id=4034 (accessed on 21 June 2018).

19. Sisk, R. Trump Signs $55 Billion Bill to Replace VA Choice Program. *Military.com*, 6 June 2018.

20. Tiefer, C. *Veterans Sustain Two Serious Defeats from Trump and the House to VA Health Care*; Forbes: New York, NY, USA, 2018.

21. Quinn, J.B. Strategic Change: Logical Incrementalism. *Sloan Manag. Rev.* **1989**, *30*, 45–60.

22. Kauffman, T. New Poll Shows Veterans Oppose Privatizing VA Health Care. 2015. Available online: https://www.afge.org/publication/new-poll-shows-veterans-oppose-privatizing-va-health-care/ (accessed on 21 June 2018).

23. Lee, M.Y.H.; Rein, L.; Weigel, D. How a Koch-Backed Veterans Group Gained Influence in Trump's Washington. *Chicago Tribune*, 7 April 2018.

24. Pew Research Center. Public Support for Increased Spending on Veterans at Highest Level in Two Decades. 2017. Available online: http://www.people-press.org/2017/04/24/with-budget-debate-looming-growing-share-of-public-prefers-bigger-government/attachment/42/ (accessed on 21 June 2018).

25. III, L.S. Vets Groups and Lawmakers Say They're Against It—But What Does 'Privatization' of Veterans Affairs Really Mean? *MilitaryTimes*, 10 April 2018.

26. GOP. Republican Platform. 2018. Available online: https://www.gop.com/platform/ (accessed on 21 June 2018).

27. Buchanan, L. After 12 Months of Trump, Here's What 100 CEOs Are Saying About His Effect on Business. *Inc.*, 30 January 2018.

28. Zurawik, D. CNN's VA Scandal Coverage Reminder of What Cable News Can be. *Baltimore Sun*, 24 May 2014.

29. MacRae, D.; Wilde, J.A. *Policy Analysis for Public Decisions*; University Press of America: Lanham, MD, USA, 1985; p. 325.

30. Baltussen, R.; Niessen, L. Priority Setting of Health Interventions: The Need for Multi-Criteria Decision Analysis. *Cost Effect. Resour. Alloc.* **2006**, *4*, 14–19. [CrossRef] [PubMed]

31. Kissick, W. *Medicine's Dilemmas*; Yale University Press: New Haven, CT, USA, 1994.

32. Weber, D.J. Analyzing Political Feasibility: Political Scientists unIque Contribution to Policy Analysis. *Policy Stud. J.* **1986**, *14*, 545–553. [CrossRef]

33. Government Accounting Office. *VA Health Care: Improvements Needed in Data and Monitoring of Clinical Productivity and Efficiency*; Government Accounting Office: Washington, DC, USA, 2017.

34. Slack, D. Illegal VA Policy Allows Hiring Since 2002 of Medical Workers with Revoked Licenses. *USA Today*, 21 December 2017.

35. Data.Medicare.Gov. Hospital Compare Datasets. 2018. Available online: https://data.medicare.gov/data/hospital-compare (accessed on 21 June 2018).
36. Cleary, P.D.; Meterko, M.; Wright, S.M.; Zaslavsky, A.M. Are comparisons of patient experiences across hospitals fair? A study in Veterans Health Administration hospitals. *Med. Care* **2014**, *52*, 619–625. [CrossRef] [PubMed]
37. O'Hanlon, C.; Huang, C.; Sloss, E.; Price, R.A.; Hussey, P.; Farmer, C.; Gidengil, C. Comparing VA and Non-VA Quality of Care: A Systematic Review. *J. Gen. Int. Med.* **2017**, *32*, 105–121. [CrossRef] [PubMed]
38. Blay, E., Jr.; DeLancey, J.O.; Hewitt, D.B.; Chung, J.W.; Bilimoria, K.Y. Initial Public Reporting of Quality at Veterans Affairs vs Non-Veterans Affairs Hospitals. *JAMA Int. Med.* **2017**, *177*, 882–885. [CrossRef] [PubMed]
39. Veterans Health Administration. Patient Access Data. 2018. Available online: https://www.va.gov/health/access-audit.asp (accessed on 21 June 2018).
40. TRICARE. TRICARE Health Plan Costs. 2018. Available online: https://www.tricare.mil/Costs/HealthPlanCosts (accessed on 21 June 2018).
41. CBO. Comparing the Costs of the Veteran's Health Care System with Private Sector Costs. 2014. Available online: https://www.cbo.gov/publication/49763 (accessed on 21 June 2018).
42. Government Accounting Office. *Report to Congressional Committees High Risk Series: Progress on Many High-Risk Areas While Substantial Efforts Needed on Others*; Government Accounting Office: Washington, DC, USA, 2017.
43. Slack, D. Secret VA Nursing Home Ratings Hide Poor Quality Care from the Public. *USA Today*, 17 June 2018.
44. VA Office of the Inspector General. *Critical Deficienciess at the Washington DC VA Medical Center*; VA Office of the Inspector General: Washington, DC, USA, 2018.
45. Krause, B. Veteran Forced to Pay for Own Surgery Despite Choice Program Approval Due to HealthNet Hangups. 2018. Available online: https://www.disabledveterans.org/2017/09/07/veteran-forced-pay-surgery-despite-choice-program-healthnet/ (accessed on 21 June 2018).
46. Nugent, G.N.; Hendricks, A.; Nugent, L.; Render, M.L. Value for taxpayers' dollars: What VA care would cost at medicare prices. *Med. Care Res. Rev.* **2004**, *61*, 495–508. [CrossRef] [PubMed]
47. Holtz-Eakin, D.; Book, R. Competition and the Medicare Part D Program. 2013. Available online: https://www.americanactionforum.org/research/competition-and-the-medicare-part-d-program/ (accessed on 21 June 2018).
48. Howard, C.B.; Blau, R. *Legal Settlements at Veterans Affairs More than Tripled Since 2011, Many due to Medical Malpractices*; New York Daily News: New York, NY, USA, 2018.
49. Kaiser Foundation. Medicare Spending per Enrollee, by State. 2014. Available online: https://www.kff.org/medicare/state-indicator/per-enrollee-spending-by-residence/?currentTimeframe=0&sortModel=%7B%22colId%22:%22Location%22,%22sort%22:%22asc%22%7D (accessed on 21 June 2018).
50. Bureau of Labor Statistics Databases, Tables, and Calculators by Subject. Available online: https://data.bls.gov/timeseries/CUUR0000SA0L1E?output_view=pct_12mths (accessed on 21 June 2018).
51. R Core Team. *R: A Language and Environment for Statistical Computing*; R Foundation for Statistical Computing: Vienna, Austria, 2018.
52. CBO. Approaches to Reducing Federal Spending on Military Health Care. 2014. Available online: https://www.cbo.gov/sites/default/files/113th-congress-2013-2014/reports/44993-militaryhealthcare.pdf (accessed on 21 June 2018).
53. Kaiser Foundation. Primary Physicians Accepting Medicare: A Snapshot. 2015. Available online: https://www.kff.org/medicare/issue-brief/primary-care-physicians-accepting-medicare-a-snapshot/ (accessed on 21 June 2018).
54. Government Accounting Office. *TRICARE Multiyear Surveys Indicate Problems with Access to Care for Nonerolled Beneficiaries*; Government Accounting Office: Washington, DC, USA, 2013.
55. Health Net Federal Services. Veterans Choice Program. 2018. Available online: https://www.hnfs.com/content/hnfs/home/va/provider/resources/faqs/vcp.html (accessed on 21 June 2018).
56. Health Net Federal Services. TRICARE West. 2018. Available online: https://www.tricare-west.com/ (accessed on 21 June 2018).

9

Development and Psychometric Properties of The Delayed Childbearing Questionnaire (DCBQ-55)

Samira Behboudi-Gandevani [1], Saeideh Ziaei [1,*], Anoshirvan Kazemnejad [2], Farideh Khalajabadi Farahani [3] and Mojtaba Vaismoradi [4]

[1] Department of Midwifery & Reproductive Health, Medical Sciences Faculty, Tarbiat Modares University, 14115-111 Tehran, Iran; behboudi@endocrine.ac.ir
[2] Department of Biostatistics, Medical Sciences Faculty, Tarbiat Modares University, 14115-111 Tehran, Iran; kazem_an@modares.ac.ir
[3] National Population Studies & Comprehensive Management Institute, 1531635711 Tehran, Iran; farideh.farahani@psri.ac.ir
[4] Faculty of Nursing and Health Sciences, Nord University, 8049 Bodø, Norway; mojtaba.vaismoradi@nord.no
*   Correspondence: ziaei_sa@modares.ac.ir

Abstract: The comprehensive assessment of delayed childbearing needs a valid and reliable instrument. Therefore, the aim of the present study was to develop an instrument to evaluate factors influencing delayed childbearing among women and to assess its psychometric properties. The current methodological study was performed in two phases of (i) qualitative instrument development, and (ii) quantitative psychometric assessment of the developed instrument. Face and content validity of the instrument was assessed by eligible women and a panel of experts. Construct validity was assessed using the exploratory factor analysis (EFA). For reliability, internal consistency reliability and intra-rater reliability analysis were used. The initial instrument developed from the qualitative phase consisted of 60 items, which were reduced to 55 items after the face and content validity processes. EFA ($n = 300$) using the Kaiser criteria (Eigenvalues > 1) and the scree plot led to a six-factor solution accounting for 61.24% of the observed variance. The Cronbach's alpha coefficient, Spearman's correlation, test–retest and intra-class correlation coefficients for the whole instrument were reported as 0.83, 0.86 and 0.81, respectively. The final instrument entitled the delayed childbearing questionnaire (DCBQ-55) included 50 items with six domains of 'readiness for childbearing', 'stability in the partner relationship', 'awareness about the adverse outcomes of pregnancy in advanced maternal age', 'attitude toward delayed childbearing', 'family support', and 'social support' on a five-point Likert scale. The DCBQ-55 as a simple, valid and reliable instrument can assess factors influencing delayed childbearing. It can be used by reproductive healthcare providers and policy makers to understand factors influencing delayed childbearing and devise appropriate strategies.

Keywords: delayed childbearing; fertility; postponement; psychometric properties; questionnaire; reproductive health; women health

1. Introduction

Delayed childbearing as 'a personal choice to postpone childbearing in women over 35 years' has become a health concern in both developed and developing countries [1,2]. It is believed that the age of a woman at the first pregnancy and the number of pregnancies in women aged over 35 years are rising across the globe [2,3]. An extensive use of family planning programs, increased popularity of assisted reproductive technology (ART), occupation and education, lack of support by the society for childbearing, lack of knowledge of the negative consequences of advanced maternal age, socioeconomic uncertainties and irresponsible partners are some of the known factors underlying delayed childbearing [4–7]. However, the postponement of childbearing can lead to a wide range of adverse social, health, and demographic outcomes for the mother and child. For instance, it carries the risk of infertility, obstetric complications, pregnancy-associated chronic diseases and neonatal health issues [8–10].

Delayed childbearing is a significant risk factor for low birth weight, but some positive associations have been reported between the maternal profile and birth outcomes among women aged $\geq$ 35 years [11]. Nevertheless, it can create some challenges to maternity care in terms of the spacing of a woman's pregnancies. It is recommended to create a balance between inter-pregnancy intervals associated with higher risks for adverse pregnancy outcomes and increased maternal age at delivery [12]. In terms of psychological issues, those women who are childless after delaying childbearing experience similar feelings to those women that are childless after infertility [13]. Therefore, couples' understandings of the planning and timing of parenthood, as well as the impact of female and male age on the ability to achieve parenthood, should be improved [14].

Delayed childbearing is an evolving global issue across the world with a wide range of clinical and social outcomes. For instance, a study in the USA on the basis of national birth data showed an increasingly prominent trend of delayed childbearing from 1971 to 2016. Only in 2016, delayed childbearing accounted for 24% and 38% of multiple births for white and black women, respectively. It was predicted that by 2025, delayed childbearing would account for higher rates of multiple births [15]. Postponement of childbearing can have a tremendous effect on the total fertility rate [16,17]. In the EU-28 Member States, the total fertility rate has steadily declined from the mid-1960s, but since the 2000s, some signs of increase have been reported. In 2010, a subsequent reduction was observed, followed by a slight increase towards 2016 [18]. With regard to the Iranian fertility context, the introduction of family planning services in the 1960s and increased marriage age during the 1970s reduced the fertility rate. Socioeconomic factors including gender roles, changes in women's education and workforce participation have mainly influenced the trend of long-term fertility in Iran [19]. Since 1988, the development of the economy and living standards has led to changes in the population policy in terms of fertility control programs [20]. Fertility in Iran has been reported to be constant from 2000 to 2009 at a level of 1.8–2.0 births per woman, indicating an effort to sustain fertility at the replacement level. However, a population bill in 2013 showed that the fertility rate in Iran had fallen to a low level, and a wide range of policies were devised to increase it to 2.5 births per woman [21]. The report by the Iran's national statistics organization in the period of 2012–2016 showed that the total fertility rate was 2.01 children [22]. In a recent cross-sectional study in 2015 in Tehran on 1067 married women participating in the Tehran Lipid and Glucose Study (TLGS), the overall prevalence of lifetime primary infertility was reported as 17.3%, which was higher than its global trend [23]. Iranian women are largely unaware of the potential complications of delayed childbirth and its relationship with infertility [24]. It is believed that a short postponement of motherhood by Iranian women has occurred since 1990 onwards. An Iranian study (2013) showed that childlessness between ages 15–39 increased during 1991–2003, but was reduced from 3.8% to 2.2% in the last years of reproductive age. In addition, voluntary and involuntary childlessness among married women were reported as 8.5% and 2.0%, respectively [25]. The recent report by Iran's national statistics organization (2017) showed the highest increase in fertility was observed within the age group of 35–39 in urban areas. It was mentioned that such a change in the age pattern greatly influenced the fertility rate to the replacement level in Iran [22].

Knowledge of factors influencing delayed childbearing is important for the improvement of maternal and child care. However, there is a lack of appropriate and specific instrument for the assessment of delayed childbearing, both in the Iranian society and across the globe. A valid and reliable instrument for the assessment of delayed childbearing can cover multidimensional aspects of this phenomenon and comprehensively explore factors influencing it, given cultural and regional differences in various contexts [26]. Therefore, the aim of the present study was to develop an instrument to evaluate factors influencing delayed childbearing among women and to assess its psychometric properties.

2. Material and Methods

Devising the instrument for a comprehensive assessment of various dimensions of delayed childbearing needed a context-based study and a thorough literature search. Therefore, this methodologic study was consisted of the two phases of (i) qualitative (to define the components of delayed childbearing and develop the initial instrument) and (ii) quantitative (to assess the psychometric properties of the instrument) [27].

2.1. The Qualitative Phase

The details of this phase have been described elsewhere [2]. Briefly, subjects were 23 nulliparous married women, aged ≥ 30 years, who voluntarily postponed childbearing. They were selected using the purposive sampling method on the basis of following inclusion criteria: decided to postpone childbirth for at least five years, attended three prenatal or gynecology healthcare clinics in Tehran for various health-related reasons, and were willing to participate in this study [2]. They were informed of the aim and process of the study, and signed the written informed consent form before data collection. Next, 28 sessions of in-depth semi-structured interviews, lasting 20–40 min, were held in places convenient to them. Each woman was requested by the first author (SBG) to describe her own individual perspective and experience about all aspects of delayed childbearing with a focus on the following questions: 'What is your understanding of delayed childbearing? Why have you decided to delay childbearing? What factors influenced your decision to delay childbearing? Are you satisfied with your decision?' Also, branching questions were asked to follow their thoughts and increase the interviews' depth. A conventional content analysis approach [28,29] was used for data analysis, concurrently with data collection. The interviews were discontinued when no new data was collected and data saturation was reached. Main themes developed in this study were "personal inclination", "perceived beliefs about delayed childbearing", and "social support" [2].

In addition, the researchers conducted a thorough review of literature in Farsi and English to retrieve published articles and instruments on delayed childbearing. International academic databases such as PubMed (including Medline), Scopus, Science Direct, Cinahl, Web of Science and Iranian databases that provided the highest yield of citations on the study topic up to 2015 were searched. Furthermore, for maximizing coverage, a manual search of the reference lists of related articles were performed. The search key words included 'childbearing', 'delay', 'postponement', 'fertility', and 'childlessness'. The search yielded 2356 potentially relevant articles. The titles and abstracts of the initial list of articles were reviewed by the researchers independently and 21 articles were selected on the basis of the following inclusion criteria: focused on factors influencing delayed childbearing, published in peer-reviewed journals, and being available online. The contents of the selected articles were used for item generation. No specific instrument for the assessment of factors influencing delayed childbearing was found in the literature.

2.2. The Quantitative Phase

In the second phase, the psychometric properties of the preliminary instrument were evaluated. Validity of the instrument was established through the assessment and confirmation of content, face and construct (exploratory factor analysis (EFA)) validities. For reliability, internal consistency and test–retest analyses were performed. Details of this phase have been described as follow:

2.2.1. Initial Item Generation

An initial 60-item instrument was developed based on the extracted themes and related codes from the qualitative study and the thorough literature search [30]. It used a five-point

Likert scale (1 = strongly disagree to 5 = strongly agree) for respondents to show their level of agreement/disagreement with each item.

2.2.2. Face Validity

Face validity was performed to investigate the women's understandings of the instrument items. Qualitative and quantitative methods of face validity were used. For qualitative evaluation of face validity, 10 women with delayed childbearing were requested to assess each item in terms of 'difficulty', 'irrelevance', and 'ambiguity'. Also, they were asked to provide feedbacks and give additional suggestions for the improvement of the initial instrument and rectify potential mistakes. As such, the quantitative assessment of face validity was performed using the item impact score reflecting the subjects' perceptions of the items' importance on a five-point Likert scale. The item impact was defined as the proportion of the women who identified it as 'important' and the mean importance score attributed to the item (impact score = frequency * importance). The satisfactory score for the acceptance of each item was ≥ 1.5 [30].

2.2.3. Content Validity

Content validity helped determine whether the items adequately addressed the construct of delayed childbearing. An expert panel consisting of 15 multidisciplinary specialists in the fields of midwifery, reproductive health, obstetrics and gynecology, maternal–child health, nursing, community health, psychology, and sociology evaluated the content validity of the initial instrument using the Waltz and Bausell content validity index (CVI) [30]. They scored the 'relevancy', 'clarity', and 'simplicity' of each item using a four-point Likert scale, and the CVI for each item was calculated by dividing the number of specialists who scored items three or four by the total number of specialists. The item was accepted if the CVI was ≥ 0.79 [30]. The necessity of the items was assessed using a three-point rating scale as (i) not necessary, (ii) useful, but not essential, and (iii) essential. Following the experts' evaluation, a content validity ratio (CVR) for the total scale was also calculated. According to the Lawshe table, an acceptable CVR value for the 15-expert panel was reported as 0.49 [30].

2.2.4. Construct Validity

A cross-sectional study was performed to assess the construct validity of the initial instrument using the EFA with the principal components method and varimax rotation. The recommended number of subjects for the EFA was recommended as five times the number of items [30,31]. Therefore, 300 women aged ≥ 35 who had experienced a time in their life when they decided to postpone childbearing for at least five years on the basis of personal reasons and attended three healthcare centers were selected. Those women who suffered from chronic serious illnesses which substantially affected their ability to experience pregnancy, such as high-grade heart failure or linguistic or cognitive problems, and also those who did not provide the answer to at least 20% of all items were excluded from data analysis.

The characteristics of the women were presented in Table 1. After explaining the aim of the study and obtaining signed written informed consent, they were requested to provide responses to the instrument's items. The Kaiser-Meyer-Olkin (KMO) test was used to evaluate the sample adequacy [31], and the cut-off point of 0.40 was considered the minimum load factor required for maintaining each item of the factor being extracted [31].

Table 1. Characteristics of the subjects in this study.

Variable	Response (n = 300)
Age, mean (SD), y	36.1 (8.2)
Marital age, mean (SD), y	8.2 (3.9)
Husband's age, mean (SD), y	40.1 (5.7)
Education level, n (%)	
≥High school graduate	162 (54)
Bachelor's degree	90 (30)
Postgraduate	48 (16)
Job status, n (%)	
Employed	192 (64)
Unemployed	108 (36)
Household income *, n (%)	
Poor	54 (18)
Middle	216 (72)
Well-off	30 (10)

* Self-reported.

2.2.5. Reliability

Reliability of the instrument was examined using internal consistency and test–retest (test of stability across time) analyses. The Cronbach's alpha coefficients were calculated for subscales and the whole instrument to evaluate the internal consistency for which a value of ≥0.6 was accepted for descriptive studies [32]. Stability of the instrument was examined using the test–retest analysis conducted on 25 women with delayed childbearing who completed the questionnaire twice within a two-week interval [33]. The intra-class correlation coefficient (ICC) was also calculated and classified as follows: 0.0–0.2 as low, 0.21–0.40 as fair, 0.41–0.60 as moderate, 0.61–0.80 as substantial, and 0.81–1 as almost perfect [34].

2.2.6. Statistical Analysis

The SPSS software for Windows version 16.0 was used to perform all statistical analyses (SPSS Inc., Chicago, IL, USA, 2008). Both item- and subscale-level analyses were conducted using descriptive statistics including frequencies, means and standard deviations. The statistical analysis of construct validity was performed through the EFA with the principal component method and varimax rotation. Eigenvalues of more than one and a scree plot were used to determine the number of factors. Factor loadings equal or greater than 0.4 were considered appropriate. The Cronbach's alpha coefficient and ICC were also calculated. p-values < 0.05 were set as statistically significant.

2.3. Ethical Considerations

The Research and Ethics Committee affiliated with Tarbiat Modares University (decree code: 15-6-2014) approved the study research protocol. The women were informed of their rights and the possibility of withdrawal from the study at any time. They were also ensured that the data collection was confidential and would be used only for the research purpose. Also, the written informed consent form was signed by all women who willingly agreed to take part in this study.

3. Results

The total number of initial items generated during the qualitative phase and literature review were 82 items. After eliminating redundancies by the research team, they were reduced to 60 items. The classification of these 60 items under the three themes resulting from qualitative content analysis was as follows: personal inclination (18 items), perceived beliefs about delayed childbearing (15 items), and social support (27 items).

During face validity, some typographical errors were corrected and also all items achieved the minimum impact score required for inclusion. In content validity, the number of items was reduced from 60 to 57, since the CVR was less than 0.49. The mean CVR in this study for the total scale was reported as 0.87, indicating a satisfactory result. As such, two items did not achieve the CVI above 0.79 and were omitted from the final questionnaire. The mean CVR and CVI for the scale were 0.87 and 0.92, respectively, indicating appropriate content validity.

For the identification of the underlying factor structure of the instrument, the EFA was conducted using a principal components analysis. A total of 300 women with the experience of delayed childbearing (mean age of 37.8 years) agreed to complete the 55-item questionnaire entitled The Delayed Childbearing Questionnaire (DCBQ-55).

The KMO coefficient was reported as 0.809 ($p < 0.001$), indicating that the properties of the correlation matrix justified conducting the EFA. A varimax rotation identified six latent factors. The extraction was based on the visual interpretation of the scree plot (Figure 1) and Kaiser's criterion for Eigenvalues ≥ 1. The six factors jointly accounted for 61.24% of the observed variance. No item was deleted due to adequate loading on the factors. However, due to its further compatibility, one item from domain five was transferred to domain six. Table 2 provides the details, factors, labels and the number of items.

Scree Plot

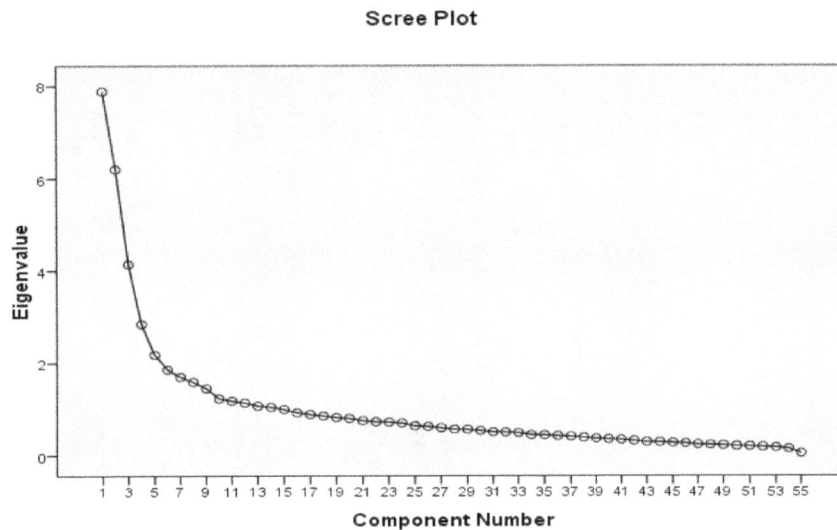

Figure 1. Scree plot for The Delayed Childbearing Questionnaire (DCBQ-55) ($n = 300$).

The Cronbach's alpha coefficient was reported as 0.836. The ICC was reported as 0.81 indicating a suitable stability of the instrument. Table 3 provides the description of the Cronbach's α coefficient and ICC for the instrument and its domains. For stability through the test–retest analysis, Spearman's correlation coefficient was reported as 0.86.

Table 2. Factors, items and factor loadings of The Delayed Childbearing Questionnaire (DCBQ-55)* (*n* = 300).

Items	Factor 1	Factor 2	Factor 3	Factor 4	Factor 5	Factor 6
Factor 1: Readiness for childbearing						
Being sure about physical health before pregnancy	0.821	0.471	0.017	0.067	0.074	0.017
Control of chronic diseases before pregnancy	0.819	0.215	0.063	0.084	0.051	0.036
Having mental peace before pregnancy	0.815	0.015	0.074	0.128	0.121	0.097
Ability to transfer mental safety and security to the spouse before pregnancy	0.798	0.122	0.005	0.014	0.224	0.215
Having concerns about being a good mother and wife at the same time	0.777	0.168	0.084	0.157	0.168	0.254
Meeting the basic necessities before pregnancy	0.763	0.101	0.054	0.108	0.185	0.135
Having suitable financial savings before pregnancy	0.755	0.020	0.035	0.114	0.117	0.136
Having a suitable and secure job before pregnancy	0.745	0.187	0.150	0.168	0.231	0.198
Ability to provide the best facilities for childcare	0.732	0.096	0.220	.0164	0.226	0.146
Completing education and studies before pregnancy	0.703	0.124	0.221	0.064	0.117	0.318
Having concerns about financial problems during pregnancy	0.620	0.183	0.012	0.134	0.091	0.018
Having concerns about losing better economic situations during pregnancy	0.581	0.163	0.187	0.078	0.107	0.015
Lack of responsibility and commitment to have a child	0.506	0.043	0.024	0.093	0.208	0.147
Lack of self-confidence to be a mother	0.506	0.123	0.014	0.215	0.018	0.095
High costs of pregnancy and childbirth	0.319	0.106	0.054	0.197	0.064	0.031
Factor 2: Stability in the partner relationship						
Achieving a comprehensive understanding of the spouse before pregnancy	0.33	0.860	0.214	0.057	0.163	0.069
Being sure of the reliability of the spouse for the rest of life	0.051	0.741	0.011	0.001	0.002	0.101
Developing strong relationships with the spouse	0.43	0.714	0.197	0.036	0.102	0.111
Feeling concerns about the ability to have enjoyable sexual relationships during pregnancy	0.33	0.707	0.72	0.128	0.114	0.022
Feeling concerns about personal attractiveness during pregnancy	0.87	0.686	0.233	0.043	0.210	0.185
Necessity of having children to achieve peace and stability in life	0.051	0.317	0.114	0.045	0.084	0.036
Factor 3: Awareness about the adverse outcomes of pregnancy in advanced maternal age						
Increased risk of infertility in women older than 35 years	0.047	0.124	0.617	0.165	0.036	0.182
Increased risk of obstetrics complications in advanced maternal age	0.088	0.065	0.611	0.109	0.062	0.126
Increased risk of neonatal complications in advanced maternal age	0.047	0.125	0.524	0.068	0.085	0.051
Presence of effective treatments for infertility to solve related problems	0.091	0.054	0.454	1.25	0.150	0.055
Losing the chance of having a second child due to delayed childbearing	0.158	0.026	0.409	0.001	1.05	0.201
Factor 4: Attitudes toward delayed childbearing						
Possibility of having a child at any age without facing any problem if God willing	0.103	0.156	0.048	0.667	0.114	0.165
Completion of the woman's identity through motherhood	0.147	0.121	0.039	0.633	0.065	0.195
Giving a meaning to the life through having a child	0.031	0.114	0.094	0.591	0.069	0.168
Importance of bringing a male or female child	0.085	0.032	0.129	0.588	0.142	0.024
Delayed childbearing as an interference in God's affairs	0.044	0.052	0.152	0.580	0.063	0.065
Creating a balance in the family decision-making between man and woman by delayed childbearing	0.163	0.098	0.231	0.572	0.117	0.096
Reduction of the women's power in the family due to early childbearing	0.047	0.187	0.011	0.570	0.016	0.048
Sufficiency of having only one child for the family	0.214	0.025	0.053	0.545	0.021	0.057
Starting a family later in life due to marriage at the old age	0.001	0.064	0.121	0.454	0.133	0.045

Table 2. *Cont.*

Items	Factor 1	Factor 2	Factor 3	Factor 4	Factor 5	Factor 6
Factor 5: Family support						
Being under pressure by the couple's families for delayed childbearing	0.062	0.147	0.036	0.080	0.656	0.037
Getting help from the couple's families for taking care of the child	0.142	0.015	0.199	0.142	0.614	0.091
Successful experiences of delayed childbearing in the couple's families	0.070	0.088	0.078	0.058	0.602	0.158
Persuasion of the couple to delay childbearing due to being raised in a small paternal family	0.018	0.011	0.148	0.046	0.581	0.036
Factor 6: Social support						
Childbearing as one of the most important social functions of the family	0.091	0.044	0.015	0.190	0.247	0.701
Being encouraged by others to delay childbearing	0.035	0.088	0.107	0.047	0.675	0.692
Limitations in the freedom for getting engaged in social activities due to childbearing	0.125	0.121	0.044	0.013	0.214	0.671
Delayed childbearing as a sign of modernity	0.017	0.014	0.125	0.166	0.118	0.657
Popularity of early childbearing in families with a lower social status	0.094	0.055	0.087	0.122	0.147	0.649
Education regarding delayed childbearing in schools and universities	0.225	0.024	0.096	0.085	0.129	0.629
Free access to modern contraceptive methods	0.019	0.035	0.067	0.101	0.155	0.625
Lack of childcare facilities at the workplace	0.195	0.128	0.088	0.032	0.138	0.624
Giving the responsibility of child care to a nursery with confidence	0.109	0.165	0.036	0.080	0.091	0.590
The high cost of childcare in a nursery	0.068	0.135	0.166	0.063	0.050	0.581
The short period of maternity leave for employed mothers	0.36	0.100	0.109	0.085	0.075	0.570
Support of delayed childbearing in mass media	0.015	0.121	0.094	0.021	0.150	0.564
Lack of special laws to support pregnant women or mothers	0.190	0.134	0.096	0.048	0.021	0.562
Being fired from work due to getting pregnant	0.087	0.087	0.148	0.046	0.107	0.513
Threating the child due to social insecurity	0.046	0.050	0.018	0.080	0.075	0.507
Lack of a bright future to start a family	0.011	0.010	0.115	0.198	0.114	0.481

* The permission to use the DCBQ-55 in future studies is granted by the authors ONLY with a full citation to this article.

Table 3. Descriptive statistics and reliability measurements of the DCBQ-50. CI = confidence interval.

Domain	Item (Number)	Cronbach's Alpha	ICC (95% CI)	Spearman's Correlation Coefficient ($n = 25$)	p-Value
Readiness for childbearing	15	0.833	0.83 (0.81–0.87)	0.71	0.001
Stability in the partner relationship	6	0.735	0.69 (0.67–0.74)	0.91	0.001
Awareness about the adverse outcomes of pregnancy in advanced maternal age	5	0.844	0.83 (0.80–0.88)	0.85	0.001
Attitude toward delayed childbearing	9	0.839	0.82 (0.79–0.89)	0.96	0.001
Family support	4	0.830	0.83 (0.79–0.85)	0.91	0.001
Social support	16	0.815	0.70 (0.68–0.84)	0.86	0.001
Total	55	0.836	0.81 (0.79–0.86)	0.86	0.001

4. Discussion

In this methodological study, both qualitative and quantitative approaches were used to design an applicable instrument for the assessment of factors influencing delayed childbearing. In addition, it was shown that the DCBQ-55 met psychometric requirements including reliability, validity, and internal consistency for use in community and clinical settings. The main characteristic of the DCBQ-55 is to directly address the perceptions and concerns of women regarding delayed childbearing. It includes 55 items in six domains of 'readiness for childbearing', 'stability in the partner relationship', 'awareness about the adverse outcomes of pregnancy in advanced maternal age', 'attitude toward delayed childbearing', 'family support', and 'social support', enabling researchers and policymakers to assess the various aspects of this phenomenon overlooked in previous studies. To our knowledge, prior to the DCBQ-55, there was no specific instruments for the assessment of factors influencing delayed childbearing. The use of qualitative and quantitative approaches and a thorough literature search have led to the development of an instrument that can help with a systematic assessment of this phenomenon. For instance, in terms of reliability, the acceptable level of internal consistency of the DCBQ-55 was reported. It meant that each item in this instrument was highly correlated with the total score, suggesting that the items were homogeneous and measured a similar overall assessment's construct.

The first domain of the DCBQ-55 was 'readiness for childbearing'. According to the international literature, lack of readiness by couples has been be linked to their awareness of the sacrifices and costs of parenthood, and the common notion that parenthood can be delayed safely. Couples need to improve their knowledge of the age-related decline in fertility and its impact on future parenthood [14]. Creating a positive atmosphere regarding childbearing can influence a couple's decision on the postponement of childbearing [35].

'Stability in the partner relationship' was another domain of the instrument developed in this study. Koert and Daniluk reported that women were delaying childbearing to seek an appropriate partner [13]. For many women, enduring marital relationships is associated with better health-related decisions and outcomes in life [36]. On the other hand, making a decision on the family size is adjusted and explained by changes in the partner. If there is a decision of childbearing postponement until the age of 30 years, it is more likely to lower the family size than if the childbearing career is started earlier [37].

With regard to 'awareness about the adverse outcomes of pregnancy in advanced maternal age', as the third dimension of the DCBQ-55, a matched case-control study in women aged over 35 years in comparison with younger mothers in Nigeria showed that delayed childbearing after 35 years was often not associated with adverse pregnancy outcomes. In other words, it could indicate women's awareness of the potential risks of pregnancy and increased use of obstetric services [38]. According to another study in Denmark, the increased risk of infertility, spontaneous abortions, ectopic pregnancies and trisomy 21 started at around 30 years of age, and the increasing risk of preterm births and stillbirths started at around 35 years of age. Therefore, increasing couples' awareness of the probable negative effects of advanced maternal age on reproductive outcomes is crucial [39].

'Attitude toward delayed childbearing' was the fourth dimension of this instrument. A recent study in Canada showed that women $\geq$ 35 years of age believed themselves to have more knowledge regarding age-related pregnancy risks than those under the age of 35 years. However, they preferred to receive further counselling about it. This study also demonstrated that women's attitudes did not correlate with their measured knowledge. Therefore, continuous and face-to-face education regarding the age-related risks of pregnancy is required to improve their health literacy [40]. It is also believed that individuals' values may directly impact behaviors related to reproductive health [41]; however, the effect of personal values and being informed and encouraged about the timing of pregnancy during young adulthood needs further longitudinal evaluations [42].

The fifth dimension of the DCBQ-55 was 'family support'. It has been stated that women's perceptions of family support may have a negative association with family planning unmet needs among women [43]. Therefore, support systems should be devised with the aim of improving women's access to maternity services, especially culturally appropriate services that encompass community, stakeholder options and respect for their cultural preferences [44].

The last dimension of the DCBQ-55 was 'social support'. It is noted that maternity-related decisions are mainly associated with conflicts and difficulties as a result of family values, religious beliefs and presence of social and healthcare support. Social and educational institutions need to become more pregnancy-friendly to encourage women to have an early pregnancy [45]. In addition, women will benefit from increased support in the workplace and from insurance systems for fertility preservation and healthy reproduction [41].

The DCBQ-55 includes the sexual-related issues of delayed childbearing that have been overlooked by previous studies. While this section is highly cultural [46], it provides important information for a more precise assessment of delayed childbearing among women. In this respect, the high prevalence of sexual-related problems among pregnant women [47], the common notion that sexual relationships are forbidden during pregnancy [48,49], prolonged sexual abstinence after childbirth for ensuring family health, and the social implications of non-adherence to sexual abstinence norms [50] can negatively impact couples' emotional and sexual life [2].

Since no appropriate and culture-contextual instrument was available to assess delayed childbearing, concurrent validity could not be examined in this study. Nevertheless, the comprehensive literature review performed in the first phase of instrument development enriched the item pool and ensured that the DCBQ-55 could be used by researchers in other cultures and contexts. Also, the study's subjects in both the qualitative and quantitative phases were female, but childbearing decision-making might be mostly a couple's decision. Therefore, future studies need to involve males in data collection to provide a more comprehensive picture of delayed childbearing. In this study, only women that postponed childbearing based on their own personal choices and in controlled situations were recruited. However, some other women may perceive that they have no ultimate control on the timing of childbearing [51]. Future studies need to consider the perspectives of such women, men and healthcare providers involved in making a decision on delayed childbearing to further revise the DCBQ-55 and improve its generalizability.

5. Conclusions

Delayed childbearing is an important contributor to women's maternity experiences and requires greater attention in clinical and policy-making decisions related to the family planning process. The DCBQ-55 as a simple, valid and reliable instrument opens the way for a more comprehensive assessment of factors influencing delayed childbearing. The average time to complete the DCBQ-55 by a participant is about 10–15 min, indicating that the DCBQ-55 is quick to complete and easy to score. The researchers suggest the incorporation of culture-contextual aspects of delayed childbearing during data collection using the DCBQ-55 and interpretation of findings. The DCBQ-55 can feed information to reproductive healthcare providers and policy makers to make appropriate decisions regarding delayed childbearing in line with population development policies.

Author Contributions: S.B.G., S.Z. and F.K.F. designed the study. The analysis process and results were assessed by S.B.G., A.K. and M.V. All authors contributed to drafting the manuscript and approved its content to be published in the journal.

Funding: This study was one part of the first author's (S.B.G.) dissertation for the fulfilment of a PhD degree in Reproductive Health in 2014 and was supported by Tarbiat Modares University, Tehran, Iran.

References

1.   Wiebe, E.; Chalmers, A.; Yager, H. Delayed motherhood: Understanding the experiences of women older than age 33 who are having abortions but plan to become mothers later. *Can. Fam. Physician* **2012**, *58*, e588–e595. [PubMed]

2.   Behboudi-Gandevani, S.; Ziaei, S.; Khalajabadi Farahani, F.; Jasper, M. The Perspectives of Iranian Women on Delayed Childbearing: A Qualitative Study. *J. Nurs. Res.* **2015**, *23*, 313–321. [CrossRef] [PubMed]

3.   Balasch, J.; Gratacós, E. Delayed childbearing: Effects on fertility and the outcome of pregnancy. *Curr. Opin. Obstet. Gynecol.* **2012**, *24*, 187–193. [CrossRef] [PubMed]

4.   Maheshwari, A.; Porter, M.; Shetty, A.; Bhattacharya, S. Women's awareness and perceptions of delay in childbearing. *Fertil. Steril.* **2008**, *90*, 1036–1042. [CrossRef] [PubMed]

5.   Mills, M.; Rindfuss, R.R.; McDonald, P.; te Velde, E. Why do people postpone parenthood? Reasons and social policy incentives. *Hum. Reprod. Update* **2011**, *17*, 848–860. [CrossRef] [PubMed]

6.   Proudfoot, S.; Wellings, K.; Glasier, A. Analysis why nulliparous women over age 33 wish to use contraception. *Contraception* **2009**, *79*, 98–104. [CrossRef] [PubMed]

7.   Sol Olafsdottir, H.; Wikland, M.; Möller, A. Reasoning about timing of wanting a child: A qualitative study of Nordic couples from fertility clinics. *J. Reprod. Infant. Psychol.* **2011**, *29*, 493–505. [CrossRef]

8.   Kenny, L.C.; Lavender, T.; McNamee, R.; O'Neill, S.; Mills, T.; Khashan, A.S. Advanced maternal age and adverse pregnancy outcome: Evidence from a large contemporary cohort. *PLoS ONE* **2013**, *8*, e56583. [CrossRef] [PubMed]

9.   Weng, Y.-H.; Yang, C.-Y.; Chiu, Y.-W. Risk assessment of adverse birth outcomes in relation to maternal age. *PLoS ONE* **2014**, *9*, e114843. [CrossRef] [PubMed]

10. Petersen, K.B.; Hvidman, H.W.; Sylvest, R.; Pinborg, A.; Larsen, E.C.; Macklon, K.T.; Andersen, A.N.; Schmidt, L. Family intentions and personal considerations on postponing childbearing in childless cohabiting and single women aged 35–43 seeking fertility assessment and counselling. *Hum. Reprod.* **2015**, *30*, 2563–2574. [CrossRef] [PubMed]

11. Varea, C.; Terán, J.M.; Bernis, C.; Bogin, B. The impact of delayed maternity on foetal growth in Spain: An assessment by population attributable fraction. *Women Birth* **2018**, *31*, e190–e196. [CrossRef] [PubMed]

12. Asgharpour, M.; Villarreal, S.; Schummers, L.; Hutcheon, J.; Shaw, D.; Norman, W.V. Inter-pregnancy interval and pregnancy outcomes among women with delayed childbearing: Protocol for a systematic review. *Syst. Rev.* **2017**, *6*, 75. [CrossRef] [PubMed]

13. Koert, E.; Daniluk, J.C. When time runs out: Reconciling permanent childlessness after delayed childbearing. *J. Reprod. Infant Psychol.* **2017**, *35*, 342–352. [CrossRef] [PubMed]

14. Sylvest, R.; Koert, E.; Birch Petersen, K.; Malling, G.M.H.; Hald, F.; Nyboe Andersen, A.; Schmidt, L. Attitudes towards family formation among men attending fertility counselling. *Reprod. Biomed. Soc. Online* **2018**, *6*, 1–9. [CrossRef] [PubMed]

15. Adashi, E.Y.; Gutman, R. Delayed Childbearing as a Growing, Previously Unrecognized Contributor to the National Plural Birth Excess. *Obstet. Gynecol.* **2018**. [CrossRef] [PubMed]

16. Te Velde, E.; Habbema, D.; Leridon, E.; Eijkemans, M. The effect of postponement of first motherhood on permanent involuntary childlessness and total fertility rate in six European countries since the 1970s. *Hum. Reprod.* **2012**, *27*, 1179–1183. [CrossRef] [PubMed]

17. Sobotka, T. Post-transitional fertility: The role of childbearing postponement in fuelling the shift to low and unstable fertility levels. *J. Biosoc. Sci.* **2017**, *49*, S20–S45. [CrossRef] [PubMed]

18. Eurostat Statistics Explained, Fertility Statistics. 2018. Available online: https://ec.europa.eu/eurostat/statistics-explained/index.php/Fertility_statistics (accessed on 15 September 2018).

19. Saadat, S.; Chowdhury, S.; Mehryar, A. Fertility Decline in the Islamic Republic of Iran, 1980–2006: A Case Study. Available online: http://siteresources.worldbank.org/INTPRH/Resources/376374-1278599377733/Iran62910PRINT.pdf (accessed on 15 September 2018).

20. Aghajanian, A. Family Planning Program and Recent Fertility Trends in Iran. Measure Evaluation, Carolina Population Center, University of North Carolina at Chapel Hill, March 1998. Available online: https://www.measureevaluation.org/resources/publications/wp-98-04 (accessed on 15 September 2018).

21. McDonald, P.; Hosseini-Chavoshi, M.; Abbasi-Shavazi, M.J.; Rashidian, A. An assessment of recent Iranian fertility trends using parity progression ratios. *Demogr. Res.* **2015**, *32*, 1581–1602. [CrossRef]

22. The Iran's National Statistics Organization. Based on the Results of the Census of 2016, the Total Fertility Rate of Iran in the Period of 2012–2016 Reached to 2.01 Children. 2017. Available online: https://www.amar.org.ir/DesktopModules/DnnForge%20-%20NewsArticles/Print.aspx?tabid=123&tabmoduleid=507&articleId=5080&moduleId=613&PortalID=0 (accessed on 15 September 2018).

23. Kazemijaliseh, H.; Tehrani, F.R.; Behboudi-Gandevani, S.; Hosseinpanah, F.; Khalili, D.; Azizi, F. The Prevalence and Causes of Primary Infertility in Iran: A Population-Based Study. *Glob. J. Health Sci.* **2015**, *7*, 226–232. [CrossRef] [PubMed]

24. Behboudi-Gandevani, S.; Ziaei, S.; Khalajabadi-Farahani, F.; Jasper, M. Iranian primigravid women's awareness of the risks associated with delayed childbearing. *Eur. J. Contracept. Reprod. Health Care* **2013**, *18*, 460–467. [CrossRef] [PubMed]

25. Nasrabad, H.B.R.; Abbasi-Shavazi, M.J.; Hosseini-Chavoshi, M.; Karegar-Shoraki, M.R. Trend and Patterns of Childlessness in Iran. In Proceedings of the XXVII International Population Conference of the IUSSP, Busan, Korea, 26–31 August 2013. Available online: https://iussp.org/sites/default/files/event_call_for_papers/Childlessness%20in%20Iran%20-%20draft.pdf (accessed on 15 September 2018).

26. Shorey, S.; Yang, Y.Y.; Ang, E. The impact of negative childbirth experience on future reproductive decisions: A quantitative systematic review. *J. Adv. Nurs.* **2018**, *74*, 1236–1244. [CrossRef] [PubMed]

27. Ivankova, N.V.; Creswell, J.W.; Stick, S.L. Using mixed-methods sequential explanatory design: From theory to practice. *Field Methods* **2006**, *18*, 3–20. [CrossRef]

28. Graneheim, U.H.; Lundman, B. Qualitative content analysis in nursing research: Concepts, procedures and measures to achieve trustworthiness. *Nurse. Educ. Today* **2004**, *24*, 105–112. [CrossRef] [PubMed]

29. Vaismoradi, M.; Turunen, H.; Bondas, T. Content analysis and thematic analysis: Implications for conducting a qualitative descriptive study. *Nurs. Health Sci.* **2013**, *15*, 398–405. [CrossRef] [PubMed]

30. Waltz, C.F.; Strickland, O.L.; Lenz, E.R. *Measurement in Nursing and Health Research*; Springer Publishing Company: New York, NY, USA, 2010.

31. Munro, B.H. *Statistical Methods for Health Care Research*; Lippincott Williams & Wilkins: Philadelphia, PA, USA, 2005.

32. Bland, J.M.; Altman, D.G. Statistics notes: Cronbach's alpha. *BMJ* **1997**, *314*, 572. [CrossRef] [PubMed]

33. Polit, D.F.; Beck, C.T. *Essential of Nursing Research: Appraising Evidence for Nursing Practice*; Lippincott Williams & Wilkins: Philadelphia, PA, USA, 2018.

34. Landis, J.R.; Koch, G.G. The measurement of observer agreement for categorical data. *Biometrics* **1977**, *33*, 159–174. [CrossRef] [PubMed]

35. Taheri, M.; Takian, A.; Taghizadeh, Z.; Jafari, N.; Sarafraz, N. Creating a positive perception of childbirth experience: Systematic review and meta-analysis of prenatal and intrapartum interventions. *Reprod Health* **2018**, *15*, 73. [CrossRef] [PubMed]

36. Williams, K.; Sassler, S.; Frech, A.; Addo, F.; Cooksey, E. Nonmarital Childbearing, Union History, and Women's Health at Midlife. *Am. Sociol. Rev.* **2011**, *76*, 465–486. [CrossRef] [PubMed]

37. Liefbroer, A.C. Changes in Family Size Intentions Across Young Adulthood: A Life-Course Perspective. *Eur. J. Popul.* **2009**, *25*, 363–386. [CrossRef] [PubMed]

38. Olusanya, B.O.; Solanke, O.A. Perinatal correlates of delayed childbearing in a developing country. *Arch. Gynecol. Obstet.* **2012**, *285*, 951–957. [CrossRef] [PubMed]

39. Schmidt, L.; Sobotka, T.; Bentzen, J.G.; Andersen, A.N.; ESHRE Reproduction and Society Task Force. Demographic and medical consequences of the postponement of parenthood. *Hum. Reprod. Update* **2012**, *18*, 29–43. [CrossRef] [PubMed]

40. Sheinis, M.; Carpe, N.; Gold, S.; Selk, A. Ignorance is bliss: Women's knowledge regarding age-related pregnancy risks. *J. Obstet. Gynaecol.* **2018**, *38*, 344–351. [CrossRef] [PubMed]

41. Simoni, M.K.; Mu, L.; Collins, S.C. Women's career priority is associated with attitudes towards family planning and ethical acceptance of reproductive technologies. *Hum. Reprod.* **2017**, *32*, 2069–2075. [CrossRef] [PubMed]

42. Maeda, E.; Nakamura, F.; Boivin, J.; Kobayashi, Y.; Sugimori, H.; Saito, H. Fertility knowledge and the timing of first childbearing: A cross-sectional study in Japan. *Hum. Fertil.* **2016**, *19*, 275–281.

43. Shah, M.A.; Shah, N.M.; Chowdhury, R.I.; Menon, I. Unmet need for contraception in Kuwait: Issues for health care providers. *Soc. Sci. Med.* **2004**, *59*, 1573–1580. [CrossRef] [PubMed]

44. Simmonds, D.M.; West, L.; Porter, J.; Davies, M.; Holland, C.; Preston-Thomas, A.; O'Rourke, P.K.; Tangey, A. The role of support person for Ngaanyatjarra women during pregnancy and birth. *Women Birth* **2012**, *25*, 79–85. [CrossRef] [PubMed]

45. Arhin, A.O.; Cormier, E. Factors influencing decision-making regarding contraception and pregnancy among nursing students. *Nurse Educ. Today* **2008**, *28*, 210–217. [CrossRef] [PubMed]

46. Allen, L.; Fountain, L. Addressing sexuality and pregnancy in childbirth education classes. *J. Perinat. Educ.* **2007**, *16*, 32–36. [CrossRef] [PubMed]

47. Jamali, S.; Mosalanejad, L. Sexual dysfnction in Iranian pregnant women. *Iran. J. Reprod. Med.* **2013**, *11*, 479–486. [PubMed]

48. Moscrop, A. Can sex during pregnancy cause a miscarriage? A concise history of not knowing. *Br. J. Gen. Pract.* **2012**, *62*, e308–e310. [CrossRef] [PubMed]

49. Andraweera, P.; Roberts, C.T.; Leemaqz, S.; McCowan, L.; Myers, J.; Kenny, L.C.; Walker, J.; Poston, L.; Dekker, G.; SCOPE Consortium. The duration of sexual relationship and its effects on adverse pregnancy outcomes. *J. Reprod. Immunol.* **2018**, *128*, 16–22. [CrossRef] [PubMed]

50. Mbekenga, C.K.; Pembe, A.B.; Darj, E.; Christensson, K.; Olsson, P. Prolonged sexual abstinence after childbirth: Gendered norms and perceived family health risks. Focus group discussions in a Tanzanian suburb. *BMC Int. Health Hum. Rights* **2013**, *13*, 4. [CrossRef]

51. Cooke, A.; Mills, T.A.; Lavender, T. Advanced maternal age: Delayed childbearing is rarely a conscious choice. A qualitative study of women's views and experiences. *Int. J. Nurs. Stud.* **2012**, *49*, 30–39. [CrossRef] [PubMed]

10

Lyme Disease Transmission Risk: Seasonal Variation in the Built Environment

Amanda Roome [1] ⓘ**, Rita Spathis** [2]**, Leah Hill** [3]**, John M. Darcy** [4] **and Ralph M. Garruto** [1,5,*]

[1] Department of Anthropology, Binghamton University, Binghamton, NY 13902, USA; aroome1@binghamton.edu

[2] School of Pharmacy and Pharmaceutical Sciences, Binghamton University, Binghamton, NY 13902, USA; rspathis@binghamton.edu

[3] Quality Control, Regeneron Pharmaceuticals, Albany, NY 12144, USA; lhill5@binghamton.edu

[4] US Clinical Development & Medical Affairs in the Division of Immunology, Hepatology and Dermatology, Novartis, East Hanover, NJ 07936, USA; jdarcyi1@binghamton.edu

[5] Department of Biological Sciences, Binghamton University, Binghamton, NY 13902, USA

* Correspondence: rgarruto@binghamton.edu

Abstract: Seasonal variation in spatial distribution and pathogen prevalence of *Borrelia burgdorferi* in blacklegged ticks (*Ixodes scapularis*) influences human population risk of Lyme disease in peri-urban built environments. Parks, gardens, playgrounds, school campuses and neighborhoods represent a significant risk for Lyme disease transmission. From June 2012 through May 2014, ticks were collected using 1 m^2 corduroy cloths dragged over low-lying vegetation parallel to walkways with high human foot traffic. DNA was extracted from ticks, purified and presence of *B. burgdorferi* assessed by polymerase chain reaction amplification. Summer is reported as the time of highest risk for Lyme disease transmission in the United States and our results indicate a higher tick density of 26.0/1000 m^2 in summer vs. 0.2/1000 m^2 to 10.5/1000 m^2 in spring and fall. However, our findings suggest that tick infection rate is proportionally higher during the fall and spring than summer (30.0–54.7% in fall and 36.8–65.6% in spring vs. 20.0–28.2% in summer). Seasonal variation in infected tick density has significant implications for Lyme disease transmission as people are less likely to be aware of ticks in built environments, and unaware of increased infection in ticks in spring and fall. These factors may lead to more tick bites resulting in Lyme infection.

Keywords: tick-borne diseases; *Borrelia burgdorferi*; tick density and infection rate; human risk factors; Northeastern United States

1. Introduction

Emerging infectious diseases (EID's) and re-emerging infectious diseases are a significant and growing problem affecting population health and place an increasingly heavy burden on public health infrastructure globally by stressing individuals, families and communities [1–5]. While many factors contribute to EID's, the intersection of ecological and environmental factors with human behavioral patterns are increasingly recognized as fundamental to the transmission of zoonotic diseases [6–9]. Currently, zoonoses represent the majority of EID's in humans [3,10,11], with vector-driven zoonoses emerging due to societal, demographic and climatic changes [12–15].

Lyme disease, caused by *Borrelia burgdorferi* sensu lato complex, a spirochetal bacterium, is the most common vector-borne disease in the United States and is transmitted to humans via the blacklegged tick, *Ixodes scapularis* (formerly known as the deer tick), in the Northeast and Upper Midwest, and transmitted by *Ixodes pacificus* on the West Coast [16–19]. The ensuing multi-systemic bacterial infection can result in flu-like symptoms, fever, fatigue, joint pain, musculoskeletal pain, headaches, sleep disturbances and depression, among other symptoms [20–23]. The disease is also known for erythema migrans (EM), a rash that sometimes resembles a "bull's eye"; however, EM is not associated with every case of Lyme, and can also manifest in a solid, spreading nontarget skin lesion [24–26]. Untreated, the disease can result in serious neurologic and cardiac complications (potentially manifesting as myocarditis, pericarditis, pancarditis, dilated cardiomyopathy, and heart failure) [21,27]. Currently, the Centers for Disease Control and Prevention estimates that 300,000 new cases of Lyme disease occur annually, with 95% of reported cases occurring in 14 states in the Northeast and Upper Midwest [28–30]. Between 2004 and 2016, tick-borne diseases more than doubled, and were the majority (77%) of all vector-borne diseases reported [31]. The continuing upward trend in cases and its geographic expansion in the United States, Canada and temperate parts of Eurasia make Lyme disease a growing concern for population health in these regions [32,33].

We define built environments, according to the criteria of Srinivasan and colleagues [34], as places where people live, work and spend their leisure time, such as parks, school campuses, neighborhood backyards and other human-made or altered external environmental space where people are regularly perambulating or congregating. These are peri-urban environments in which infectious ticks and the transmission of tick-borne diseases can occur [35,36]. These peri-urban spaces, with fragmented landscapes [32] are conducive to the transmission of zoonotic diseases to human populations and may remain overlooked in terms of Lyme disease risk and management by local communities. Unlike rural or remote hiking, camping, fishing, hunting or other outdoor activities that primarily take place during the summer months, humans within built environments interact year-round, which may leave them at a heightened risk of exposure to infected ticks during spring, summer and fall [35–37].

Ecological factors and forest fragmentation are known to have a positive correlation with tick density and infection prevalence of *B. burgdorferi* [37,38]. The initiation and duration of the tick life cycle is an important factor in the overall impact of the environment on tick populations. *Ixodes scapularis*, the blacklegged tick, has a typical life cycle of two years, during which it takes three blood meals, one at each stage of development (larval, nymphal and adult) [39,40]. As *B. burgdorferi* is not transmitted transovarially, larval stage ticks hatch from uninfected eggs [41,42]. It is worth noting, however, that another species of *Borrelia, B. miyamotoi,* which is also found in New York, can be transmitted transovarially at a rate of 6–73% [43,44]. Larval ticks take a blood meal during the summer, molt into nymphal ticks, which overwinter and take a blood meal the following spring or summer. Nymphal ticks then molt into adult ticks and take their final blood meal during the fall, with mating typically occurring on a vertebrate host. Females then drop off the host, overwinter and lay eggs the following spring. If, however, females do not mate and feed during the fall, they overwinter, emerge in the spring and take a blood meal, mate and lay eggs [40]. Once infected, a tick, whether in the nymphal or adult stage, is able to transmit the spirochetes causing Lyme disease to other hosts, including humans [45,46].

In New York and the Northeastern United States, many fragmented landscapes within built environments see high human activity during summer months, with a majority of Lyme disease cases reported between May and August [47]. However, human activities continue throughout the year, with significant exposures during the fall and spring months. Larval ticks may become infected after their first blood meal, then molt into nymphs, which are very small and hard to detect. The nymphal stage, which primarily appears between May and August, has been reported to cause most cases of Lyme disease [48–50]. Likewise, summer is when large numbers of people typically spend time outdoors, posing an increased risk of Lyme disease transmission [40]. In the present study, we determine the spatial distribution of *I. scapularis* ticks and the prevalence of the Lyme disease pathogen (*B. burgdorferi*) to assess the risk of infection during all seasons of the year, especially in built environments with fragmented landscapes. In the Northeastern United States and Upper Midwest, little data on tick infection rates within built environments across all seasons currently exists, except for the Hudson Valley and Long Island [51,52].

2. Materials and Methods

This study was conducted over the course of two years, from June 2012 to May 2014 in the Southern Tier region of upstate New York State along 50 walkways intensively used by humans on the 376.4 hectare Binghamton University campus, its adjacent Nature Preserve (73.7 ha), and in Chenango Valley State Park (460.1 ha) and Wolfe Park (73.7 ha), all within peri-urban Broome County (Figure 1). All sites encompass an assortment of ecological niches that are surrounded by residential, commercial and woodland areas with high human activity (Figure 2). These settings provide ample opportunity for community members, who are interacting with their environments, to come in contact with infected ticks. Seasonality was categorized as follows: spring; April and May, summer; June through August, and fall; September through November. Ticks were not collected December through March due to snow and cold weather and thus low tick activity.

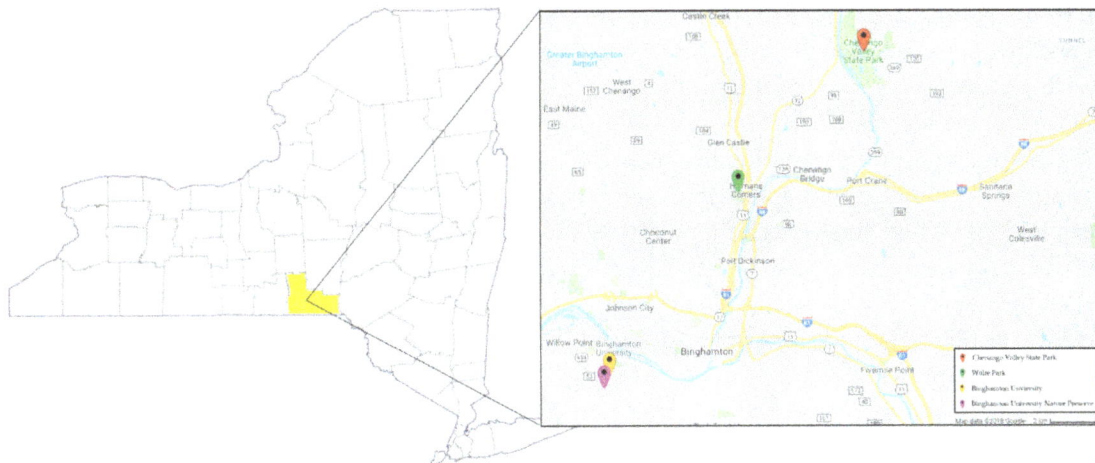

Figure 1. Map of New York State with Broome County (study location) highlighted in yellow. On the right side of the figure are each of the four field sites.

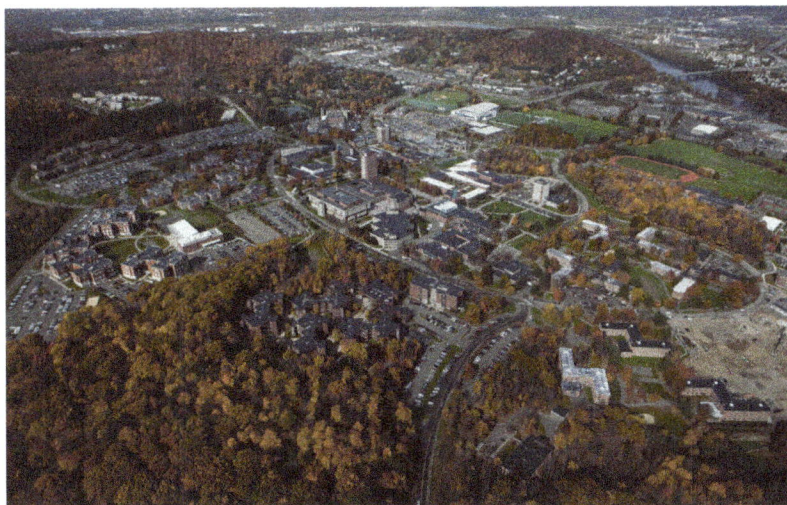

Figure 2. An aerial view of peri urban Broome County, representing a built environment, with interspersed fragmented landscapes and microecologies.

2.1. Tick Collection

Along 50 walkways with high human foot traffic on the Binghamton University campus (two sites) and in two parks within Broome County, we designed a specific methodology to assess tick density by collecting ticks three consecutive meters on both sides of and parallel to walkways and paths [53] by dragging a 1 m^2 white corduroy cloth over low lying vegetation and leaf litter [54–56]. Tick collection took place between June 2012 and May 2014, with each walkway being dragged 2–3 times per month. Questing ticks (in search of a blood meal) were removed from the cloth with forceps, placed into sterile cryovials containing 70% ethanol and stored at −20 °C until DNA extraction.

Density for nymphal and adult ticks was determined by calculating the total area dragged in square meters, either from direct path and walkway measurements, or from existing known path and walkway distances. The number of ticks collected was divided by the total area dragged and multiplied by 1000, resulting in the density of ticks per 1000 m^2.

2.2. Prevalence of B. burgdorferi in Ticks

For each tick species, life cycle stage, sex and collection location were identified. Ticks were then flash frozen in liquid nitrogen and were physically disrupted using chrome steel beads (Biospec Products, Bartlesville, OK, USA) with a TissueLyser LT bead mill (Qiagen, Germantown, MD, USA). DNA was extracted using a Qiagen DNeasy Blood and Tissue Kit according to the manufacturer's instructions. The presence of *B. burgdorferi* in 1200 ticks was assessed using LD1/LD2 pathogen specific primers targeting the 16S rRNA sequence [57]. For 195 tick samples, *B. burgdorferi* was assessed by *OspC* polymerase chain reaction amplification as a means of determining specific genotypes [58]. When cross checking positivity rates in a sub-sample of 51 ticks between *OspC* and LD1/LD2 primers, infection rates were 98% similar, therefore, there was not a noticeable difference between primer sets.

PCR amplification was performed in 12.5 µL reaction containing 0.5 units HotStar Taq (Qiagen, Germantown, MD, USA), 1.5 mM MgCl$_2$, 0.2 mM dNTPs, and 200 nM of each of the primers. The primers sets used were either LD1 and LD2 (LD1: ATGCACACTTGGTGTTAACTA, LD2: GACTTATCACCGGCAGTCTTA [58], or OPSC_4F and OSPC_693R (OPSC_4F: GAAAAAGA ATACATTAAGTG, OSPC_693R: GACTTTATTTTTCCAGTTACTTTTT [59]). Thermal cycling was performed using a GeneAmp® PCR System 9700 (Applied Biosystems, Foster City, CA, USA) with the following program: 15 min at 94 °C, 45 cycles of 94 °C for 15 s, 55 °C for 30 s, and 72 °C for 45 s, followed by 5 min at 72 °C. The presence of PCR product was assessed by agarose gel electrophoresis.

2.3. Statistical Analyses

Logistic Regression analyses were conducted using IBM SPSS Statistics Version 19.0 (IBM Corp., Armonk, NY, USA). A Logistic Regression Model was used to determine which variables predicted the outcome of tick infection rates. Z-tests for proportions were used to determine significance between tick infection rates and chi-square tests used to determine significance between overall tick densities.

3. Results

Along walkways from four sites in Broome County over the two-year period (June 2012–May 2014), a total of 1375 ticks (481 nymphs and 894 adults) were collected by dragging an area equivalent to 12.7 hectares (126,612.6 m^2) (Table 1).

3.1. Tick Density

Along walkways with high human foot traffic, 1375 ticks were collected, with an overall density of 10.9/1000 m^2. The highest tick density was found in nymphal ticks during the summer of 2013 at 26.0/1000 m^2 (Table 1). Summer 2012 density data is not available as walkways and paths were not measured during this initial phase of the study. Adult tick density was slightly higher in fall 2012 at 10.5/1000 m^2 compared to fall 2013 at 8.6/1000 m^2.

Table 1. Tick density and infection rate along 50 heavily traveled walkways by season, month and life cycle stage over a two-year period, from June 2012 through May 2014.

Season	Month	Total Ticks Collected		Total Area Dragged	Tick Density per 1000 m²		# Ticks Tested		% Ticks Infected	
		Nymphs	Adults	Square Meters	Nymphs (95% CI)	Adults (95% CI)	Nymphs	Adults	Nymphs (95% CI)	Adults (95% CI)
Summer 2012	June			Data not collected			15	3	46.7	66.7
	July						54	12	14.8	8.3
	Overall						69	15	21.7	20.0
Fall 2012	October	4	68	5304.4	0.8	12.8	4	68	50.0	47.1
	November	0	20	3051.6	0.0	6.6	0	18	n/a	83.3
	Overall	4	88	8356.0	0.5	10.5	4	86	50.0	54.7
Spring 2013	April	0	32	3172.1	0.0	10.1	0	29	n/a	37.9
	May	0	9	4829.0	0.0	1.9	0	9	n/a	33.3
	Overall	0	41	8001.1	0.0	5.1	0	38	n/a	36.8
Summer 2013	June	467	1	17,958.9	26.0	0.1	419	1	28.2	0.0
	Overall	467	1	17,958.9	26.0	0.1	419	1	28.2	0.0
Fall 2013	September	0	13	11,286.3	0.0	1.2	0	13	n/a	30.8
	October	10	525	53,048.4	0.2	9.9	10	521	30.0	38.2
	November	0	24	927.0	0.0	25.9	0	24	n/a	50.0
	Overall	10	562	65,261.7	0.2	8.6	10	558	30.0	38.5
Spring 2014	April	0	131	20,627.9	0.0	6.4	0	130	n/a	62.3 [a]
	May	0	71	6407.1	0.0	11.1	0	65	n/a	72.3 [a]
	Overall	0	202	27,035.0	0.0	7.5	0	195	n/a	65.6 [a]
Summer 2012–Spring 2014		481	894	126,612.6	3.8 (±3.1)	7.1 (±3.1)	502	893	27.5 (±4.38)	45.5 (±2.83)
Overall		1375 *		126,612.6	10.9 (±2.19)		1395 *		39.0 (±2.38)	

[a] Tick DNA was amplified using OspC primers and was 98% similar to LD1/LD2 primers; * Total ticks collected differ from total ticks tested so as not to alter density calculations because area dragged was not determined in Summer 2012.

3.2. Tick Infection Rate

Along walkways with high human use, DNA analyses revealed an overall *B. burgdorferi* infection rate of 39.0%, with 27.5% infection rate in nymphal ticks and 45.5% in adult ticks for the time period spanning summer 2012 through summer 2014 (Table 1). Tick infection rates were also calculated by season. The two seasons with the lowest tick infection rates were summer 2012 with a nymphal infection rate of 21.7% and an adult infection rate of 20.0% and summer 2013, with a nymphal infection rate of 28.2%. Only one adult tick was collected during summer of 2013. The highest infection rates were observed in fall 2012, with nymphal and adult infection rates of 50.0% and 54.7%, respectively, and in spring 2014, with an adult infection rate of 65.6% (Table 1). However, the nymphal tick infection rate in fall 2012 was based on only 4 ticks.

3.3. Seasonality

Density of infected ticks was also determined by season (Table 2, Figure 3).

Table 2. Density of infected ticks per 1000 m^2 along heavily traveled walkways by season and life cycle stage based on 502 nymphal ticks and 893 adult ticks collected from fall 2012 to spring 2014. Overall figures were determined by calculating the sum of positive ticks and the sum of area dragged from all months and determining density of infected ticks per 1000 m^2. ((Is the bold necessary?) (Is the capital necessary?)

Season	Month	Density of Infected Ticks	
		Nymphs	**Adults**
Fall 2012	October	0.4	6.6
	November	0.0	4.9
	Ovearll	0.2	5.5
Spring 2013	April	0.0	3.5
	May	0.0	0.6
	Overall	0.0	1.7
Summer 2013	June	6.6	0.0
	July	Data not collected for July and August. Cannot be calculated	
	August		
	Overall	6.6	0.0
Fall 2013	September	0.0	0.4
	October	0.1	3.8
	November	0.0	12.9
	Overall	0.1	3.3
Spring 2014	April	0.0	3.9
	May	0.0	7.3
	Overall	0.0	4.7
Fall 2012–Spring 2014		1.1 (±3.1)	3.2 (±3.1)
Total Ticks Fall 2012–Spring 2014		4.3 (±3.1)	

To statistically determine the impact of life cycle stage and season on infection rate, a logistic regression was run. Infection rates in both fall 2013 and spring 2014 were significantly higher than summer 2013 ($p = 0.02$ and $p = 0.01$, respectively). The overall likelihood ratio of the effect of season on the outcome of infection rate was statistically significant at $p < 0.01$.

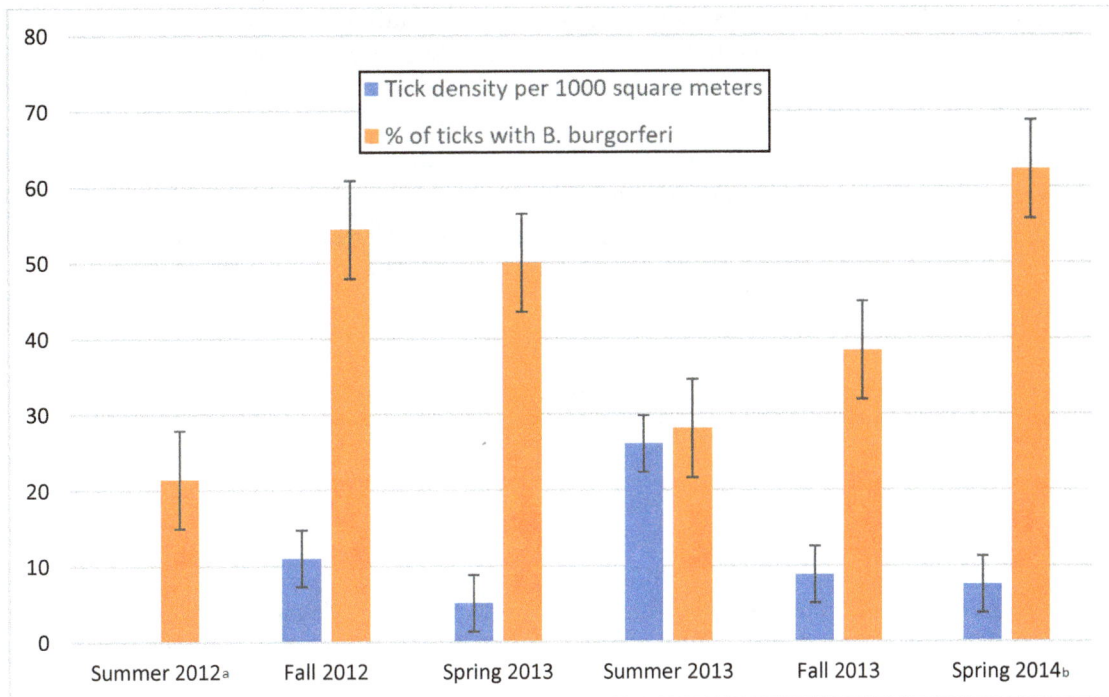

Figure 3. Tick density and infectivity (nymphal and adult) by season during the period Summer 2012 through Spring 2014 with standard error bars. [a] Density data for summer 2012 was unavailable, as distances dragged were not determined during that time. [b] Spring 2014 infectivity data in this figure represents *OspC* primer sets.

4. Discussion

The rise in incidence of Lyme disease in the Northeastern United States is said to be associated with a myriad of factors, including landscape modification, due in part to suburbanization, climate change, and migratory bird routes [12,15,48,60–63]. The continued expansion of built environments creates fragmented landscapes where human exposure to infected tick populations is more likely [35,36].

Our study finds that overall tick infection rates in both nymphal and adult ticks with *B. burgdorferi* along walkways of high human use in built environments with fragmented landscapes is as high, or higher than many endemic Hudson Valley counties [64] with the highest reported incidence of Lyme disease in New York State and among the highest in the nation [64,65]. Using the number of ticks tested and percent infected with *B. burgdSorferi* from data presented in Prusinski et al. [64], we calculated overall prevalence rate of infected ticks at 17.6% and 45.2% in nymphs and adults, respectively, among Hudson Valley counties, compared to infection rates of 27.5% and 45.5% for nymphs and adults, respectively, for the current study in Broome County (Table 1). All sites surveyed in this study are of high human use. The Binghamton University campus and the adjacent Nature Preserve are heavily used by faculty, staff, students, and the community. Wolfe Park and Chenango Valley State Park are heavily used by the community for recreational purposes. Many walkways have questing height vegetation growing onto the path or walkway, making it inevitable for walkway users to come in contact with vegetation, and thus, potentially with infected ticks.

Summer is considered the highest risk season for Lyme disease transmission [54,61], and health departments often stress that people should take appropriate precautions when entering forested environments [49]. However, it is worth noting that many cases diagnosed in the summer were transmitted in the spring, as symptoms do not usually occur for 3–30 days after a bite [40]. Our results show that although there is a higher density of ticks throughout the summer months (June through August) when smaller nymphal ticks are most active and less likely to be detected [48,49], tick infection and the density of infected ticks is proportionally much higher during spring (April and May) and fall (September to November). It is likely that public health precautions during summer months may cause people to infer that spring and fall pose less of a risk of infection. Yet, our data suggest that high tick density and infection rate in spring and fall months represent a significant population health risk (Tables 1 and 2, Figure 3), a risk compounded by behavioral attitudes informed by the notion that built environments provide a safe haven from contact with potentially infected ticks. Seasonal variation in risk of transmission within built environments may also be influenced by local and regional climatic patterns associated with global climate change. Such influences have resulted in warmer wetter shorter winters in higher latitudes and earlier longer warmer seasons. These changes have contributed to the geographic expansion and growth of tick populations into more northerly areas of the US, Canada and Eurasia impacting areas not previously known for tick-bone disease [12].

Adult ticks have a higher infection rate than nymphal ticks, as they have two opportunities to take a blood meal, thus two opportunities to be infected with *B. burgdorferi* and it has been shown that transmission of infection to humans can occur in less than 24 h, with other tick-borne pathogens being transmitted in as few as 15 min [66] supporting the view that adult ticks in spring and fall months are a significant threat to human health [67–69]. Studies of seasonal variations in tick density and infection in Switzerland and Sweden show that adult ticks have a higher prevalence of infection than nymphal ticks, that density and infection are higher during spring [69], and that tick infection is reduced during summer months and early autumn [70], findings consistent with our results in this newly emerging Lyme endemic area in Upstate New York.

Although Lyme disease is the most common vector-borne disease in the Northeastern United States, other co-infections should not be overlooked. A study in New York State by Tokarz et al. [71] determined that 71% of all ticks tested harbored at least one tick-borne pathogen and our data indicate that precautions should be taken during all seasons in which ticks are active to avoid tick bites using permethrin treated clothing, DEET, IR3535, wearing light colored clothing with long sleeves and long pants, tucking pant legs into socks, doing frequent tick checks while outdoors, removing clothing immediately upon coming indoors and putting clothing through the dryer, as well as showering after outdoor activities [72–74].

5. Conclusions

We conclude that the high density of ticks infected with *B. burgdorferi* found in built environments with fragmented landscapes and high human activity presents an increased population risk of contact with infected ticks throughout all seasons in which ticks are active. Awareness of this increased risk within built environments will assist with health intervention and education programs directed at mitigating the increase in Lyme disease cases in human populations in current and emerging endemic areas. Future studies will include assessing multiple tick-borne pathogens to determine human risk in upstate New York.

Author Contributions: Conceptualization, J.M.D. and R.M.G.; Methodology, R.S., J.M.D. and R.M.G.; Formal Analysis, A.R. and L.H.; Investigation, A.R., L.H. and R.S.; Resources, A.R., L.H. and R.M.G. Data Curation, A.R. and R.S.; Writing–Original Draft Preparation, A.R.; Writing–Review and Editing, L.H., R.S., J.M.D., R.M.G.; Visualization, A.R.; Supervision, R.M.G.; Project Administration, R.M.G.; Funding Acquisition, R.M.G.

Funding: This research was funded in part by a grant to the State University of New York at Binghamton from the Howard Hughes Medical Institute, the Binghamton University Foundation, and the Binghamton University's Harpur College Undergraduate Research Center.

Acknowledgments: We would like to thank all of the undergraduate researchers who took part in tick collections, without whom this project would not be possible.

References

1. Binder, S.; Levitt, A.M.; Sacks, J.J.; Hughes, J.M. Emerging infectious diseases: Public health issues for the 21st century. *Science* **1999**, *284*, 1311–1313. [CrossRef] [PubMed]
2. Jones, K.E.; Patel, N.G.; Levy, M.A.; Storeygard, A.; Balk, D.; Gittleman, J.L.; Daszak, P. Global trends in emerging infectious diseases. *Nature* **2008**, *451*, 990–993. [CrossRef] [PubMed]
3. King, D.A.; Peckham, C.; Waage, J.K.; Brownlie, J.; Woolhouse, M.E.J. Infectious diseases: Preparing for the future. *Science* **2006**, *313*, 1392–1393. [CrossRef] [PubMed]
4. Morens, D.M.; Folkers, G.K.; Fauci, A.S. The challenge of emerging and re-emerging infectious diseases. *Nature* **2004**, *430*, 242–249. [CrossRef] [PubMed]
5. Smolinski, M.S.; Hamburg, M.A.; Lederberg, J. *Microbial Threats to Health: Emergence, Detection and Response*; The National Academies Press: Washington, DC, USA, 2003; p. 367, ISBN 0-309-50730-8.
6. Daszak, P.; Cuningham, A.A.; Hyatt, A.D. Emerging infectious diseases of wildlife threats to biodiversity and human health. *Science* **2000**, *287*, 443–449. [CrossRef] [PubMed]
7. Patz, J.A.; Daszak, P.; Tabor, G.M.; Aquirre, A.A.; Pearl, M.; Epstein, J.; Wolfe, N.D.; Kilpatrick, A.M.; Foufopoulos, J.; Molyneux, D.; et al. Unhealthy landscapes: Policy recommendations on land use change and infectious disease emergence. *Environ. Health Perspect.* **2004**, *112*, 1092–1098. [CrossRef] [PubMed]
8. Taylor, L.H.; Latham, S.M.; Woolhouse, M.E.J. Risk factors for human disease emergence. *Philos. Trans. R. Soc. Lond.* **2001**, *356*, 983–989. [CrossRef] [PubMed]
9. Woolhouse, M.E.J.; Gowtage-Sequeria, S. Host range and emerging and reemerging pathogens. *Emerg. Infect. Dis.* **2005**, *11*, 1842–1847. [CrossRef] [PubMed]
10. Lederberg, J.; Shope, R.E.; Oakes, S.C.J. *Emerging Infections: Microbial Threats to Health in the United States*; Institute of Medicine, The National Academies Press: Washington, DC, USA, 1992; p. 294, ISBN 0-309-04741-2.
11. Weiss, R.A.; McMichael, A.J. Social and environmental risk factors in the emergence of infectious diseases. *Nat. Med.* **2004**, *10*, S70–S76. [CrossRef] [PubMed]
12. Altizer, S.; Ostfeld, R.S.; Johnson, T.J.; Kutz, S.; Harvell, C.D. Climate Change and Infectious Diseases: From Evidence to a Predictive Framework. *Science* **2013**, *341*, 514–519. [CrossRef] [PubMed]
13. Gubler, D.J. Resurgent vector-borne diseases as a global health pattern. *Emerg. Infect. Dis.* **1998**, *4*, 442–450. [CrossRef] [PubMed]
14. Kilpatrick, A.M.; Randolph, S.E. Drivers, dynamics, and control of emerging vector-borne zoonotic diseases. *Lancet* **2012**, *380*, 1946–4955. [CrossRef]
15. McMichael, A.J.; Woodruff, R.E.; Hales, S. Climate change and human health: Present and future risks. *Lancet* **2006**, *367*, 859–869. [CrossRef]
16. Burgdorfer, W.A.; Barbour, A.G.; Hayes, S.F.; Benach, J.L.; Grunwaldt, E.; Davis, J.P. Lyme disease—A tick-borne spirochetosis? *Science* **1982**, *216*, 1317–1319. [CrossRef] [PubMed]
17. Eisen, R.J.; Piesman, J.; Zielinski-Gutierrez, E.; Eisen, L. What do we need to know about disease ecology to prevent Lyme disease in the Northeastern United States? *J. Med. Entomol.* **2012**, *49*, 11–22. [CrossRef] [PubMed]
18. Rudenko, N.; Golovchenko, M.; Grubhoffer, L.; Oliver, J.H., Jr. Updates on *Borrelia burgdorferi* sensu lato complex with respect to public health. *Ticks Tick Borne Dis.* **2011**, *2*, 123–128. [CrossRef] [PubMed]
19. Burgdorfer, W.; Lane, R.S.; Barbour, A.G.; Gresbrink, R.A.; Anderson, J.R. The Western Black-Legged Tick, *Ixodes pacificus*: A Vector of *Borrelia Burgdorferi*. *Am. J. Trop. Med. Hyg.* **1985**, *34*, 925–930. [CrossRef] [PubMed]
20. Shadick, N.A.; Phillips, C.B.; Shangha, O.; Logigian, E.L.; Kaplan, R.F.; Wright, E.A. Musculoskeletal and Neurological Outcomes in Patients with Previously Treated Lyme Disease. *Ann. Intern. Med.* **1999**, *131*, 919–926. [CrossRef] [PubMed]
21. Shadick, N.A.; Phillips, C.B.; Logigian, E.L.; Steere, A.C.; Kaplan, R.F.; Berardi, V.P.; Duray, P.H.; Larson, M.G.; Wright, E.A.; Katz, J.N.; et al. The long-term clinical outcomes of Lyme disease. A population-based retrospective cohort study. *Ann. Intern. Med.* **1994**, *121*, 560–567. [CrossRef] [PubMed]
22. Citrea, M.; Freeman, P.R.; Horowitz, R.I. Empirical validation of the Horowitz Multiple Systemic Infectious Disease Syndrome Questionnaire for suspected Lyme disease. *Int. J. Intern. Med.* **2017**, *10*, 249–273. [CrossRef] [PubMed]

23. Rebman, A.W.; Bechtold, K.T.; Yang, T.; Mihm, E.A.; Soloski, M.J.; Novak, C.B.; Aucott, J.N. The Clinical, Symptom, and Quality-of-Life Characterization of a Well-Defined Group of Patients with Posttreatment Lyme Disease Syndrome. *Front. Med.* **2017**, *4*, 224. [CrossRef] [PubMed]

24. Aucott, J.N.; Crowder, L.A.; Yedlin, V.; Kortte, K.B. Bull's-Eye and Nontarget Skin Lesions of Lyme Disease: An Internat Survey of Identification of Erythema Migrans. *Dermatol. Res. Pract.* **2012**, *2012*, 451727. [CrossRef] [PubMed]

25. Steere, A.C.; Bartenhagen, N.H.; Craft, J.E.; Hutchinson, G.J.; Newman, J.H.; Rahn, D.W.; Sigal, L.H.; Spieler, P.N.; Stenn, K.S.; Malawista, S.E. The early clinical manifestations of Lyme disease. *Ann. Intern. Med.* **1983**, *99*, 76–82. [CrossRef] [PubMed]

26. Steere, A.C.; Sikand, W.V. The presenting manifestations of Lyme disease. *Ann. Intern. Med.* **2003**, *348*, 2472–2474. [CrossRef]

27. Kostic, T.; Momcilovic, S.; Perisic, Z.D.; Apostolovic, S.R.; Cvetkovic, J.; Jovanovic, A.; Barac, A.; Salinger-Martinovic, S.; Tasic-Otasevic, S. Manifestations of Lyme carditis. *Int. J. Cardiol.* **2017**, *232*, 24–32. [CrossRef] [PubMed]

28. Kuehn, D.M. CDC estimates 300,000 cases of Lyme disease annually. *J. Am. Med. Assoc.* **2013**, *310*, 1110. [CrossRef] [PubMed]

29. Hinckley, A.F.; Connally, N.P.; Meek, J.I.; Johnson, B.J.; Kemperman, M.M.; Feldman, K.A.; White, J.L.; Mead, P.S. Lyme disease testing by large commercial laboratories in the United States. *Clin. Infect. Dis.* **2014**, *59*, 676–681. [CrossRef] [PubMed]

30. Nelson, C.A.; Saha, S.; Kugeler, K.J.; Delorey, M.J.; Shankar, M.B.; Hinckley, A.F.; Mead, P.S. Incidence of Clinician-Diagnosed Lyme Disease, United States, 2005–2010. *Emerg. Infect. Dis.* **2015**, *21*, 1625–1631. [CrossRef] [PubMed]

31. Rosenberg, R.; Lindsey, N.P.; Fischer, M.; Gregory, C.J.; Hinckley, A.F.; Mead, P.S.; Paz-Bailey, G.; Waterman, S.H.; Drexler, N.A.; Kersh, G.J.; et al. Vital Signs: Trends in Reported Vectorborne Disease Cases- United States and Territories, 2004–2016. *Morb. Mortal. Wkly. Rep.* **2018**, *67*, 496–501. [CrossRef] [PubMed]

32. Eisen, R.J.; Eisen, L. The Blacklegged Tick, Ixodes scapularis: An Increasing Public Health Concern. *Trends Parasitol.* **2018**, *34*, 295–309. [CrossRef] [PubMed]

33. McMichael, A.J. The urban environment and health in a world of increasing globalization: Issues for developing countries. *Bull. World Health Organ.* **2000**, *78*, 1117–1126. [CrossRef] [PubMed]

34. Srinivasan, S.; O'Fallon, L.R.; Dearry, A. Creating healthy communities, healthy homes, healthy people: Initiating a research agenda on the built environment and public health. *Am. J. Public Health* **2003**, *93*, 1446–1450. [CrossRef] [PubMed]

35. Cruz, T.; Keppler, H.; Thomas, J.; Kommareddy, D.; Hempstead, S.; Valentine, E.; Spathis, R.; Darcy, J.M., II; Garruto, R.M. Assessing prevalence of tick-borne infectious agents on a university campus. *Am. J. Hum. Biol.* **2013**, *25*, 254–255.

36. Darcy, J.M., II; Spathis, R.; Schmidt, J.; Keppler, H.; Hempstead, S.; Cruz, T.; Kommareddy, D.; Thomas, J.; Riddle, M.; Sayama, H.; et al. Emergence, transmission and risk of Lyme disease and other tick-borne infections: A community based natural experimental model. *Am. J. Hum. Biol.* **2013**, *25*, 255.

37. Allan, B.F.; Keesing, F.; Ostfeld, R.S. Effect of Forest Fragmentation on Lyme Disease Risk. *Conserv. Biol.* **2003**, *17*, 267–272. [CrossRef]

38. Brownstein, J.S.; Skelly, D.K.; Holford, T.R.; Fish, D. Forest fragmentation predicts local scale heterogeneity of Lyme disease risk. *Oecologia* **2005**, *146*, 469–475. [CrossRef] [PubMed]

39. Anderson, J.F.; Magnarelli, L.A. Biology of ticks. *Infect. Dis. Clin. N. Am.* **2008**, *22*, 195–215. [CrossRef] [PubMed]

40. Hengge, U.R.; Tannapfel, A.; Tyring, S.K.; Erbel, R.; Arendt, G.; Ruzicka, T. Lyme borreliosis. *Lancet Infect. Dis.* **2003**, *3*, 489–500. [CrossRef]

41. Ostfeld, R.S.; Keesing, F. Biodiversity and disease risk: The case of Lyme disease. *Conserv. Biol.* **2000**, *14*, 722–728. [CrossRef]

42. Rollend, L.; Fish, D.; Childs, J.E. Transovarial transmission of Borrelia spirochetes by Ixodes scapularis: A summary of the literature and recent observations. *Ticks Tick-Borne Dis.* **2013**, *4*, 46–51. [CrossRef] [PubMed]

43. Crowder, C.D.; Carolan, H.E.; Rounds, M.A.; Honig, V.; Mothes, B.; Haag, H.; Nolte, O.; Luft, B.J.; Grubhoffer, L.; Ecker, D.J.; et al. Prevalence of *Borrelia miyamotoi* in *Ixodes* Ticks in Europe and the United States. *Emerg. Infect. Dis.* **2014**, *20*, 1678–1682. [CrossRef] [PubMed]

44. Salkeld, D.J.; Cinkovich, S.; Nieto, N.C. Tick-borne Pathogens in Northwestern California, USA. *Emerg. Infect. Dis.* **2014**, *20*, 493–494. [CrossRef] [PubMed]

45. Kurtenbach, K.; Hanincova, K.; Tsao, J.I.; Margos, G.; Fish, D.; Ogden, N.H. Fundamental processes in the evolutionary ecology of Lyme borreliosis. *Nat. Rev. Microbiol.* **2006**, *4*, 660–669. [CrossRef] [PubMed]

46. Martinez, A.; Salinas, A.; Martinez, F.; Cantu, A.; Miller, D.K. Serosurvey for selected disease agents in white-tailed deer from Mexico. *J. Wildl. Dis.* **1999**, *35*, 799–803. [CrossRef] [PubMed]

47. A History of Lyme Disease, Symptoms, Diagnosis, Treatment and Prevention. Available online: http://www.niaid.nih.gov/topics/lymeDisease/understanding/Pages/intro.aspx (accessed on 8 August 2017).

48. Barbour, A.G.; Fish, D. The biological and social phenomenon of Lyme disease. *Science* **1993**, *260*, 1610–1616. [CrossRef] [PubMed]

49. LoGuidice, K.; Ostfeld, R.S.; Schmidt, K.A.; Keesing, F. The ecology of infectious disease: Effects of host diversity and community composition on Lyme disease risk. *Proc. Natl. Acad. Sci. USA* **2003**, *100*, 567–571. [CrossRef] [PubMed]

50. Be Tick Free—A Guide for Preventing Lyme Disease. Available online: http://www.health.ny.gov/publications/2825/ (accessed on 8 August 2017).

51. Diuk-Wasser, M.A.; Hoen, A.G.; CIslo, P.; Brinkerhoff, R.; Hamer, S.A.; Rowland, M.; Cortinas, R.; Vourc'h, G.; Melton, F.; Hickling, G.J.; et al. Human risk of infection with *Borrelia burgdorferi*, the Lyme disease agent, in Eastern United States. *Am. J. Trop. Med. Hyg.* **2012**, *86*, 320–327. [CrossRef] [PubMed]

52. Hamer, S.A.; Tsao, J.I.; Walker, E.D.; Hickling, G.J. Invasion of the Lyme disease vector *Ixodes scapularis*: Implications for *Borrelia burgdorferi* endemicity. *EcoHealth* **2010**, *7*, 47–63. [CrossRef] [PubMed]

53. Roome, A.; Bower, K.; Murnock, C.G.; Hill, L.; Ho, B.; Tyurin, S.; Al-Feghali, V.; Zeitz, H.; Rios, D.; Parwez, R.; et al. Prevalence of tick-borne pathogens and human behavioral risk factors in built environments of upstate New York suggest a necessity for the development of risk management models. *Am. J. Hum. Biol.* **2014**, *26*, 279.

54. Daniels, T.J.; Ralco, R.C.; Fish, D. Estimating population size and drag sampling efficiency for the blacklegged tick (Acari: Ixodidae). *J. Med. Entomol.* **2000**, *37*, 357–363. [CrossRef] [PubMed]

55. Falco, R.C.; Fish, D. A comparison of methods for sampling the deer tick, Ixodes dammini, in a Lyme disease endemic area. *Exp. Appl. Acarol.* **1992**, *14*, 165–177. [CrossRef] [PubMed]

56. Hersh, M.H.; Ostfeld, R.S.; McHenry, D.J.; Tibbett, M.; Brunner, J.L.; Killilea, M.E.; LoGiudice, K.; Schmidt, K.A.; Keesing, F. Co-infection of blacklegged ticks with Babesia microti and *Borrelia burgdorferi* is higher than expected and acquired from small mammal hosts. *PLoS ONE* **2014**, *9*, e99348. [CrossRef] [PubMed]

57. Marconi, R.T.; Garon, C.F. Development of polymerase chain reaction primer sets for diagnosis of Lyme disease and for species-specific identification of Lyme disease isolates by 16S rRNA signature nucleotide analysis. *J. Clin. Microbiol.* **1992**, *30*, 2830–2834. [PubMed]

58. Lee, S.H.; Vigliotti, V.S.; Vigliotti, J.S.; Jones, W.; Pappu, S. Increased Sensitivity of *Borrelia burgdorferi* 16S Ribosomal DNA Detection. *Am. J. Clin. Pathol.* **2010**, *133*, 569–576. [CrossRef] [PubMed]

59. Vuong, H.B.; Canham, C.D.; Fonesca, D.M.; Brisson, D.; Morin, P.J.; Smouse, P.E.; Ostfeld, R.S. Occurrence and transmission efficiencies of *Borrelia burgdorferi* OspC types in avian and mammalian wildlife. *Infect. Genet. Evolut.* **2014**, *27*, 594–600. [CrossRef] [PubMed]

60. Frank, D.H.; Fish, D.; Moy, F.H. Landscape features associated with Lyme disease risk in a suburban residential environment. *Landsc. Ecol.* **1998**, *13*, 27–36. [CrossRef]

61. Maupin, G.O.; Fish, D.; Zultowsky, J.; Campos, E.G.; Piesman, J. Landscape ecology of Lyme disease in a residential area of Westchester County, New York. *Am. J. Epidemiol.* **1991**, *133*, 1105–1113. [CrossRef] [PubMed]

62. Communicable Disease in New York State—Rate Per 100,000 Population: Lyme Disease to Shigellosis: 2000. Available online: https://www.health.ny.gov/statistics/diseases/communicable/2000/rates3.htm (accessed on 8 August 2017).

63. Newman, E.A.; Eisen, L.; Eisen, R.J.; Fedorova, N.; Hasty, J.M.; Vaughn, C.; Lane, R.S. *Borrelia burgdorferi* sensu lato spirochetes in wild birds in northwestern California: Associations with ecological factors, bird behavior and tick infestation. *PLoS ONE* **2015**, *10*, e0118146. [CrossRef] [PubMed]

64. Prusinski, M.A.; Kokas, J.E.; Hukey, K.T.; Kogut, S.J.; Lee, J.; Backenson, P.B. Prevalence of *Borrelia burgdorferi* (Spirochaetales: Spirochaetaceae), Anaplasma phagocytophilum (Rickettsiales: Anaplasmataceae), and Babesia microti (Piroplasmida: Babesiidae) in Ixodes scapularis (Acari: Ixodidae) collected from recreational lands in the Hudson Valley Region, New York State. *J. Med. Entomol.* **2014**, *51*, 226–236. [PubMed]

65. Lyme Disease Incidence per 100,000. Available online: https://www.health.ny.gov/statistics/chac/general/g40.htm (accessed on 8 August 2017).

66. Ebel, G.D.; Kramer, L.D. Short report: Duration of tick attachment required for transmission of Powassan virus by deer ticks. *Am. J. Trop. Med. Hyg.* **2004**, *71*, 268–271. [PubMed]

67. Hynote, E.D.; Mervine, P.C.; Stricker, R.B. Clinical evidence for rapid transmission of lyme disease following a tickbite. *Diagn. Microbiol. Infect. Dis.* **2012**, *72*, 188–192. [CrossRef] [PubMed]

68. Piesman, J.; Schneider, B.S.; Zeidner, N.S. Use of quantitative PCR to measure density of *Borrelia burgdorferi* in the midgut and salivary glands of feeding tick vectors. *J. Clin. Microbiol.* **2001**, *39*, 4145–4148. [CrossRef] [PubMed]

69. Cook, M.J. Lyme borreliosis: A review of data on transmission time after tick attachment. *Int. J. Gen. Med.* **2015**, *8*, 1–8. [CrossRef] [PubMed]

70. Jouda, F.; Perret, J.L.; Gern, L. Density of questing *Ixodes ricinus* nymphs and adults infected by *Borrelia burgdorferi* sensu lato in Switzerland: Spatio-temporal pattern at a regional scale. *Vector Borne Zoonotic Dis.* **2004**, *4*, 23–32. [CrossRef] [PubMed]

71. Tälleklint, L.; Jaenson, T.G. Seasonal variations in density of questing *Ixodes ricinus* (Acari: Ixodidae) nymphs and prevalence of infection with *B. burgdorferi* s.l. in south central Sweden. *J. Med. Entomol.* **1996**, *33*, 592–597. [CrossRef] [PubMed]

72. Tokarz, R.; Jain, K.; Bennett, A.; Briese, T.; Lipkin, W.I. Assessment of polymicrobial infections in ticks in New York state. *Vector Borne Zoonotic Dis.* **2010**, *10*, 217–221. [CrossRef] [PubMed]

73. Couch, P.; Johnson, C.E. Prevention of Lyme disease. *Am. J. Health-Syst. Pharmacy.* **1992**, *49*, 1164–1173.

74. Vazquez, M.; Muehlenbein, C.; Cartter, M.; Hayes, E.B.; Ertel, S.; Shapiro, E.D. Effectiveness of Personal Protective Measures to Prevent Lyme Disease. *Emerg. Infect. Dis.* **2008**, *14*, 210–216. [CrossRef] [PubMed]

11

Physical Activity on Prescription with Counsellor Support: A 4-Year Registry-Based Study in Routine Health Care in Sweden

Pia Andersen [1,2,*], Sara Holmberg [1,3], Lena Lendahls [1,4], Per Nilsen [2] and Margareta Kristenson [2]

[1] Department of Research and Development, Region Kronoberg, 351 88 Växjö, Sweden; sara.holmberg@kronoberg.se (S.H.); lena.lendahls@lnu.se (L.L.)

[2] Division of Community Medicine, Department of Medical and Health Sciences, Linköping University, 581 83 Linköping, Sweden; per.nilsen@liu.se (P.N.); margareta.kristenson@liu.se (M.K.)

[3] Division of Occupational and Environmental Medicine, Institute of Laboratory Medicine, Lund University, 221 00 Lund, Sweden

[4] Department of Health and Caring Sciences, Faculty of Health and Life Sciences, Linnaeus University, 391 82 Kalmar, Sweden

* Correspondence: pia.andersen@kronoberg.se

Abstract: *Background*: Public health gains from physical activity on prescription (PAP) depend on uptake in routine care. We performed an evaluation of the implementation, in a Swedish county council, of counsellors who give personalized support to PAP recipients aimed at facilitating PAP delivery. The aim was to compare characteristics between PAP recipients and the health care population as well as between PAP recipients who used and did not use counsellor support. We also investigated professional belonging and health care setting of health care professionals who prescribed PAP. *Methods:* All patients' ≥18 years who received PAP during 2009–2012 in primary and secondary care in the County Council of Kronoberg were included (*n* = 4879). Data were retrieved from electronic medical records. Main outcome measures were patient and professional characteristics. *Results:* A third of the PAP recipients had diseases in ≥5 diagnostic groups and more than half had ≥11 office visits the year before receiving PAP. Counsellor support was used by one-third and PAP recipients who used counsellor support had more multiple diagnoses and office visits compared with non-users. Physicians issued 44% of prescriptions and primary care was the predominant setting. The amount of PAP did not change over time, but the proportion of physicians' prescriptions decreased while the proportion of nurses' prescriptions increased. *Conclusions:* PAP recipients had high morbidity and were frequent health care attenders, indicating that PAP was predominantly used for secondary or tertiary prevention. PAP rates did not increase as intended after the implementation of counsellor support.

Keywords: physical activity prescription; implementation; counselling; primary care; secondary care

1. Background

Insufficient physical activity contributes considerably to premature mortality and is a risk factor for a broad range of non-communicable diseases, including cardiovascular diseases, cancer, diabetes, as well as musculoskeletal and mental health disorders [1,2]. Globally, one in four adults report physical activity below recommended levels, and the proportion is even higher in Sweden: one in three adults [3]. Hence, policies and interventions to achieve increased physical activity levels in the population are of utmost importance for public health [1,2].

The concept of physical activity on prescription (PAP) has been developed for health care services mainly to support patients in primary care who might benefit from increased physical activity [4–9]. The Swedish PAP concept (referred to as FaR in Sweden) was introduced in 2001 as a part of the national project "Sweden on the move" and is now used by all Swedish county councils (which are responsible for provision of health care in Sweden). The concept consists of patient-centred counselling, written prescription of individualized physical activity using the FYSS manual (the meaning of "FYSS" is Physical Activity in the Prevention and Treatment of Disease, English version) [10], collaboration with local organizations and follow-up assessments of the recipient's physical activity [11]. The FYSS manual is an evidence-based handbook for health care professionals and it describes how physical activity can be used in prevention and treatment of several types of diseases and conditions. The PAP concept in Sweden is used in the prevention and treatment of diseases [10] with the aim to support the recipients to incorporate physical activity into their everyday life [11].

Several studies have demonstrated the effectiveness of PAP to achieve increased physical activity levels in adults at 6 [5,12], 12 [12,13], 16 [8] and 24 months' follow-up [14]. However, public health gains are affected by the uptake of PAP in routine care. Study findings suggest that PAP concepts tend to reach relatively few patients, more female recipients than male and primarily patients over the age of 45 [6,15]. In a Swedish county council-based study in 2004–2005, Leijon et al. [6] found that PAP was delivered to less than 1.5% of all primary care patients in one year. In 2007–2010, the amount of PAP in Sweden doubled, although there was a large variation in prescriptions between county councils [16]. Harrison et al. [15] estimated that 4% of the sedentary adult residents in a primary care district in northwestern England received an exercise referral in 2000–2004.

Barriers for delivery of PAP in routine care include perceived time constraints [17–19], reservations about the effectiveness of PAP as a treatment or preventive intervention and the lack of clear routines concerning how to integrate PAP into regular practice [18]. A Swedish study found that simplifying routines of PAP delivery for primary care physicians prescription rates increased over two years (2006–2007) [20]. Multi-professional PAP concepts that involve physical activity counsellors who provide personalized support to PAP recipients to achieve increased physical activity have been proposed as a possible means to facilitate health care delivery of PAP [18,21]. Furthermore, the use of physical activity counsellors in primary care has been proposed as a possible means to raise the quality of physical activity counselling [21,22]. However, long-term evaluations of the reach and effectiveness of multi-professional PAP concepts in routine care are lacking and there are no studies covering both primary and secondary health care settings.

Addressing important knowledge gaps with regard to PAP delivery in routine health care, this study provides a registry-based long-term evaluation of a multi-professional PAP concept with counsellor support implemented in a Swedish county council. The aim was to investigate differences in characteristics between PAP recipients and the total health care population and between PAP recipients who used counsellor support and PAP recipients who did not use this support. The aim was also to investigate health care professionals who prescribe PAP in terms of professional belonging and health care setting. The use of medical record registry data allowed for analyses of previous morbidity in all PAP recipients, which has not been done in earlier routine health care studies of PAP delivery. Furthermore, data allowed for comparisons of characteristics between PAP recipients and the total health care population.

2. Methods

2.1. Study Design and Setting

This registry-based study involved patients who received PAP in routine primary and secondary care in the County Council of Kronoberg, a predominantly rural district in southern Sweden. Health care in Sweden is primarily publicly funded. All residents are insured by the state and have equal access to health care. Out-of-pocket fees are low and regulated by law.

Primary care in the County Council of Kronoberg consists of 22 public and 11 privately operated (publicly funded) units; secondary care is provided in two public hospitals. All primary and secondary care units have used the same electronic medical record system (Cambio Cosmic, Cambio Healthcare System AB, Linköping, Sweden) since 2005.

Since 2009, patients who receive PAP in the County Council of Kronoberg are offered counselling support by appointed physical activity counsellors. Patients who want this support can contact a counsellor; there is no formal referral system. The support is free of charge and can be utilized for one year after the PAP is issued. The counsellors are health care professionals, e.g., nurses and physiotherapists, who are trained in motivational interviewing counselling techniques [23]. An important rationale for implementing the concept was to reduce the clinical work load as a means of enabling higher numbers of prescriptions of physical activity.

2.2. Data Collection

All patients aged 18 years or older receiving PAP in primary or secondary care in the County Council of Kronoberg in 2009–2012 were identified via the electronic medical record system using specific registry codes. The only exception was PAP delivered in two privately operated primary care centres, which were not included because of lack of consent from the managers of the centres.

In total, 5864 prescriptions were registered. Of these, 985 prescriptions were excluded because they were repeated, duplicated or erroneously registered prescriptions, such as prescriptions in home care of the elderly. Only the first prescription of each PAP recipient during the study period was selected. This left 4879 PAP recipients to be included for analysis.

The characteristics of the PAP recipients were retrieved from the electronic medical record: sex, age and all registered diagnoses for the 12 months before PAP, the number of office visits (including visits to all professions in primary and secondary care), the number of secondary inpatient care occasions, PAP-prescribing profession and prescribing health care unit.

Several measures were used to capture morbidity: registered diagnoses, office visits (to primary and/or secondary care) and inpatient (secondary) care. Diagnostic groups have previously been used to describe morbidity among frequent health care attendees [24]. The European General Practice Research Network states that any combination of at least two diseases (acute or chronic) can be used as a definition of multi-morbidity [25].

Diagnoses were grouped according to the International Classification of Diseases (ICD) system version 10 [26]. Patients were categorized according to (a) having any diagnosis versus not having any diagnosis within each diagnostic group of diseases (yes/no), and (b) the number of diagnostic groups of diseases (0–2, 3–4, ≥5). The diagnostic groups pregnancy, childbirth/puerperium and factors influencing health status and contact with health services were excluded.

The total health care population in the County Council of Kronoberg in 2009 was used as a reference population for the PAP recipients in 2009. For the reference group, data on sex, age, diagnoses and inpatient care were retrieved using the same registry codes for capturing registry data as for the PAP recipients.

2.3. Statistical Analysis

Data are presented using numbers and proportions (%), means and standard deviation (SD), and median and 25th and 75th percentiles. Differences between groups were tested with the chi-squared test. A p-value ≤ 0.05 was regarded statistically significant. All statistical analyses regarding PAP recipients were performed with IBM SPSS Statistics for Windows, version 23.0 (IBM Corp., Armonk, NY, USA).

2.4. Ethical Considerations

The Regional Ethical Review Board in Linköping approved the project (Ref. No. 2013/51-31). The data were delivered in such a way that the patients and prescribers of PAP could not be identified by the researchers.

3. Results

3.1. Characteristics of PAP Recipients over Time

The 4879 adult patients who received a first PAP in primary or secondary care during 2009–2012 represents 3% of all primary and secondary care adult patients (186,117 patients) during these four years.

Approximately 60% of prescribed patients were female. The age group 45–64 years dominated (Table 1). The proportion of PAP recipients aged 65 years or older increased somewhat over time (from 26% to 33%). The mean age of the PAP recipients for the study period was 53.6 years (SD 16.1 years).

Table 1. Patients receiving PAP (Physical Activity on Prescription) in primary and secondary care and differences between years of prescription.

Patient Characteristics	Year				p-Value *
	2009	2010	2011	2012	
	n = 1148	n = 1341	n = 1242	n = 1148	
	% (n)	% (n)	% (n)	% (n)	
Sex					0.100
Female	58 (668)	63 (843)	60 (746)	62 (707)	
Male	42 (480)	37 (498)	40 (496)	38 (441)	
Age					≤0.001
18–29 years	9 (101)	9 (126)	11 (132)	11 (122)	
30–44 years	18 (209)	22 (296)	18 (221)	18 (207)	
45–64 years	48 (546)	43 (571)	43 (528)	39 (446)	
65+ years	25 (292)	26 (348)	29 (361)	33 (373)	
Diagnoses ** and health care consumption *** in the 12 months before PAP					
Musculoskeletal diseases (yes)	47 (541)	45 (602)	46 (573)	50 (574)	0.089
Endocrine diseases (yes)	52 (549)	41 (550)	38 (469)	37 (421)	≤0.001
Circulatory diseases (yes)	45 (510)	40 (529)	43 (538)	43 (497)	0.088
Mental health disorders (yes)	23 (265)	31 (412)	30 (370)	34 (391)	≤0.001
Respiratory diseases (yes)	24 (272)	26 (344)	24 (303)	27 (307)	0.298
Other diagnostic groups (yes)	76 (866)	77 (1027)	81 (999)	81 (921)	0.004
Number of diagnostic groups					0.034
0–2 diagnostic groups	35 (405)	34 (447)	33 (414)	31 (356)	
3–4 diagnostic groups	37 (425)	37 (493)	36 (442)	35 (396)	
≥5 diagnostic groups	28 (315)	29 (387)	29 (387)	34 (390)	
Number of office visits					0.054
0–5 office visits	22 (253)	23 (312)	25 (307)	27 (310)	
6–10 office visits	22 (250)	21 (282)	20 (247)	22 (255)	
≥11 office visits	56 (645)	56 (747)	55 (688)	51 (583)	
≥1 occasion of inpatient care (yes)	27 (310)	28 (376)	28 (352)	21 (245)	≤0.001

* Tested by chi-squared test. ** 24 ICD- (International Classification of Diseases) 10 diagnostic groups of diseases assessed by the first coding character, i.e., letter, excluding O (pregnancy, childbirth and the puerperium) and Z (factors influencing health status and contact with health services). Analysis of patients with (yes) or without (no) assessed diagnostic group of diseases. *** Office visits in primary and secondary care, and inpatient somatic and/or psychiatric care. Inpatient care analysis includes patients with (yes) or without (no) inpatient care.

The most frequent diagnostic groups were musculoskeletal disease, circulatory disease, endocrine disease and mental health disorders (Table 1). The proportion with endocrine disease decreased from 52% in 2009 to 34% in 2012, whereas the proportion with mental health disorders increased from 23% in 2009 to 34% in 2012. The number of diagnostic groups per patient ranged from 0 to 16, with an average of 3.7 (SD 2.6). The proportion of patients with five or more diagnostic groups increased over the period, from 28% in 2009 to 34% in 2012.

During the year before PAP, more than half of the PAP recipients had 11 or more registered office visits to primary and/or secondary care and approximately 25% had been hospitalized (inpatient care) (Table 1).

Compared with the total health care population of the County Council of Kronoberg, a larger proportion of the PAP recipients were female and over 45 years old. The PAP recipients had almost twice the proportion of registered diagnoses for the majority of diagnostic groups. More PAP recipients had at least one occasion with inpatient (hospital) care, 27% compared with 14% for the total health care population (Table 2).

Table 2. Differences in characteristics between PAP recipients and the total health care population in 2009.

Patient Characteristics	PAP Recipients	Total Health Care Population	p-Value *
	n = 1148 % (n)	n = 121,869 % (n)	
Sex			0.027
Female	58 (668)	55 (66926)	
Male	42 (480)	45 (54943)	
Age			≤0.001
18–29 years	9 (101)	18 (22515)	
30–44 years	18 (209)	29 (35392)	
45–64 years	48 (546)	24 (29752)	
65+ years	25 (292)	28 (34210)	
Diagnostic groups **			
Musculoskeletal diseases (yes)	47 (541)	25 (30753)	≤0.001
Endocrine diseases (yes)	48 (549)	13 (15443)	≤0.001
Circulatory diseases (yes)	45 (510)	21 (26089)	≤0.001
Mental health disorder (yes)	23 (265)	11 (13464)	≤0.001
Respiratory diseases (yes)	24 (272)	18 (22372)	≤0.001
Other diagnostic groups (yes)	76 (866)	65 (79366)	≤0.001
Inpatient care ***			≤0.001
≥1 occasion of inpatient care	27 (310)	14 (2399)	

* Tested by chi-squared test. ** 24 ICD-10 diagnostic groups of diseases assessed by the first coding character, i.e., letter, excluding O (pregnancy, childbirth and the puerperium) and Z (factors influencing health status and contact with health services). Analysis of patients with (yes) or without (no) assessed diagnostic group of diseases. PAP recipients' diagnoses were measured in the 12 months before PAP. *** Somatic and/or psychiatric inpatient care within a year before PAP. PAP recipients' inpatient care was measured in the 12 months before PAP. Analysis includes patients with (yes) or without (no) inpatient care.

3.2. Characteristics of PAP Recipients Using Counsellor Support

One-third of all PAP recipients (n = 1555; 32%) used support from a physical activity counsellor in the year after prescription (Table 3). PAP recipients using support compared with non-users were more often female and over 45 years of age. The support users more often had an endocrine diagnosis and a mental health disorder, and had higher frequency of multiple diagnoses (≥5 diagnostic groups of diseases) and office visits (≥11) compared with non-users. Prescriptions by physicians were more common among counsellor support users, but no difference according to health care setting was seen.

Table 3. Differences in characteristics between patients using versus not using counsellor support after receiving a PAP (*n* = 4879).

Patient Characteristics	Counsellor Support		*p*-Value *
	Yes (*n* = 1555) % (*n*)	No (*n* = 3324) % (*n*)	
Sex			≤0.001
Female	66 (1024)	58 (1940)	
Male	34 (531)	42 (1384)	
Age			≤0.001
18–29 years	8 (125)	11 (356)	
30–44 years	20 (316)	19 (617)	
45–64 years	46 (712)	41(1379)	
65+ years	26 (402)	29 (972)	
Diagnoses ** and health care consumption * in the 12 months before PAP**			
Musculoskeletal diseases (yes)	49 (749)	47 (1541)	0.221
Endocrine diseases (yes)	44 (683)	39 (1306)	0.002
Circulatory diseases (yes)	42 (645)	43 (1429)	0.337
Mental health disorder (yes)	31 (487)	29 (951)	0.050
Respiratory diseases (yes)	27 (409)	25 (817)	0.187
Other diagnostic groups (yes)	79 (1218)	79 (2595)	0.773
Number of diagnostic groups			0.011
0–2 diagnostic groups	29 (450)	34 (1102)	
3–4 diagnostic groups	37 (566)	36 (1190)	
≥5 diagnostic groups	33 (509)	30 (965)	
Number of office visits			0.002
1–5 office visits	23 (354)	25 (828)	
6–10 office visits	19 (295)	22 (739)	
≥11 office visits	58 (906)	53 (1757)	
≥1 occasion of inpatient care	25 (389)	27 (893)	0.171
Prescribing professional			≤0.001
Physician	49 (767)	41(1356)	
Nurse	23 (357)	28 (935)	
Physiotherapist	19 (295)	24 (799)	
Other professionals ****	9 (136)	7 (234)	
Prescribing setting			0.082
Primary care	70 (1093)	70 (2345)	
Secondary somatic care	25 (392)	24 (783)	
Secondary psychiatric care	5 (70)	6 (196)	

* Tested by chi-squared test. ** 24 ICD-10 diagnostic groups of diseases assessed by the first coding character, i.e., letter, excluding O (pregnancy, childbirth and the puerperium) and Z (factors influencing health status and contact with health services). Analysis of patients with (yes) or without (no) assessed diagnostic group of diseases. *** Office visits in primary and secondary care, and inpatient somatic and/or psychiatric care. Inpatient care analysis includes patients with (yes) or without (no) inpatient care. **** Psychologists, behavioural therapists, midwifes, dieticians and occupational therapists.

3.3. PAP Delivery by Health Care Professional and Setting over Time

The total number of prescriptions increased by 20% from 2009 to 2010, but, in the fourth year, 2012, the number of prescribed patients was the same as in 2009 (Table 4). Physicians prescribed the largest proportion of PAPs, but with a decreasing proportion over the years (from 49% to 39%). In contrast, the proportion of nurses prescribing PAP increased from 22% to 30%. Physiotherapists prescribed about one-fourth of the PAP recipients in all four years. The individual variation of prescriptions was large, ranging from 1 to 135 prescriptions per prescriber (median 19, —25th to 75th percentiles (9–37). Primary care was the dominant setting with 64% to 75% of the prescriptions.

Table 4. PAP delivery by health care professional and setting over time ($n = 4879$).

Professional Groups and Health Care Setting	Year of Prescription				p-Value *
	2009 $n = 1148$ % (n)	2010 $n = 1341$ % (n)	2011 $n = 1242$ % (n)	2012 $n = 1148$ % (n)	
Professional group					≤0.001
Physician	49 (566)	47 (626)	39 (483)	39 (448)	
Nurse	22 (253)	24 (322)	30 (374)	30 (343)	
Physiotherapist	22 (254)	21 (280)	23 (286)	24 (274)	
Other professionals **	7 (75)	8 (113)	8 (99)	7 (83)	
Health care setting					≤0.001
Primary care	74 (850)	70 (941)	64 (791)	75 (856)	
Secondary somatic care	24 (277)	23 (308)	31 (391)	17 (199)	
Secondary psychiatric care	2 (21)	7(92)	5 (60)	8 (93)	

* Tested by chi-squared test. ** Psychologists, behavioural therapists, midwifes, dieticians, occupational therapists.

4. Discussion

This registry-based study investigated the characteristics of patients who received PAP and the health care professionals who issued these prescriptions in a multi-professional PAP concept with counselling support. The concept was implemented in primary and secondary care in a county council in Sweden and was studied over four years. We found higher prevalence of morbidity in terms of more diagnoses and more inpatient care among PAP recipients compared with a reference population of all patients visiting health care. Morbidity was even higher among PAP recipients who used support by PAP counsellors compared to non-users. Slightly more than half of prescriptions were by professionals other than physicians and about one-quarter were prescribed in secondary care.

All information in this registry-based study was based on data captured in electronic medical records from primary and secondary care. The very high coverage of data (almost 100%) and the length of the study period are strengths of the study. The four-year study period ensured that the results were not only an effect of enthusiasm about a new organisational structure for PAP. However, medical records are structured for use in clinical care, which means that there might be quality problems when using these data for research purposes [27]. To ensure completeness, validity, consistency and accuracy of the data, the researchers had an ongoing dialogue with health care professionals familiar with registration of codes, data analysts familiar with how to capture the specific data codes and with quality control of the county councils' health care data, and with statisticians with experience of using health care data.

External validity, i.e., generalizability, of the study findings to other settings is somewhat restricted. Aside from sex and age, we have limited information about the PAP recipients that could facilitate comparisons between PAP populations, e.g., socio-economic variables, reason for receiving PAP, PAP recipients' level of physical activity and motivation. Generalizability may also be restricted due to different strategies used by health care organisations to support uptake of PAP in routine care, e.g., strategies involving pay for performance of PAP, and different organisational structures for PAP delivery. On the other hand, external validity is enhanced by the fact that the study was conducted in routine care. Unlike most routine care PAP studies, the study allowed for analyses of long-term real-life health care delivery of PAP in an unselected total health care population with no selection bias.

Data were collected in a way that did not require effort or even awareness of the study by the health care professionals and PAP recipients.

Furthermore, it is difficult to determine the extent to which the patients in our study differ from PAP recipients in other PAP studies with regard to morbidity because previous studies have not investigated prevalence of morbidity in terms of medical diagnoses among PAP recipients in health care populations. The high prevalence of morbidity among the PAP recipients in this study suggests that the PAP concept was predominantly applied as a secondary or tertiary preventive strategy, i.e., aimed at reducing the impact of a diagnosed disease or softening the impact of an ongoing illness [28]. The benefit of physical activity has been demonstrated in both primary (i.e., no evidence of disease) and secondary prevention [10]. However, our findings indicate that PAP is not viewed as a primary prevention strategy by the health care professionals, who instead predominantly prescribed physical activity to patients with a broad range of diseases.

The uptake of PAP in the total health care population was found to be broadly similar to what has been reported from previous population-based primary health care studies [6,15]. One-third of the PAP recipients used counsellor support. The reasons why the PAP recipients sought or did not seek counsellor support were not investigated. It is difficult to determine whether the use by one-third was a small or large proportion since there are no comparative studies. Still, the proportion of users of counsellor support was lower than expected among the health care practitioners who were involved in implementing the concept. The patients' reasons for choosing to use, or not to use, this support will be investigated in a forthcoming study. Our findings of an association between morbidity and use of counsellor support are in line with results from a recently published study of PAP recipients with chronic musculoskeletal pain, which found that they experienced obstacles to increasing their physical activity and needed individually tailored information and support when prescribed physical activity [21].

Two-thirds of the prescriptions were issued by physicians and nurses, which is in line with a previous Swedish primary care study of PAP [6]. Persson et al. [20] found that simplified routines increased the physicians' prescription rate over two years. In our study, in line with Leijon et al. [6], we found decreasing proportion of PAP by physicians over time. This finding suggests that the physicians' interest or enthusiasm for the PAP concept declined over time. Physicians in Sweden have expressed some scepticism about the practice of issuing PAP [18]. Other studies have noted that physicians feel confident in providing advice about physical activity [29], but a Canadian study [7] observed that physicians were more likely to provide verbal counselling on physical activity than use PAP.

Despite the expressed ambition to achieve higher PAP rates by means of the multi-professional concept with counselling support, the prescription rates for 2012 were similar to those for 2009. However, the rates could have been even lower without the concept. Our study did not investigate the reasons for decreasing rates of prescription over time, but implementation research has shown that adoption or uptake of new practices in routine health care is influenced by a combination of several interdependent factors. These factors include the characteristics of the practices (e.g., perceived complexity and compatibility with existing routines), the health care professionals (e.g., their attitudes, beliefs, motivation and self-efficacy concerning the new practice), strategies used to facilitate the implementation and the context of the implementation [30]. Numerous factors associated with the wider context may have influenced our results. A trend towards increasing the amount of PAP in Sweden has been seen at the national level [16]. The studied PAP concept was new and it is possible that the strategies used to enhance implementation in 2009–2010, e.g., information and education targeting health care professionals, contributed to increased prescription in the initial years. However, no comparative data at the national level exist for 2011 and 2012. In 2011, the Swedish National Board of Health and Welfare introduced guidelines for disease prevention, which included recommendations for management of insufficient levels of physical activity. The effects of these guidelines on prescription rates have not been studied.

While the aim of the counsellor support was to reduce the clinical workload as a means of enabling higher numbers of prescriptions of physical activity, overall PAP rates did not increase as intended. However, it is not possible to determine how the rates would have developed without the implementation of the concept. Qualitative studies are warranted to explore some of the unanswered "why" questions of quantitative PAP research.

5. Conclusions

In this four-year registry-based study of a multi-professional PAP concept with counsellor support implemented in a Swedish county council, we found that PAP recipients had high morbidity and were frequent attenders in health care. Counsellor support was used by approximately one-third of all PAP recipients, and morbidity was even higher in this group. The PAP concept therefore seems predominantly to have been used as a secondary or tertiary prevention strategy. The overall prescription rate was similar to prescription rates found in other PAP studies.

Acknowledgments: Statisticians Lars Valter, Linköping University, and Anna Lindgren, Lund University, contributed statistical assistance. IT analysts Quan Nguyen and Thomas Frisk, Region Kronoberg, contributed to data collection and quality control of data.

Author Contributions: All authors (Pia Andersen, Sara Holmberg, Lena Lendahls, Per Nilsen and Margareta Kristenson) conceived and designed the study; Pia Andersen collected data; Pia Andersen, Sara Holmberg and Lena Lendahls analyzed the data; Pia Andersen drafted the manuscript and Sara Holmberg, Lena Lendahls, Per Nilsen and Margareta Kristenson participated in preparation of the manuscript; all authors read and approved the final manuscript.

References

1. World Health Organization. Global Recommendations on Physical Activity for Health. 2010. Available online: http://www.who.int/dietphysicalactivity/factsheet_recommendations/en/ (accessed on 18 August 2017).
2. World Health Organization. Global Action Plan for the Prevention and Control of Noncommunicable Diseases 2013–2020. 2013. Available online: http://www.who.int/nmh/events/ncd_action_plan/en/ (accessed on 18 August 2017).
3. World Health Organization. Global Health Observatory Data Repository. Prevalence of Insufficient Physical Activity among Adults. 2015. Available online: http://apps.who.int/gho/data/view.main.2482?lang=en (accessed on 18 August 2017).
4. Aittasalo, M.; Miilunpalo, S.; Ståhl, T.; Kukkonen, H.K. From innovation to practice: Initiation, implementation and evaluation of a physician-based physical activity promotion programme in Finland. *Health Promot. Int.* **2007**, *22*, 19–27. [CrossRef] [PubMed]
5. Harrison, R.A.; Roberts, C.; Elton, P.J. Does primary care referral to an exercise programme increase physical activity one year later? A randomized controlled trial. *J. Public Health* **2005**, *27*, 25–32. [CrossRef] [PubMed]
6. Leijon, M.E.; Bendtsen, P.; Nilsen, P.; Ekberg, K.; Ståhle, A. Physical activity referrals in Swedish primary health care—Prescriber and patient characteristics, reasons for prescriptions, and prescribed activities. *BMC Health Serv. Res.* **2008**, *8*, 201. [CrossRef] [PubMed]
7. Petrella, R.J.; Lattanzio, C.N.; Overend, T.J. Physical activity counseling and prescription among Canadian primary care physicians. *Arch. Intern. Med.* **2007**, *167*, 1774–1781. [CrossRef] [PubMed]
8. Sorensen, J.; Sorensen, J.B.; Skovgaard, T.; Skovgaard, T.; Bredahl, T.; Puggaard, L. Exercise on prescription: changes in physical activity and health-related quality of life in five Danish programmes. *Eur. J. Public Health* **2011**, *21*, 56–62. [CrossRef] [PubMed]
9. Swinburn, B.A.; Walter, L.G.; Arroll, B.; Tilyard, M.W.; Russell, D.G. The green prescription study: A randomized controlled trial of written exercise advice provided by general practitioners. *Am. J. Public Health* **1998**, *88*, 288–291. [CrossRef] [PubMed]

10.   Professional Associations for Physical Activity. Physical Activity in the Prevention and Treatment of Disease. 2010. Available online: https://www.folkhalsomyndigheten.se/contentassets/5de033c2c75a494a99cbba2407594c22/physical-activity-prevention-treatment-disease-webb.pdf (accessed on 4 April 2018).

11.   FaR. Individanpassad Skriftlig Ordination av Fysisk Aktivitet. Statens Folkhälsoinstitut. 2011. Available online: https://www.folkhalsomyndigheten.se/contentassets/c6e2c1cae187431c86c397ba1beff6f0/r-2011-30-far-individanpassad-skriftlig-ordination-av-fysisk-aktivitet.pdf (accessed on 14 April 2018).

12.   Rödjer, L.; Jonsdotter, I.H.; Börjesson, M. Physical activity on prescription (PAP): Self-reported physical activity and quality of life in a Swedish primary care population, 2-year follow-up. *Scand. J. Prim. Health Care* **2016**, *34*, 443–452. [CrossRef] [PubMed]

13.   Leijon, M.E.; Bendtsen, P.; Stahle, A.; Ekberg, K.; Festin, K.; Nilsen, P. Factors associated with patients self-reported adherence to prescribed physical activity in routine primary health care. *BMC Fam. Pract.* **2010**, *11*, 38. [CrossRef] [PubMed]

14.   Lawton, B.A.; Rose, S.B.; Elley, C.R.; Dowell, A.C.; Fenton, A.; Moyes, S.A. Exercise on prescription for women aged 40–74 recruited through primary care: Two year randomised controlled trial. *BMJ* **2008**, *337*, a2509. [CrossRef] [PubMed]

15.   Harrison, R.A.; McNair, F.; Dugdill, L. Access to exercise referral schemes—A population based analysis. *J. Public Health* **2005**, *27*, 326–330. [CrossRef] [PubMed]

16.   Kallings, L.V. Physical activity on prescription—An underutilized resource. Statistics on prescription shows large variations between counties. *Läkartidningen* **2012**, *109*, 2348–2350. Available online: http://www.lakartidningen.se/Functions/OldArticleView.aspx?articleId=19030 (accessed on 4 April 2018). [PubMed]

17.   Din, N.U.; Moore, G.F.; Murphy, S.; Wilkinson, C.; Williams, N.H. Health professionals' perspectives on exercise referral and physical activity promotion in primary care: Findings from a process evaluation of the national exercise referral scheme in Wales. *Health Educ. J.* **2015**, *74*, 743–757. [CrossRef] [PubMed]

18.   Persson, G.; Ovhed, I.; Hansson, E.E. Simplified routines in prescribing physical activity can increase the amount of prescriptions by doctors, more than economic incentives only: An observational intervention study. *BMC Res. Notes* **2010**, *3*, 304. [CrossRef] [PubMed]

19.   Swinburn, B.A.; Walter, L.G.; Arroll, B.; Tilyard, M.W.; Russell, D.G. Green prescriptions: Attitudes and perceptions of general practitioners towards prescribing exercise. *Br. J. Gen. Pract.* **1997**, *47*, 567–569. [PubMed]

20.   Persson, G.; Brorsson, A.; Ekvall, H.E.; Troein, M.; Strandberg, E.L. Physical activity on prescription (PAP) from the general practitioner's perspective—A qualitative study. *BMC Fam. Pract.* **2013**, *14*, 128. [CrossRef] [PubMed]

21.   Joelsson, M.; Bernhardsson, S.; Larsson, M.E.H. Patients with chronic pain may need extra support when prescribed physical activity in primary care: A qualitative study. *Scand. J. Prim. Health Care* **2017**, *35*, 64–74. [CrossRef] [PubMed]

22.   O'Sullivan, T.L.; Fortier, M.S.; Faubert, C.; Culver, D.; Blanchard, C.; Reid, R.; Hogg, W.E. Interdisciplinary physical activity counseling in primary care: A qualitative inquiry of the patient experience. *J. Health Psychol.* **2010**, *15*, 362–372. [CrossRef] [PubMed]

23.   William, R.; Miller, S.R. *Motivational Interviewing: Helping People Change*, 3rd ed.; Guilford Press: New York, NY, USA, 2012; pp. 1–482. ISBN 9781609182274.

24.   Bergh, H.; Marklund, B. Characteristics of frequent attenders in different age and sex groups in primary health care. *Scand. J. Prim. Health Care* **2003**, *21*, 171–177. [CrossRef] [PubMed]

25.   Le Reste, J.Y.; Nabbe, P.; Rivet, C.; Lygidakis, C.; Doerr, C.; Czachowski, S.; Lingner, H.; Argyriadou, S.; Lazic, D.; Assenova, R.; et al. The European general practice research network presents the translations of its comprehensive definition of multimorbidity in family medicine in ten European languages. *PLoS ONE* **2015**, *10*, e0115796. [CrossRef] [PubMed]

26.   Swedish National Board of Health and Welfare. Swedish Version of International Statistical Classification of Diseases and Related Health Problems, Tenth Revision (ICD-10). 2011. Available online: http://www.socialstyrelsen.se/Lists/Artikelkatalog/Attachments/20199/2016-5-17.pdf (accessed on 18 August 2017).

27.   Terry, A.L.; Chevendra, V.; Thind, A.; Stewart, M.; Marshall, J.N.; Cejic, S. Using your electronic medical record for research: A primer for avoiding pitfalls. *Fam. Pract.* **2010**, *27*, 121–126. [CrossRef] [PubMed]

28. Groene, O.; Garcia-Barbero, M. Health Promotion in Hospitals: Evidence and Quality Management. Country Systems, Policies and Services Division of Country Support WHO Regional Office for Europe. 2005. Available online: http://www.euro.who.int/__data/assets/pdf_file/0008/99827/E86220.pdf (accessed on 21 August 2017).

29. Buffart, L.M.; van der Ploeg, H.P.; Smith, B.J.; Kurko, J.; King, L.; Bauman, A.E. General practitioners' perceptions and practices of physical activity counselling: Changes over the past 10 years. *Br. J. Sports Med.* **2009**, *43*, 1149–1153. [CrossRef] [PubMed]

30. Nilsen, P. Making sense of implementation theories, models and frameworks. *Implement. Sci.* **2015**, *10*, 53. [CrossRef] [PubMed]

12

Comparison of Perceived and Observed Hand Hygiene Compliance in Healthcare Workers in MERS-CoV Endemic Regions

Modhi Alshammari *, Kelly A. Reynolds[ID], Marc Verhougstraete[ID] and Mary Kay O'Rourke[ID]

Mel and Enid Zuckerman College of Public Health, Department of Community, Environment and Policy, University of Arizona, Tucson, AZ 85719, USA; reynolds@email.arizona.edu (K.A.R.); mverhougstraete@email.arizona.edu (M.V.); MKOR@email.arizona.edu (M.K.O.)
* Correspondence: alshammari@email.arizona.edu

Abstract: This study investigated healthcare workers' perceptions of hand hygiene practices by comparing personal reports, as assessed by questionnaires, to direct observations of the workers' hand hygiene practices. The study employed a cross-sectional research design. Observations were made using a 16-item checklist, based on three sources: Centers for Disease Control and Prevention (CDC), World Health Organization (WHO), and Boyce and Pittet's guidelines of hand hygiene. The checklist was used for both direct-observation and self-reported data collection purposes. Pearson correlation and Multivariate Analysis of Covariance (MANCOVA) were utilized to statistically determine the relationship between healthcare workers' reports of hand hygiene practices and observed hand hygiene behaviors. The study was conducted in the outpatient examination rooms and emergency departments of three types of hospitals in the Eastern region of Saudi Arabia where Middle East respiratory syndrome coronavirus (MERS-CoV) is endemic and is observed in routine cases and outbreaks. The total sample size included 87 physicians and nurses recruited while on duty during the scheduled observation periods, with each healthcare worker being observed during individual medical examinations with at least three patients. No statistically significant correlations between the healthcare workers' perceptions of hand hygiene practices and healthcare workers' actual behaviors were evident. Based on the self-report questionnaires, significant differences were found between physicians' and nurses' hand hygiene practices reports. Healthcare workers clearly understand the importance of careful hand hygiene practices, but based on researchers' observations, the medical personnel failed to properly implement protocol-driven hand hygiene applications. However, the significant differences between physicians' and nurses' self-reports suggest further inquiry is needed to fully explore these discrepancies.

Keywords: hand hygiene; healthcare; viruses

1. Introduction

1.1. Middle East Respiratory Syndrome (MERS)

Middle East respiratory syndrome (MERS) is a type of coronavirus first discovered in Saudi Arabia in 2012 [1,2]. The virus causes a range of respiratory and gastrointestinal symptoms including fever, cough, shortness of breath, and diarrhea. Infections may progress to pneumonia and organ failure leading to approximately 35% reported mortality rate [3].

MERS in the region was previously attributed to local bats. Recent studies indicated that animal to human transmission is a cause, but with camels, instead of bats, as the most likely source [4]. Per an August 2017 Ministry of Health Report 4, the MERS coronavirus has infected a total of 1609 people with 685 fatalities in Saudi Arabia [5]. Chowell et al. conclude that a significant number of MERS cases are linked to healthcare settings, ranging from 43.5% for the outbreak in Jeddah, Saudi Arabia, in 2014, to 100% for the outbreaks in Al-Hasa, Saudi Arabia, in 2013 [6].

1.2. Transmission of Virus in Hospitals

MERS, a droplet-transmitted virus, is primarily transmitted by contact with surfaces or patients already infected with the virus. Patients with MERS can present with mild and atypical symptoms, making it hard to identify the virus from the initial medical visit. Healthcare workers, in order to protect themselves and other patients, should practice standard precautions, including hand-washing hygiene before and after patient contact, use of personal protective equipment, adequate sterilization of patient care equipment before subsequent use, and respiratory etiquette (giving masks to patients with coughs and encouraging patients to appropriately cover their mouths) [7].

The World Health Organization proclaimed hand hygiene to be the major component of standard precaution and one of the most effective methods to prevent transmission of pathogens. Specifically, hand hygiene practice refers to washing hands with plain soap and water, using water alone, or rubbing hands with an alcohol-based solution [8]. The MERS outbreak in Saudi Arabia raised questions about the potential exposure to the virus, as well as the hygiene protocols followed by healthcare workers. Numerous researchers concur that effective hand hygiene practices could significantly limit the transmission of MERS and other emerging viruses in endemic regions [2,7,9]. In Western medical practice, patients enter a waiting room and check in at the reception. They wait and are eventually escorted to a small exam room. Healthcare providers usually use either hand sanitizer or wash hands when entering the room with a new patient. In Saudi Arabia, a doctor is assigned a stationary examination room where he/she waits at a desk and successive patients enter the room. The physician may not move and lacks the physical prompt to implement hand hygiene practices between patients. Hand hygiene compliance among healthcare workers has been thoroughly studied by questionnaire [10,11] and direct observations [12,13]. Additionally, a few studies have examined a combination of questionnaires and observations [14,15]. The current research investigates the differences noted between healthcare workers' self-reports of hand hygiene practices and researcher observations of actual hand hygiene behavior.

2. Materials and Methods

Quantitative data was collected using a dichotomous scale, with questionnaire data utilizing a five-level Likert scale [16] to measure each participant's hand hygiene reports and behavior.

2.1. Setting

The study took place in three types of hospitals, i.e., public, security forces, and private, in Eastern Saudi Arabia, with approval of the study design and instruments granted by the University of Arizona Institutional Review Board (UA-IRB) as well as approvals obtained from each hospital, including the general directory of health affairs in Eastern Saudi Arabia. Each hospital had specific characteristics as follows.

2.1.1. Public Hospital

This hospital is one of the main public hospitals in the region, with a capacity of 500 beds. The facility has several other outpatient clinics, such as dermatologic, internal medicine, and orthopedics, and committees established to address infection control and organ transplants.

2.1.2. Security Forces Hospital

This hospital serves security force personnel and their families. It has 132 beds and some outpatient clinics and other departments created to manage infection and environmental controls.

2.1.3. Private Clinic

This clinic serves people who have insurance or pay for services *out-of-pocket*. It is a large facility with many outpatient clinics such as internal medicine, maternity, and otorhinolaryngology (ENT), but no hospitalization. Also, at the time of this study, it operated a 24-h emergency room in addition to its treatment room.

2.2. Participant Recruitment

Nurses and medical doctors were recruited from the outpatient and emergency room departments of each of the three hospital types. At each setting, the outpatient clinic supervisor provided a list of all the physicians and nurses assigned to work during the requested observation periods. Then, the sample population was selected through meetings with each healthcare worker on duty at each of the designated hospitals. During a weeklong visit at each setting, the premise of the study was explained to all healthcare workers, and participant permission was obtained to observe hand hygiene practices and to administer the self-report questionnaires. All doctors and nurses on duty in the emergency room were asked to participate. At the Security Forces hospital, infection control personnel assisted in providing access to healthcare workers on duty. Ultimately, 87 participants (46 medical doctors, 21 from the public hospital, 9 from the private clinic, and 16 from the Security Forces; and 41 nurses, 14 from the public hospital, 9 from the private clinic, and 18 from the security forces hospital) were recruited. Of the 87 participants who completed the questionnaire, 83 participants were observed during exams with at least three patients and hand hygiene practices were recorded using the checklist. No data were collected regarding patient behaviors, characteristics, reason for hospital visit, or diagnosis. Hand hygiene practices of healthcare workers (i.e., physicians and nurses) were evaluated before, during, and after interactions with patients, devices, and/or surrounding surfaces in each of the three Saudi Arabian hospitals.

2.3. Data Collection

Two instruments were utilized for this study, an Observation Checklist and Self-report Questionnaire.

2.3.1. Observation Checklist

Direct observations of healthcare workers' hand hygiene practices were conducted during work hours using a questionnaire, which contained 16 items, and was developed by the primary researcher's application of the following three sources: CDC standards [17], WHO's Five Moments for Hand Hygiene in Health Care [18], and Boyce and Pittet's (2002) guidelines [19]. Items were grouped into three patient-related time-dependent categories: (a) contact with a patient prior to entrance into an examination room (Before), (b) contact during the exam (During), and (c) contact with a patient upon exit from an examination room (After).

2.3.2. Self-Report Questionnaire

For the self-assessments, the questionnaire was reworded with the same 16 items from the observation sheet, making the statements active with a five-point Likert scale (i.e., 'Never', 'Rarely', 'Every once in a while', 'Sometimes', and 'Always') to allow healthcare workers to report their perceptions about their own hand hygiene practices after each scheduled observation in this study.

2.4. Data Analysis

2.4.1. Person Correlation

Pearson correlation was used to examine data by the questionnaire regarding healthcare workers' beliefs about hand hygiene practices obtained and their actual observed behavior of hand hygiene practices. In order to minimize the likelihood of missing data, all healthcare workers were provided work time to complete the questionnaire after being informed of the importance of the research. Data lacking both self-assessment and observations were excluded when testing the primary hypothesis, as a result, only data from the healthcare workers who were actually observed by the researcher and who had questionnaires completed were analyzed.

2.4.2. *t*-test

Two independent sample *t*-tests were used to examine differences between hand hygiene practices among healthcare workers, two hospital types, and gender. A multivariate analysis of covariance (MANCOVA) was used to further assess the relationship. When using MANCOVA, the healthcare worker (physician or nurse) was the independent variable. The practice of hand hygiene measured under three conditions (before, during, and after) was the dependent variable. Statistical analysis controlled for department (emergency rooms or outpatient department), hospital type (public, private, or security forces), and gender (male and female) of the care provider.

3. Results

Sixty-four (53/83) percent of the observed participants completed the questionnaire, four completed the questionnaire without being observed. The participants selected for the study are summarized in Table 1.

Table 1. Participant Information.

Hospital	Observation			Questionnaire		
	Physicians	Nurses	Total	Physicians	Nurses	Total
Public	20	14	34	12	3	15
Private	8	9	17	5	5	10
Security Forces	16	16	32	12	16	28
Total	44	39	83	29	24	53

3.1. Descriptive Statistics

An overview of the data in descriptive statistics for selective variables is presented. Table 2 (observations) and Table 3 (self-reports) include minimum scores, maximum scores, means, and standard deviations of all variables, based on the observation and questionnaire data. Visual representations of the overall findings are shown in Figures 1 and 2. The figures also indicate the percentage of observed hand hygiene compliance for physicians (27%) and nurses (29%) among the three time frames. In general, hand hygiene compliance scores before contacting patients among all variables were lower than compliance scores during and after contact with patients. Moreover, compliance scores during and after contact with patients were comparable to each other, except for the mean compliance score observed in the private clinic. In addition, the mean scores derived from the self-report questionnaire data were compared across conditions of patient contact. Based on the questionnaire data, all healthcare workers generally believed that they were compliant with hand hygiene procedures. Figures 1 and 2 show that physicians appear to be more self-aware about their hand hygiene practices than nurses.

Table 2. Two Independent Sample *t*-Tests of the Observational Data on Hand-Hygiene Practices. (Observations)

| Hand Hygiene | Physicians and Nurses | | | | | | |
| | Physicians Descriptive Statistics | | Nurses Descriptive Statistics | | | | |
	M	SD	M	SD	df	t	p
Before	0.06	0.14	0.04	0.12	81	0.69	0.49
During	0.10	0.11	0.14	0.13	81	−1.32	0.19
After	0.10	0.16	0.11	0.15	81	−0.17	0.87
Total	0.27	0.27	0.29	0.26	81	−0.37	0.72

Note: M = Mean; SD = Standard Deviation; *df* = Degree of Freedom; *t* = *t*-statistic; *p* = probability value

Table 3. Two Independent Sample *t*-Tests of the Questionnaire Data on Hand-Hygiene Practices. (Self-reports)

| Hand Hygiene | Physicians and Nurses | | | | | | |
| | Physicians Descriptive Statistics | | Nurses Descriptive Statistics | | | | |
	M	SD	M	SD	df	t	p
Before	3.68	1.13	4.47	0.63	51	−3.04	0.004
During	3.74	0.94	4.53	0.48	51	−3.72	0.000
After	4.17	1.01	4.65	0.54	51	−2.10	0.041
Total	10.19	4.57	13.65	1.51	51	−3.56	0.001

Note: M = Mean; SD = Standard Deviation; *df* = Degree of Freedom; *t* = *t*-statistic; *p* = probability value.

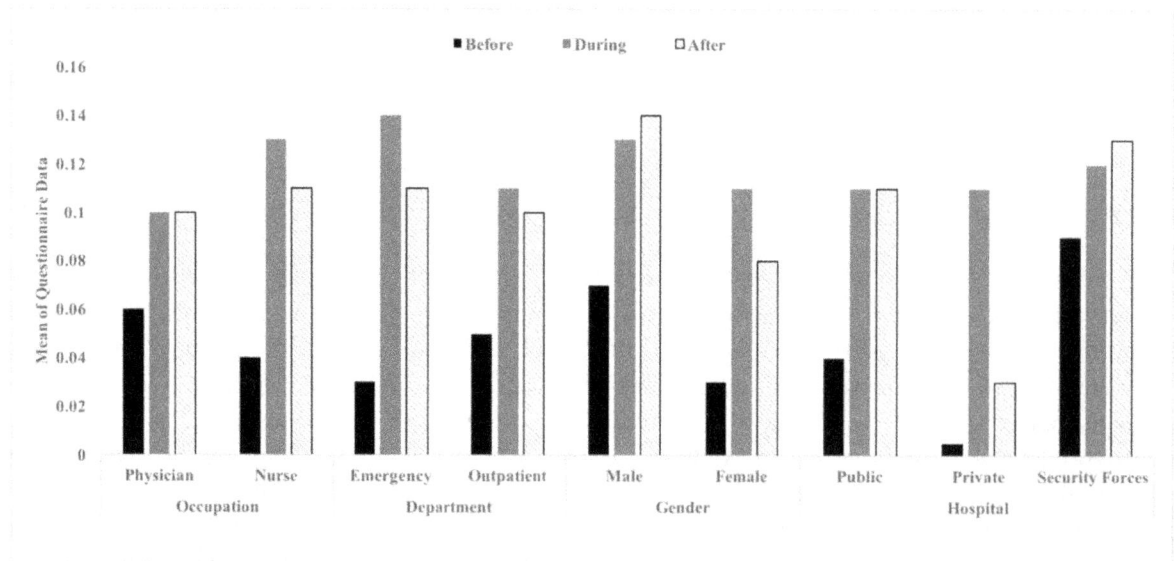

Figure 1. Comparing the mean scaled compliance scores of all variables based on the observation data. Note: Mean observation scores range from 0 to 1, with 1 being compliance 100% of the time.

3.2. Person Correlation

The results of the Pearson correlation indicated that the healthcare workers' beliefs of hygiene practices and the healthcare workers' actual behaviors did not correlate, ranging from $r = -0.01$ to $r = -0.20$.

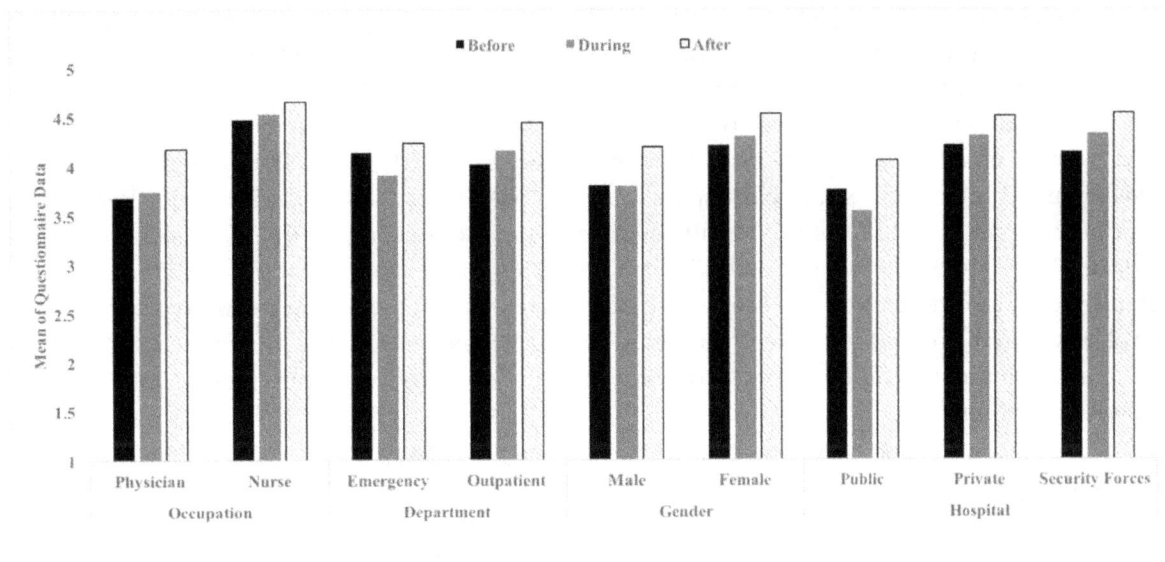

Figure 2. Comparing the means of all variables based on the questionnaire data. Note: Mean questionnaire scores range between 0 and 5, with 5 meaning compliance 100% of the time.

4. Discussion

The results of this study are robust and relevant to clinical practice in general and specifically in Saudi Arabia. First, the study design employed two observation methods (i.e., direct observation and self-report questionnaires). Second, conduct of this study increased the awareness of hand hygiene issues in healthcare settings in Saudi Arabia. Third, this study evaluated compliance with hospital hand hygiene policy in multiple types of Saudi Arabian hospitals in Eastern Saudi Arabia and considered the role played by healthcare settings and practice differences, since doctors tend to stay in a single office and patients rotate through each doctor's office.

The study had three main findings. First, hand hygiene compliance was considered low among healthcare workers in Saudi Arabia for physicians (27%) and nurses (29%), with no statistical difference observed between the two. This finding is consistent with the literature. According to Caglar et.al [14], an extensive literature review about hand hygiene practices among healthcare workers indicated that only 12.9% to 56% were compliant. For the self-report questionnaires, nurses reported higher hand hygiene compliance than physicians. Similarly, Harris et al. [20] found that non-physicians reported a higher compliance with hand hygiene when compared to physicians. Healthcare workers' beliefs, based on self-report questionnaire responses, and actual behaviors, as noted by the primary researcher's observations, did not correlate. This element of the data implied that the healthcare workers believed themselves to be more compliant with hand hygiene procedures than they actually were. A possible explanation for this discrepancy could be ignorance of hand hygiene protocols or failure to be aware of their own hand hygiene behavior.

When comparing the results from data collected in the public hospital to the data from the security forces hospital, no statistical differences existed. This is of note because the public hospital had a dedicated MERS hand hygiene intervention campaign, while the security forces hospital only had an annual seminar regarding hand hygiene procedures. This suggests that the campaign to increase hand hygiene in the public hospital needs to be rethought with a different implementation strategy. Antoniak's findings supported this idea that changes in hand hygiene behavior were not sustained beyond the period of educational intervention, demonstrating that education is not significantly effective [21]. Results from the private clinic showed the lowest compliance rates, possibly due to absence of hygiene practice materials and resources, like alcohol-based hand sanitizers in the examination rooms.

In this study, a single person was assigned to observe the hand hygiene practices of each healthcare worker. While the design used in this study minimized inconsistencies among observations, it was difficult for just one observer to fully measure the proper protocol of hand hygiene (i.e., duration and technique). Future researchers could use either video recordings or two or more observers to collect a more accurate representation of the behaviors of each participant. The premise of the study was explained fully to the study participants prior to observation sessions. This prior knowledge could have added bias to the study results by increasing rates of compliance. However, the results indicated very low hand hygiene compliance rates. This could signify that either the participants actually performed their usual practices with patient exams or that though they tried to comply due to the observer in the room they were unsuccessful because they had not had proper training. Neither of these explanations would be conclusive unless future studies of the participants' hand hygiene knowledge are conducted.

Scientific research has proven that hand hygiene is an important tool and the most effective way to prevent the spread of infectious diseases [11]. Unfortunately, prior to this study, hand hygiene practices in Saudi hospitals had not been investigated and no published articles were found. Throughout the study, the primary researcher observed many unexpected behaviors that infection control personnel at all hospitals should note and address. For example, in one observation, a healthcare worker washed her hands, then used a tissue to close the water handle, and then used the same tissue to clean nearby surfaces. On other observations, a few healthcare workers were observed not implementing proper alcohol application protocol, by using a tissue to dry excess alcohol on their hands. In other cases, some healthcare workers used alcohol wipes to clean their hands, not after hand-washing, as deemed in the proper protocol, clearly contributing to the lack of hand hygiene compliance. These behaviors should be further documented and referenced in order to improve the education of healthcare workers in the practice of proper hand hygiene.

5. Conclusions

In summary, no statistically significant correlations were found between healthcare workers' reports of hand hygiene practices and the observed behaviors of hand hygiene practices. Additionally, there were no statistically significant differences among the two types of healthcare workers (i.e., nurses and physicians) when observed. However, there were statistically significant differences when comparing the self-reported questionnaire data to observations of physicians' and nurses' hand hygiene practices. These results demonstrate that healthcare workers likely understand the importance of hand hygiene, but in practice fail to implement appropriate hand hygiene in routine activities.

Future research should utilize surrogate viral tracers to appropriately track virus transmission and portability in healthcare environments in Saudi Arabia. This is crucial for public health researchers to fully understand exposure probabilities and infection risks as well as the role of hand hygiene in the reduction of infection in order to create more focused and effective interventions. Additionally, the significant differences between physicians' and nurses' self-reports regarding hand hygiene compliance suggest further targeted inquiry and experimental research is needed to fully explore these large discrepancies.

Author Contributions: M.A. developed and identified the study topic, goals, and the methodology; she submitted applications for internal review board approval at both the University of Arizona and the hospitals in Saudi Arabia; she recruited the participants, made all observations, conducted the analysis and generated the first draft of the paper. K.A.R. contributed to the instrument development, methodology and provided expertise related to hospital based infections. M.V. contributed to data interpretation and study review. M.K.O. contributed to all aspect of the project including; the study design, IRB approvals, weekly meetings, data analysis and interpretation. All authors edited and reviewed the study repeatedly.

Funding: This research received no external funding.

Acknowledgments: The researchers of this study thank the general directory of health affairs in Eastern Saudi Arabia, each hospital's administrative staff, and most importantly all the healthcare workers who agreed to participate in this study. All authors in this study have no conflicts of interest relevant to this article. No financial support was provided to this study. None of the institutes or personal in this study were involved in any part of writing the article.

References

1. Kharma, M.Y.; Alalwani, M.S.; Amer, M.F.; Tarakji, B.; Aws, G. Assessment of the awareness level of dental students toward Middle East Respiratory Syndrome-coronavirus. *J. Int. Soc. Prev. Community Dent.* **2015**, *5*, 163–169. [CrossRef] [PubMed]

2. Pavli, A.; Tsiodras, S.; Maltezou, H.C. Middle East respiratory syndrome coronavirus (MERS-CoV: Prevention in travelers. *Travel Med. Infect. Dis.* **2014**, *12*, 3–5. [CrossRef] [PubMed]

3. Badawi, A.; Ryoo, S.G. Prevalence of comorbidities in the Middle East respiratory syndrome coronavirus (MERS-CoV): a systematic review and meta-analysis. *Int. J. Infect. Dis.* **2016**, *49*, 129–133. [CrossRef] [PubMed]

4. Mohd, H.A.; Al-Tawfiq, J.A.; Memish, Z.A. Middle East Respiratory Syndrome Coronavirus (MERS-CoV) origin and animal reservoir. *Virol. J.* **2016**, *13*, 87. [CrossRef] [PubMed]

5. Statistics - Statistics. Available online: https://www.moh.gov.sa/en/CCC/PressReleases/Pages/default.aspx (accessed on 12 June 2018).

6. Chowell, G.; Abdirizak, F.; Lee, S.; Jung, E.; Nishiura, H.; Viboud, C. Transmission characteristics of MERS and SARS in the healthcare setting: A comparative study. *BMC Med.* **2015**, *13*, 210. [CrossRef] [PubMed]

7. Sampathkumar, P. Middle East respiratory syndrome: What clinicians need to know. *Mayo Clin. Proc.* **2014**, *89*, 1153–1158. [CrossRef] [PubMed]

8. World Health Organization. Infection control standard precautions in health care. 2006. Available online: http://www.who.int/csr/resources/publications/4EPR_AM2.pdf (accessed on 5 October 2018).

9. Al-Tawfiq, J.A.; Memish, Z.A. Middle East respiratory syndrome coronavirus: Transmission and phylogenetic evolution. *Trends Microbiol.* **2014**, *22*, 573–579. [CrossRef] [PubMed]

10. Sax, H.; Uçkay, I.; Richet, H.; Allegranzi, B.; Pittet, D. Determinants of Good Adherence to Hand Hygiene Among Healthcare Workers Who Have Extensive Exposure to Hand Hygiene Campaigns. *Infect. Control Hosp. Epidemiol.* **2007**, *28*, 1267–274. [CrossRef] [PubMed]

11. Darawad, M.W.; Al-Hussami, M.; Almhairat, I.I.; Al-Sutari, M. Investigating Jordanian nurses' handwashing beliefs, attitudes, and compliance. *Am. J. Infect. Control.* **2012**, *40*, 643–647. [CrossRef] [PubMed]

12. Bischoff, W.E.; Reynolds, T.M.; Sessler, C.N.; Edmond, M.B.; Wenzel, R.P. Handwashing compliance by health care workers: The impact of introducing an accessible, alcohol-based hand antiseptic. *Arch. Intern Med.* **2000**, *160*, 1017–1021. [CrossRef] [PubMed]

13. Duggan, J.M.; Hensley, S.; Khuder, S.; Papadimos, T.J.; Jacobs, L. Inverse Correlation Between Level of Professional Education and Rate of Handwashing Compliance in a Teaching Hospital. *Infect. Control Hosp. Epidemiol.* **2008**, *29*, 534–538. [CrossRef] [PubMed]

14. Caglar, S.; Yıldız, S.; Savaser, S. Observation results of handwashing by health-care workers in a neonatal intensive care unit. *Int. J. Nurs. Pract.* **2010**, *16*, 132–137. [CrossRef] [PubMed]

15. Creedon, S.A. Healthcare workers' hand decontamination practices: Compliance with recommended guidelines. *J. Adv. Nurs.* **2005**, *51*, 208–216. [CrossRef] [PubMed]

16. Allen, I.E.; Seaman, C.A. Likert Scales and Data Analyses. *Qual. Prog.* **2007**, *40*, 64–65.

17. Siegel, J.D.; Rhinehart, E.; Jackson, M.; Chiarello, L.; Health Care Infection Control Practices Advisory Committee. 2007 Guideline for isolation precautions: Preventing transmission of infectious agents in healthcare settings. **2007**, *35*, S65–S164. [CrossRef] [PubMed]

18. Programme, I.C. Clean hands are safer hands. World Health, 2006. Available online: http://www.who.int/gpsc/5may/background/5moments/en/ (accessed on 5 October 2018).

19. Boyce, J.M.; Pittet, D.; Healthcare Infection Control Practices Advisory Committee; HICPAC/SHEA/APIC/IDSA Hand Hygiene Task Force. Guideline for Hand Hygiene in Health-Care Settings. Recommendations of the Healthcare Infection Control Practices Advisory Committee and the HICPAC/SHEA/APIC/IDSA Hand Hygiene Task Force. Society for Healthcare Epidemiology of America. *MMWR Recomm. Rep.* **2002**, *51*, 1–45. [CrossRef] [PubMed]

20. Harris, A.; Samore, M.; Nafziger, R.; DiRosario, K.; Roghmann, M.; Carmeli, Y. A survey on handwashing practices and opinions of healthcare workers. *J. Hosp. Infect.* **2000**, *45*, 318–321. [CrossRef] [PubMed]

21. Antoniak, J. Handwashing compliance. *Can. Nurse* **2004**, *100*, 21–25. [PubMed]

13

Quantifying and Trending the Thermal Signal as an Index of Perfusion in Patients Sedated with Propofol

Surender Rajasekaran [1,2,*], **Mark Pressler** [2], **Jessica L. Parker** [3], **Alex Scales** [4], **Nicholas J. Andersen** [3], **Anthony Olivero** [1,2], **John R. Ballard** [5] and **Robert McGough** [6]

[1] Department of Pediatric Critical Care Medicine, Helen DeVos Children's Hospital, 100 Michigan Street NE, Grand Rapids, MI 49503, USA; Anthony.Olivero@helendevoschildrens.org

[2] Department of Pediatrics, Michigan State University College of Human Medicine, 15 Michigan Street NE, Grand Rapids, MI 49503, USA; pressler92.mark@gmail.com

[3] Office of Research Administration, Spectrum Health, 100 Michigan Street NE, Grand Rapids, MI 49503, USA; Jessica.Parker2@spectrumhealth.org (J.L.P.); Nicholas.Andersen@spectrumhealth.org (N.J.A.)

[4] Department of Emergency Medicine, Helen DeVos Children's Hospital, 100 Michigan Street NE, Grand Rapids, MI 49503, USA; scalesalex0@gmail.com

[5] Design Solutions, Inc., 1266 Park Road, Chanhassen, MN 55317, USA; john.ballard@design-solutions.com

[6] Department of Electrical and Computer and Engineering, Michigan State University, 2120 Engineering Building, East Lansing, MI 48824, USA; mcgough@egr.msu.edu

* Correspondence: Surender.Rajasekaran@spectrumhealth.org

Abstract: We examined the feasibility of a thermal imager smart phone attachment as a potential proxy of skin perfusion by assessing shifts in skin temperature following administration of the vasodilatory anesthetic propofol. Four limb distal extremity thermal images were taken before propofol administration and at 5-min intervals thereafter during monitored anesthesia. The study enrolled 60 patients with ages ranging from 1.3 to 18 years (mean 10.7 years old) from April 2016 to January 2017. Five minutes following propofol administration, the median temperature differential (delta temperature) between the core and extremity skin significantly decreased in both upper and lower extremities, 7.9 to 3.6 °C ($p < 0.0001$) and 12.1 to 6.9 °C ($p < 0.0001$), respectively. By 10 min, the median delta temperatures further decreased significantly in the upper ($p = 0.0068$) and lower extremities ($p = 0.0018$). There was a concordant decrease in mean blood pressure (MBP). These trends reverted back when the subject awoke. There was no significant difference between the four operators who used the camera ($p = 0.0831$). Blood pressure and time temperature change was the only value of significance. Mobil thermal imaging represents a non-invasive modality to assess perfusion in real time. Further studies are required to validate the clinical utility.

Keywords: hemodynamics; monitored anesthesia care; perfusion; propofol; thermal imaging

1. Introduction

Monitored anesthesia care (MAC) with propofol requires intensive monitoring, as its hemodynamic effects may significantly alter the patient's cardiovascular state [1]. In clinical practice, it is essential to promptly identify cardiovascular decompensation early so as to initiate appropriate interventions. Presently, serial blood pressure and heart rate monitoring are the gold standards in routine anesthetic monitoring, but vasodilation and vasoplegia may precede changes in blood pressure and heart rate [2]. Health care professionals also use physical exam findings such as distal extremity capillary refill and arterial pulse palpation. These procedures are subjective and often inaccurate. Changes in vasomotor tone caused by propofol such as vasodilation also lead to increased cutaneous heat exchange between the skin and the immediate environment [3].

Infrared imager devices are already being used to measure radiant biological signals in a variety of settings and could serve as an innovation in the hemodynamic monitoring of pediatric patients [4]. The thermal imager in this study is an attachment to standard cell phones that converts the infrared radiation emitted from the patient into digital data to generate a temperature map through an infrared focal plane array device [5]. This allows users to quantify and trend radiant heat loss over time.

Distal extremity vasodilation is a hallmark of propofol sedation. Propofol is a potent vasodilator that increases vessel capacitance and decreases resistance by inhibiting sympathetic tone [2]. We posit that propofol-mediated vasodilation would lead to immediate changes in skin temperature quantifiable by thermal imaging. The goal of the present study was to assess the ability of the thermal imager to trend heat loss that registers as skin temperature from propofol-mediated vasodilation and study reversibility as propofol levels drop and vascular tone returns. This study will serve as a proof of concept of a handheld device to monitor changes in skin temperature as a surrogate to perfusion.

2. Materials and Methods

2.1. Study Design

This is a prospective observational study without any interventions. We enrolled 65 patients <18 years undergoing esophagogastroduodenoscopy (EGD) in our pediatric sedation unit from April 2016 to January 2017. All subjects underwent propofol-induced sedation. Five subjects were excluded from the analysis secondary due to missing data points. The study was performed with respect to the Declaration of Helsinki. The study and consent were reviewed and approved by the Spectrum Health Institutional Review Board.

2.2. Subjects

The study included pediatric patients who were undergoing propofol sedations for EGDs. Patients were excluded from the study if they had a pre-existing cardiovascular co-morbidity, gastro-intestinal bleeding, if drugs other than propofol were used in the sedation, or if the patient was scheduled to undergo an additional procedure.

Pediatric intensivists at Helen DeVos Children's Hospital (HDVCH) provide MAC through a dedicated pediatric sedation program. Loading doses of 2–2.5 mg of propofol were administered by the physician, and afterwards smaller doses were titrated to maintain monitored anesthesia. Oxygen via nasal cannula is administered to all patients undergoing MAC. Additional interventions, dosages, and procedure times were extracted from the sedation record. The sedation nurse assessed the quality of sedation and recovery using the modified Aldrete sedation scale [6–8].

2.3. Thermal Imaging

The FLIR One thermal imaging camera attachment is a modular attachment to any commercially available smart phone (Figure 1A). The thermal camera used was a FLIR ONE First Generation (s/n FEB5000AAN) (FLIR Systems, Wilsonville, OR, USA), a portable version that attaches to an iPhone 5/5s (Apple Inc., Cupertino, CA, USA). The temperature sensitivity is 0.1 °C with a range of 0–100 °C. We used the FLIR Research IR data acquisition system, which provides the digital tools for image creation and temperature measurement.

Validation of the camera was done using a VWR Sheldon 1226 water bath (VWR International, Radnor, PA, USA) set to an assigned temperature. The temperature was verified with a Thermalert TH5 digital thermometer (Physitemp Instruments Inc., Clifton, NJ, USA). Water temperature was increased in increments of 0.1 °C, 0.2 °C, 0.4 °C, 0.8 °C, 1.6 °C; at 30 °C, temperature was increased by 5 °C to 40 °C. After the TH5 measured the temperature, an image was taken with the FLIR One camera. The investigator waited one minute between equivalent temperature readings, for a total of two images per temperature. The water bath validation results demonstrated a strong linear correlation between camera readings and a digital thermometer ($r = 0.99$) (Figure 1B).

A

B

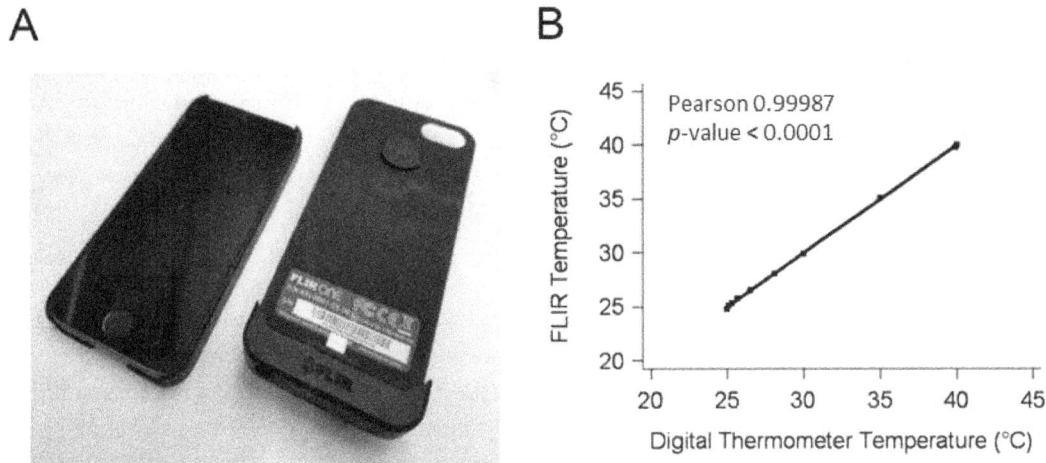

Figure 1. (**A**) The mobile thermal imager (FLIR ONE camera) on the right, and the compatible smartphone on the left (owner name and contact information was blurred from the image). The mobile thermal imager attaches to the back of the smartphone to create a single cohesive device. (**B**) Comparison between the infrared readings of a water bath taken by the mobile thermal imager and a digital thermometer.

All patients who underwent sedation for an EGD had an oral temperature taken by an electronic thermometer before and after the procedure. Those values were not significantly different (data not shown). The patients were then positioned on their left lateral side prior to sedation with the similarly trained personnel (intensivist, sedation registered nurse, sedation tech) situated in a consistent formation near the bedside, thus allowing for the camera placement and angle to be consistently maintained throughout the procedure. Prior to, and serially during the procedure, a single operator obtained thermal imaging pictures of the soles of the feet and palms of the hand, including all digits using a folded sheet of A4 paper lengthwise (28 cm) to maintain a constant distance. The images were later associated with blood pressure readings taken by the non-invasive oscillometric technique every three minutes. Vital signs and patient demographic data were abstracted from the patient's record. An ambient room temperature of approximately 21 °C was maintained in each procedure suite. Thermal values were compared with the blood pressure values taken temporally closest to the time of image acquisition. Thermal imaging is not approved by the United States Food and Drug Administration for the purpose of hemodynamic monitoring. In this manuscript, the use of thermal imaging was entirely investigational and not used to change therapy or modify care during MAC.

2.4. Data Analysis

Distal extremity thermal imaging data was collected using infrared software as part of the FLIR One thermal imaging camera attachment package. An ellipse was drawn to fit around the entire pad of the big toe and thumb using the digital photo as a guide to define the region of interest (ROI). The captured pixels each represent an average temperature value, which then generates the average for the entire elliptical region (Figure 2A). Measurement ranges were gathered from each extremity individually and over time. The right and left thumb were averaged and subtracted from the initial core temperature to calculate the delta (core minus distal extremity) temperature for each time point. Four time points were used for collecting thermal images: baseline just prior to propofol administration (pre), five minutes post-propofol administration (P5), 10 min post-propofol administration (P10), and the last image was obtained immediately after when the patient awoke and had purposeful movement (post). Blood pressure readings were collected every three minutes and were compared to the thermal readings.

2.5. Statistical Analysis

Descriptive statistics were used to summarize various patient characteristics and outcome measures. Continuous variables were expressed as mean ± standard deviation for normally distributed data and median interquartile range (IQR) for non-normally distributed data. Categorical variables were expressed as frequency (percent). *p*-values for determining the difference between core temperature and mobile thermal imager generated skin temperature were produced from a Friedman's analysis, since the data was not normally distributed across the four time points. Mixed models examine the relationship between a fixed variable and a variable that represents a random selection from the population. A mixed model was utilized to investigate differences among the four investigators over time. The interaction between the two was not included in the final model because it was not significant. A multivariate regression model was utilized to identify contributing variables that were predictive of delta temperature. To test the validation results, a Pearson correlation coefficient was used. To determine if various variables were correlated with each other, a Spearman correlation coefficient was used, since the data was not normally distributed. All statistical analyses were generated using SAS (SAS Enterprise Guide software, Version 7.1, SAS Institute Inc., Cary, NC, USA).

3. Results

3.1. Demographics

There were a total of 60 pediatric study participants. Study subject ages ranged from 1.3 to 18 years (mean 10.7 years old). Gender was split with 31 boys and 29 girls. Mean body surface area was 1.3 m^2 with a 0.4 standard deviation (Table 1). This study was performed on sedated subjects undergoing a scheduled EGD procedure. Patients had no known co-morbidities and were healthy aside from the gastrointestinal troubles that required an endoscope. Total propofol dose ranged from 2.1 to 26.7 mg/kg with a mean of 5.8 mg/kg (Table 1).

Table 1. Demographics of the subject population.

Variable	All $n = 60$
Age (years) *	10.7 ± 4.6
Sex, *n* (%)	
Male	31 (51.7)
Female	29 (48.3)
Weight (kg)	44.3 ± 20.2
BSA (m^2)	1.3 ± 0.4
Sedation length (min)	12.9 ± 3.9
Propofol dose (mg/kg)	5.8 ± 3.4

Analyses are the corresponding mean ± standard deviation. * 49 subjects. BSA: body surface area.

3.2. Median Peripheral Temperature Changes during Propofol Administration

We normalized surface temperature by subtracting the thermal readings from the initial core temperature at each time point (delta temperature). A normalized delta temperature allowed us to compare temperature changes at each time point across study subjects. To establish a delta temperature baseline (pre), investigators took thermal images of each participant's hands and feet while lying down prior to propofol administration (Figure 2A). Average temperature within the region of interest was subtracted from the patient's core temperature. All subjects had similar total (hand and foot) median pre-delta temperature (10.2 °C) (Figure 2B).After propofol induction, the surface hand temperature rose. By five minutes post-propofol (P5), the hand delta temperature decreased significantly from 7.9 °C to 3.6 °C (54.4%) as surface temperature increased. The median hand delta temperature further significantly decreased 19.4% to 2.9 °C by 10 min post-propofol (P10). The temperature change was reversible. The post-median delta temperature rose significantly to 5.9 °C 5 min after the patients awoke from sedation (post) (Figure 2). At post, patients failed to fully recover to the pre-delta temperature; skin retained elevated thermal emission (Figure 2B).

Lower extremity temperatures showed the same trend, but the normalized pre-median delta difference was 4.2 °C higher than the upper extremities (Figure 2B). This is because the pre feet temperatures were cooler than the hands. By P5, feet median delta temperature significantly decreased by 42.7% to 6.9 °C. By P10, median feet temperature significantly decreased another 26.0% to 5.1 °C. As seen in the upper extremities, the post-median feet delta temperature significantly increased but did not reach pre-level (Figure 2).

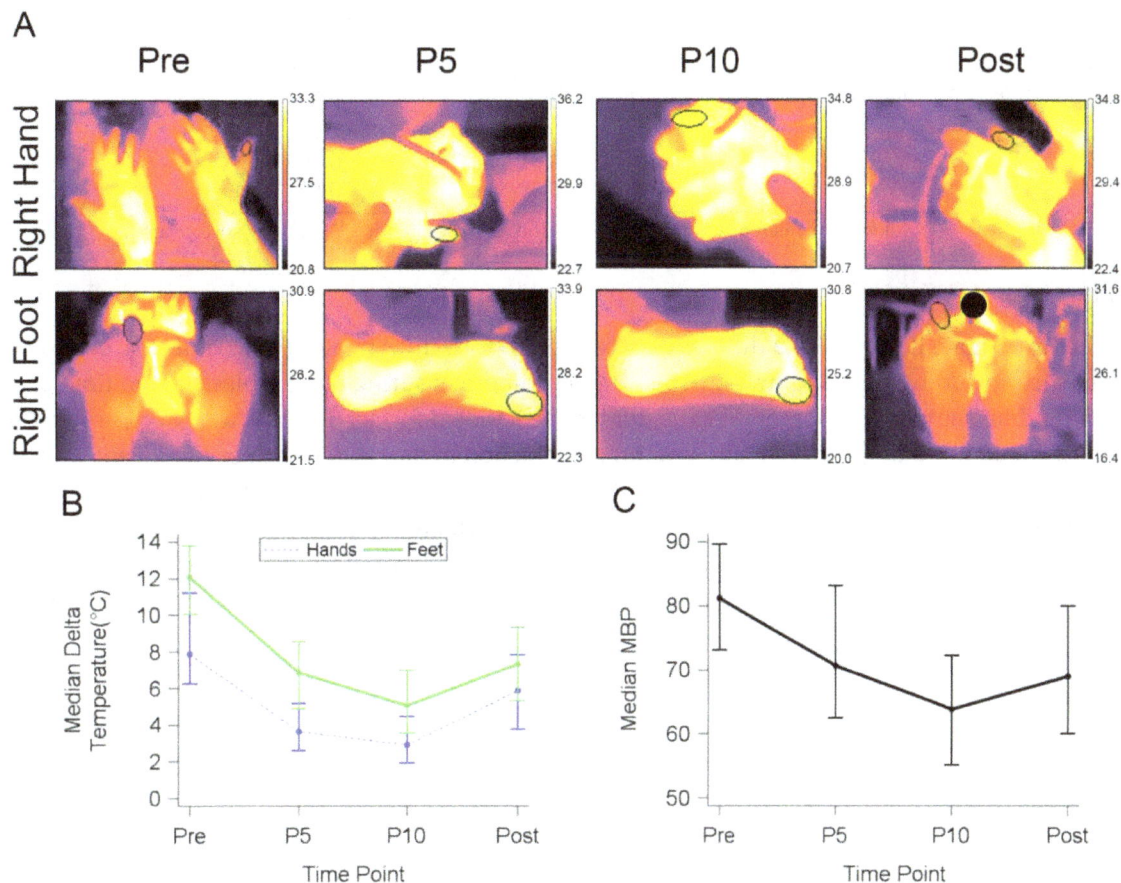

Figure 2. Median delta temperature decreases during propofol sedation. (A) Representative serial images before propofol (Pre), at 5 (P5) and 10 (P10) min post-propofol administration, and as the patient awakes (Post). Each row represents one patient over time. Region of interest (ROI; oval) marked during through the pre- and post-sedation time periods. Each image has the corresponding temperature legend in °C. (B) Median delta temperature (difference between average ROI reading and initial core) at each time point (Pre, P5, P10, Post). (C) Median of all patients' mean blood pressure (MBP) during propofol sedation and as the patient awakes.

Compared with the extremity median delta temperature, there was a concordant drop and rise in the subjects' mean blood pressure (MBP). Prior to propofol the MBP was 81.2 mm/Hg; MBP gradually decreased by 10 mm/Hg by both P5 and P10. By post, blood pressure significantly increased compared with P10, even though the mean blood pressure never reached pre-level prior to discharge (Figure 2C). Correlation analysis did not reveal any correlation between delta temperature and MBP at any time point such as the lowest MBP (P10) $r = 0.24$, $p = 0.0636$. Mean propofol dose (mg/kg) did not correlate with pre ($r = -0.17$, $p = 0.20$), P5 ($r = -0.12$, $p = 0.34$), P10 ($r = -0.13$, $p = 0.34$), or post-delta temperature ($r = 0.02$, $p = 0.8869$).

3.3. Multivariate Regression

We performed a multivariate regression to identify contributing variables. The model included the four time points, propofol dose, gender, age, and body surface area (BSA). The only significant predictor was the time point variable (Table 2).

Table 2. Regression model predicting differential between core temperature and mobile thermal imager.

Variable	Estimate	p-Value
Time (5 min) *	−5.12	<0.0001
Time (10 min) *	−6.23	<0.0001
Time (post) *	−3.36	<0.0001
Propofol dose (mg/kg)	0.07	0.38
Gender (Female) #	0.78	0.14
Age	0.01	0.96
BSA	0.88	0.55

* Pre propofol was the reference point, # male was the reference gender. BSA: body surface area.

3.4. Investigator Differences

To investigate if there was a difference between the four investigators over time, a mixed model was created including time and investigator. The repeated measuring of variables at fixed time points plus a random sample of different investigators made a mixed model the most appropriate statistical analysis. We found that the investigator and time interaction in the model was not significant, so it was removed ($p = 0.2471$). Investigator intra-study variation was insignificant between all four investigators for all time points, although Investigator 1's pre-median delta temperature was higher than the other investigators (Figure 3). The P5, P10, and post-median delta temperature were all similar between investigators. We also found that the specific investigator did not matter. There were no significant differences in the variability between investigators ($p = 0.0831$).

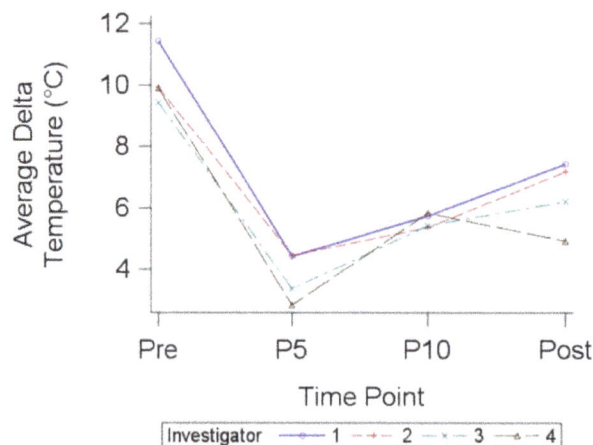

Figure 3. Longitudinal median delta temperatures for each investigator. No significant differences were found between investigators taking thermal readings. Investigator 1 ($n = 24$), Investigator 2 ($n = 25$), Investigator 3 ($n = 5$), Investigator 4 ($n = 6$).

4. Discussion

In this study, distal extremity temperature rapidly increased longitudinally during propofol sedation. Infusion of propofol preceded a drop in the median delta temperature as the skin warmed and reduced the difference between skin and initial core temperatures. Discontinuation of propofol reversed this trend; delta temperature increased as mean blood pressure trended to normal. Temperature was the only variable that significantly changed after controlling for gender, body size, and propofol dose.

This study provides the possibility of real-time monitoring of skin temperature and that such technique may act as a surrogate for perfusion and pattern recognition during anesthesia. Propofol increases tissue perfusion by inhibiting the sympathetic vasoconstrictive nerve cells resulting in vessel dilation and thermal radiation [2,3,9]. Volatile anesthetic gases exert their effect through similar mechanisms and, as such, their vasodilatory effects could be similarly trended [10]. We found a linear increase in surface temperature that was concordant with a decrease in blood pressure. As propofol's effect on sedation is relieved, surface temperature begins to fall and mean blood pressure rises. That reversal further substantiates the observation that these effects are due to propofol's effect on vasculature. Other investigators have shown the concept of skin to core temperature differential to be useful in monitoring circulatory changes [9,11–13]. In patients with vascular disease, extremity skin temperature positively correlated with tissue perfusion [13,14]. Researchers monitored thermal radiation to evaluate extremity perfusion in vascular diseases using smart phone attachments [13]. Continuous thermal imagery offers the potential to monitor the real-time therapeutic response to vasoactive agents to improve peripheral tissue perfusion or to immediately discontinue ineffective modalities in other clinical settings [13,14]. As such, the trend the device detects may be more important than the absolute temperature.

Propofol elimination does not follow a one compartment pharmacokinetic model. Propofol disperses into a deep compartment, thereby extending the terminal elimination half-life to greater than 100 minutes [15]. It is still debated whether propofol clearance adheres to a two or three compartment pharmacokinetics [15–18]. Nevertheless, propofol is detectable hours after administration. Propofol pharmacokinetics may explain that neither the temperature nor the mean blood pressure returned to pre-study levels even though the patient was awake.

This study is distinct from others in that we used a handheld thermal imaging device to map skin surface radiation under anesthesia rather than a thermistor probe that measures only the temperature at the point of contact. This technology allows the capture of a wide thermal emission field and converts it to a single image with several thousand temperature points, recorded in a fraction of a second. Continuous thermal imagery offers the potential to monitor the real-time therapeutic response of vasodilators to improve peripheral tissue perfusion or to immediately discontinue ineffective modalities [19]. We found the device to be reproducible. The device also requires little training, reducing the administrative burden; we recruited four medical students to take the thermal images. Furthermore, the cordless nature of the device does not impede provider access to the patient, as the thermal camera does not require direct patient contact.

The study does have limitations in that the patients were cared for in a setting where ambient temperature was not tightly controlled. Furthermore, not all the patients had a similar baseline blood pressure and heart rate. The patient's anxiety, discomfort, and stress of being in unfamiliar settings such as sedation suites differentially affect these. However, in studies such as this that measure hemodynamic changes, the patients often serve as their own controls. A further limitation is the variation of propofol dosing prevented a true dose response analysis. Physicians determined the appropriate propofol dose on a case-by-case basis depending on an individual patient's response and reception of the procedure. Because of this limitation, we were unable to correlate either propofol dose or blood pressure with changes in peripheral temperature.

5. Conclusions

This study reveals the feasibility of using a mobile thermal imager to assess temperature changes in patients receiving intravenous propofol. We showed that the measured skin temperature from a mobile thermal imager may serve as a potential surrogate for perfusion. The thermal bio-signal showed promise for use as a novel mode of pattern recognition during anesthesia and hemodynamic monitoring in sedated children, but further verification and validation is required.

Author Contributions: Conceptualization and Methodology: S.R., A.O., J.R.B. and R.M.; Investigation: M.P. and A.S.; Formal Analysis and Data Curation: J.L.P.; Visualization: N.J.A.; Resources: J.R.B.; Writing-Original Draft: S.R., M.P., J.L.P. and N.J.A.; Writing-Review and Edit: all authors; Supervision: S.R. and A.O.

Funding: This research received no external funding.

Acknowledgments: We would like to acknowledge Jenna Stoeken and Reena Pullikat for serving as operators for the device.

References

1. Das, S.; Ghosh, S. Monitored anesthesia care: An overview. *J. Anaesthesiol. Clin. Pharmacol.* **2015**, *31*, 27–29. [CrossRef] [PubMed]

2. Robinson, B.J.; Ebert, T.J.; O'Brien, T.J.; Colinco, M.D.; Muzi, M. Mechanisms whereby propofol mediates peripheral vasodilation in humans. Sympathoinhibition or direct vascular relaxation? *Anesthesiology* **1997**, *86*, 64–72. [CrossRef] [PubMed]

3. Hynson, J.M.; Sessler, D.I.; Moayeri, A.; McGuire, J.; Schroeder, M. The effects of preinduction warming on temperature and blood pressure during propofol/nitrous oxide anesthesia. *Anesthesiology* **1993**, *79*, 219–228. [CrossRef] [PubMed]

4. Lee, F.F.; Chen, F.; Liu, J. Infrared thermal imaging system on a mobile phone. *Sensors* **2015**, *15*, 10166–10179. [CrossRef] [PubMed]

5. Yap Kannan, R.; Keresztes, K.; Hussain, S.; Coats, T.J.; Bown, M.J. Infrared cameras are potential traceable "fixed points" for future thermometry studies. *J. Med. Eng. Technol.* **2015**, *39*, 485–489. [CrossRef] [PubMed]

6. Diaz, M.; Becker, D.E. Thermoregulation: Physiological and clinical considerations during sedation and general anesthesia. *Anesth. Prog.* **2010**, *57*, 25–32. [CrossRef] [PubMed]

7. Hertzog, J.H.; Dalton, H.J.; Anderson, B.D.; Shad, A.T.; Gootenberg, J.E.; Hauser, G.J. Prospective evaluation of propofol anesthesia in the pediatric intensive care unit for elective oncology procedures in ambulatory and hospitalized children. *Pediatrics* **2000**, *106*, 742–747. [CrossRef] [PubMed]

8. Rajasekaran, S.; Hackbarth, R.M.; Davis, A.T.; Kopec, J.S.; Cloney, D.L.; Fitzgerald, R.K.; Hassan, N.E.; Ndika, A.N.; Cornelius, K.; McCullough, A.; et al. The safety of propofol sedation for elective nonintubated esophagogastroduodenoscopy in pediatric patients. *Pediatr. Crit. Care Med.* **2014**, *15*, e261–e269. [CrossRef] [PubMed]

9. Noguchi, I.; Matsukawa, T.; Ozaki, M.; Amemiya, Y. Propofol in low doses causes redistribution of body heat in male volunteers. *Eur. J. Anaesthesiol.* **2002**, *19*, 677–681. [CrossRef] [PubMed]

10. Longnecker, D.E.; Harris, P.D. Microcirculatory actions of general anesthetics. *Fed. Proc.* **1980**, *39*, 1580–1583. [PubMed]

11. Brigitte, W.F.Y.; Childs, C. A systematic review on the role of extremity skin temperature as a non-invasive marker for hypoperfusion in critically ill adults in the intensive care setting. *JBI Libr. Syst. Rev.* **2012**, *10*, 1504–1548. [CrossRef]

12. Joly, H.R.; Weil, M.H. Temperature of the great toe as an indication of the severity of shock. *Circulation* **1969**, *39*, 131–138. [CrossRef] [PubMed]

13. Wallace, G.A.; Singh, N.; Quiroga, E.; Tran, N.T. The use of smart phone thermal imaging for assessment of peripheral perfusion in vascular patients. *Ann. Vasc. Surg.* **2018**, *47*, 157–161. [CrossRef] [PubMed]

14. Kelechi, T.J.; Michel, Y. A descriptive study of skin temperature, tissue perfusion, and tissue oxygen in patients with chronic venous disease. *Biol. Res. Nurs.* **2007**, *9*, 70–80. [CrossRef] [PubMed]

15. Doze, V.A.; Shafer, A.; White, P.F. Propofol-nitrous oxide versus thiopental-isoflurane-nitrous oxide for general anesthesia. *Anesthesiology* **1988**, *69*, 63–71. [CrossRef] [PubMed]

16. Cockshott, I.D. Propofol ('diprivan') pharmacokinetics and metabolism—An overview. *Postgrad. Med. J.* **1985**, *61* (Suppl. 3), 45–50. [PubMed]

17. Gepts, E.; Camu, F.; Cockshott, I.D.; Douglas, E.J. Disposition of propofol administered as constant rate intravenous infusions in humans. *Anesth. Analg.* **1987**, *66*, 1256–1263. [CrossRef] [PubMed]

18. Simons, P.J.; Cockshott, I.D.; Douglas, E.J.; Gordon, E.A.; Hopkins, K.; Rowland, M. Disposition in male volunteers of a subanaesthetic intravenous dose of an oil in water emulsion of 14c-propofol. *Xenobiotica* **1988**, *18*, 429–440. [CrossRef] [PubMed]

19. Grossi, G.; Mariotti, A.; Di Donato, L.; Amerio, P.; Tulli, A.; Romani, G.L.; Merla, A. Functional infrared imaging of paroxysmal ischemic events in patients with raynaud's phenomenon. *Int. J. Immunopathol. Pharmacol.* **2010**, *23*, 627–632. [CrossRef] [PubMed]

14

"That Guy, Is He Really Sick at All?" An Analysis of How Veterans with PTSD Experience Nature-Based Therapy

Dorthe Varning Poulsen [1,* iD], **Ulrika K. Stigsdotter** [1 iD] and **Annette Sofie Davidsen** [2 iD]

[1] Department of Geosciences and Natural Resource Management, University of Copenhagen, Rolighedsvej 23, 1958 Frederiksberg C, Denmark; uks@ign.ku.dk

[2] The Research Unit for General Practice, University of Copenhagen, Øster Farimagsgade 5, 1014 København K, Denmark; adavid@sund.ku.dk

* Correspondence: dvp@ign.ku.dk

Abstract: Serving in the military leads to mental diseases, such as post-traumatic stress disorder (PTSD), for a percentage of soldiers globally. The number of veterans with PTSD is increasing and, although medication and psychological treatments are offered, treatment results could be improved. Historically, different forms of nature-based therapy have been used for this target group. However, in spite of anecdotally good results, studies measuring the effect of this form of therapy are still lacking. The aim of this study is to explore how veterans with PTSD manage their everyday lives during and after a ten-week nature-based intervention in a therapy garden. Methods: Eight veterans participated in qualitative interviews, which were conducted during a one-year period and were analyzed using interpretative phenomenological analysis (IPA). Results: Five themes emerged from the IPA analysis: Bodily symptoms; relationships; building new identities; the future; and lessons learned. All the participating veterans gained a greater insight into and mastering of their condition, achieved better control of their lives, and developed tools to handle life situations more appropriately and to build a new identity. This improved their ability to participate in social activities and employment. Conclusion: The results should be considered in the future treatment of veterans with PTSD.

Keywords: veterans; post-traumatic stress disorder; nature-based therapy; Interpretative Phenomenological Analysis; qualitative study

1. Introduction

Historically, nature has been used as part of a healing process for soldiers who have been mentally wounded in World War l. The first systematic use of nature in the shape of horticultural activities was developed during World War I [1,2] for soldiers suffering from shell-shock (later referred to as post-traumatic stress disorder), a prevalent condition in soldiers returning from the battlefield. These horticultural activities were first introduced as a voluntary treatment option, but gradually they became more professionalised, and today they are integrated into the treatment of occupational injuries [3,4]. Even though many programmes exist today, containing different kinds of nature elements, such as the wilderness, horticulture, and ecotherapy, scientific studies in this area remain sparse. To gain more knowledge, this study examines the effects of nature-based therapy (NBT) on a group of Danish veterans and shows that this form of treatment may be useful as part of the treatment offered to veterans with post-traumatic stress disorder (PTSD).

1.1. PTSD Diagnosis and Prevalence among Veterans

According to the *Diagnostic and Statistical Manual of Mental Disorders* (DSM-V) [5], a person diagnosed with PTSD must have been exposed to a traumatic event personally, or have witnessed a threat of death or serious injury, and subsequently experiences symptoms such as: Re-experiencing the trauma, for example, in flashbacks and nightmares; avoidance of places or activities that trigger memories of the traumatic event; arousal and reactivity associated with negative thoughts; aggressive behaviour that occurs with little or no provocation; and concentration problems.

Exposure to traumatic experiences during military service that leads to developing PTSD is the reality for many soldiers around the world, and the symptoms of the condition may cause extensive changes in the lives of veterans after homecoming. According to figures from the U.S. Department of Veteran Affairs, 15.8 per cent of veterans reported PTSD symptoms after having served in Iraq and Afghanistan [6]. An Australian study found that 8.3 per cent of veterans reported symptoms comparable with PTSD [7], while studies of British military personnel showed a lower prevalence, varying between 2.5 per cent and 6 per cent [8]. According to Richardson et al. [9], this large variability in prevalence may be explained by differences in the sampling strategies and diagnostic criteria used in the studies. The DSM-III-R criteria did not require 'clinically significant impairment' for the diagnosis of PTSD to be made. However, this criterion was introduced in the DSM-IV, which ultimately decreased the prevalence rate of PTSD. Richardson et al. [9] also suggested that the duration and intensity of combat exposure during deployment may influence the prevalence of PTSD. Furthermore, the prevalence of veterans reporting PTSD symptoms after homecoming is expected to increase [10–12]. The reasons for this increase have not been fully documented, but a greater awareness of PTSD and more focus on breaking down the stigma surrounding mental health issues may be underlying causes [13].

In accordance with DSM-V [5], symptoms of PTSD must be present within six months after the traumatic experience. However, there is growing awareness of the condition called 'delayed-onset PTSD', where the symptoms appear later than six months after the trauma. A review by Andrews et al. [14] found that delayed-onset PTSD is 33 per cent more common in veterans compared with in the civilian population, and that the delayed onset of symptoms is likely to occur within 18 months after leaving the military. A recent study from Australia found the prevalence of delayed-onset PTSD among Australians veterans who served in Iraq or Afghanistan to be as high as 16.5 per cent [15]. In the UK, the prevalence of delayed-onset PTSD [16] in veterans increased from 3.6 per cent in 2007 to 6.9 per cent in 2009. The same tendency is found in Denmark, where 2.4 per cent of veterans who served in Afghanistan were identified with symptoms compatible with PTSD immediately after homecoming. This number had increased to 9.7% three years after homecoming [12]. Therefore, it can be assumed that in the future, the numbers of veterans suffering from PTSD will increase over time.

1.2. How Living with PTSD Affects Veterans' Lives

PTSD symptoms may affect the lives of the veterans themselves and their families at a physical, emotional, and relational level. Research also suggests that there is a relationship between PTSD and general health. Hoge et al. [17] found that, in war veterans, the PTSD diagnosis was significantly associated with lower ratings of general health and more missed work days, as well as a higher incidence of physical symptoms and pain [18,19]. Several studies [20,21] have also found alcohol and drug abuse, depression, and anxiety disorders to be prevalent comorbidities to PTSD. Milliken et al. [22] stated that 12 to 15 per cent of veterans reported problematic alcohol use three to six months after returning from combat.

In addition to these health-related problems, social and family problems are also related to living with the PTSD diagnosis [9,23]. A review from 2004 [24] found that the individual's traumatic stress had a negative effect on family members. In a recent study, Vogt et al. [25] found that PTSD was associated with poorer work and family functioning and satisfaction, and that the most consistent negative effects were on intimate relationships. Moreover, numbing, high arousal levels, and anger have been found to be associated with secondary traumatization and troubled families [26,27], and veterans suffering from PTSD have been shown to be four times more likely to contemplate suicide than non-PTSD veterans [24].

In addition to causing significant problems for the individual, PTSD involves massive economic challenges for society. The RAND report from 2008 [27] estimated that PTSD, major depression, and traumatic brain injury two years after deployment can cost up to $25,000 per case in the US. Providing evidence-based treatment to everyone could reduce these costs by up to 27 per cent [28].

1.3. Conventional Treatments for Veterans with PTSD

Medication and psychotherapy, such as behavioural and cognitive therapy, are conventional and common treatments for veterans diagnosed with PTSD. For example, Puetz et al. [29] found that SSRIs (selective serotonin reuptake inhibitors) and tricyclic antidepressants had an impact on anxiety and depressive symptoms in combat veterans. Sleep disturbances, which are common symptom of PTSD, have also been found to be alleviated by pharmacology treatment [30]. Even though many veterans feel that medication helps reduce their PTSD symptoms, the negative side effects they experience are substantial, and this leads to many of them giving up on medication [31].

Psychotherapy is a common alternative to pharmacotherapy. In a guideline from 2017 [32], the US Department of Veteran Affairs recommends: "Individual, manualized trauma-focused psychotherapy over other pharmacologic and non-pharmacologic interventions for the primary treatment of PTSD. Cognitive content and processes are seen as central to theories of understanding PTSD" [32]. In line with this, numerous studies have shown that trauma-focused cognitive behavioural therapies (CBT) such as cognitive processing therapy (CPT), prolonged exposure therapy (PE), and other cognitive therapies have a positive effect on PTSD symptoms by reducing destructive or disturbing behavioural patterns [7,33]. Moreover, a meta-analytical review [34] has shown that half of the combat veterans treated with a variety of psychotherapeutic interventions experienced an improvement in their symptoms compared with a control group.

In addition, the impact of non-trauma focused treatment has been evaluated. Present-centered therapy is an example of a non-trauma focused treatment that has been found to have a positive impact on PTSD in several studies [33,35–38]. Moreover, EMDR (eye movement desensitization and reprocessing) has been shown to have a positive effect in some studies [39,40], and mindfulness has also been shown to be effective with regard to PTSD symptoms [41–44] in a number of recent studies.

1.4. How NBT Can Be Seen as Part of a Treatment for Veterans with PTSD

Despite having a long history, NBT has, as mentioned above, only been sparsely investigated as a treatment option for war veterans. NBT may have some advantages relative to traditionally employed therapies that have high dropout rates [36,45,46] and that are sometimes experienced by veterans as reinforcing their symptoms [47]. For veterans, seeking help for mental problems is often related to perceived stigma [48–50]. Receiving therapy in nature might be an easier threshold for veterans to cross than engaging in more traditional therapy. In addition, PTSD may lead to cognitive impairment with concentration problems which might hamper the effect of the conventional therapies, and in some of the individuals, the cognitive focus could reactivate the trauma. Therefore, a therapy where the focus is not directly on thinking and reflection might be more acceptable [28,39,51]. Consequently, it would seem relevant to follow the historical thread from WWI with introduction of the first horticultural activities for war victims and offer the treatment to veterans with PTSD, along with an investigation of the participants' experiences of the intervention. NBT as a treatment for mental illness builds on a solid evidence [52–55]. NBT has been shown to be effective in the treatment of depression [56–59] and with regards to individuals with PTSD, depression is a frequent comorbidity [60,61].

1.5. Nature-Based Therapy (NBT)

NBT is often used as an umbrella term for therapy based on experiences and activities in a natural setting that are specifically identified or designed to support the treatment process. Different nature-based therapeutic activities using horticultural activities are derived from occupational therapy [62,63]. In the UK and the US, NBT developed into a discipline of its own, based on the successful rehabilitation of war veterans. The background for using nature as an important part of the intervention is grounded in attention restoration theory (ART), which was developed by Kaplan and Kaplan [64].

ART suggests that humans have two types of attention: Directed attention and soft fascination. Directed attention is used when the individual has to concentrate on important matters. This process requires effort and can cause mental fatigue over time. In contrast, soft fascination captures the individual's attention effortlessly. Soft fascination is at play when we, for example, are looking at clouds moving across the sky, and this kind of effortless brain function has been shown to lead to recovery from stress-related illnesses [65]. In relation to the treatment of war veterans suffering from PTSD, other researchers have pointed to ART as a valuable theory with which to understand the benefits for veterans of being in nature environments, e.g., [40,66,67]. Hawkins et al. [66] explained that nature, for many veterans, is experienced as emotionally calming. He refers to Kaplan's [68] descriptions of nature as having a buffering effect that reduces the adverse effects of stressors (high arousal and rapid response to sudden sensory input), in other words, nature is seen as a meaningful place. This also holds true for many veterans, who often feel related to nature because of the many hours of training they have spent there, and they experience a sense of freedom when they are in nature [69,70].

Therefore, the aim of this study is to explore how war veterans experience living with PTSD on a daily basis during and after a ten-week nature-based therapy in a therapy forest garden.

2. Materials and Methods

This is a qualitative study. Data material consisted of semi-structured individual interviews and one focus group interview with eight Danish war veterans diagnosed with PTSD. This paper is part of a larger study that explores how a nature-based intervention in a therapy garden was experienced by veterans with PTSD, with a focus on the daily experiences of living with PTSD.

2.1. Setting

The NBT took place in the University of Copenhagen's therapy forest garden, Nacadia, located in the arboretum. The garden is designed in accordance with a model for evidence-based health design [71], with activities contributing to NBT. Figure 1 gives an overview of the features in Nacadia. The design provides possibilities for nature-based activities (NBA) all year round, and its design and treatment programme are closely related. Figure 2 shows the therapy garden seen from the main wooden path just before crossing the stream.

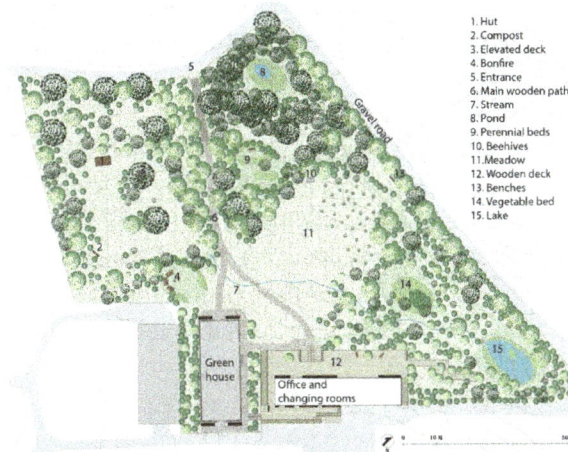

Figure 1. Figure one is a map of the therapy garden, Nacadia.

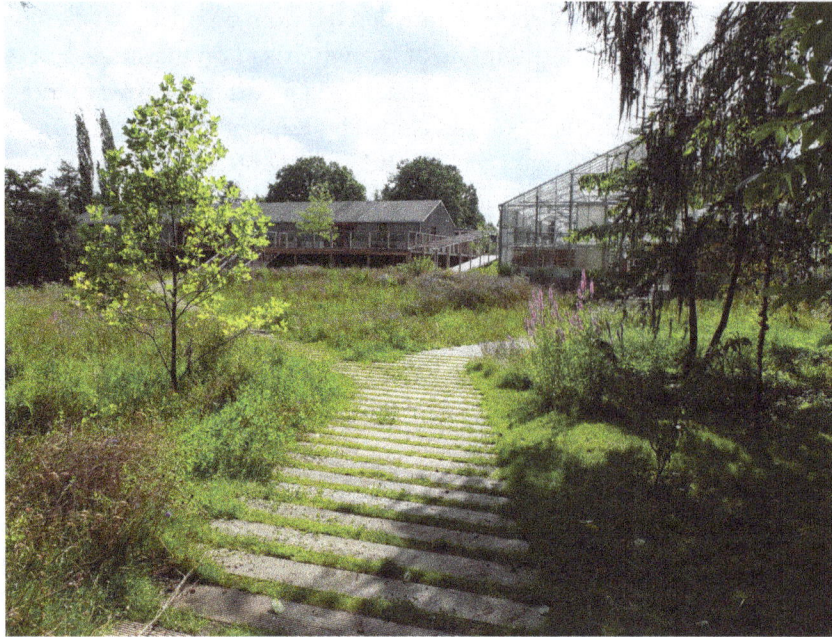

Figure 2. The picture shows a view from the therapy garden, Nacadia.

2.2. The Therapists

Two horticultural therapists with psychological backgrounds were primarily responsible for the daily programme. The arboretum supervisor initiated tasks of a more physical character. A psychiatrist and a medical doctor conducted the weekly psychotherapeutic conversations in the garden area.

2.3. Nature-Based Therapy

NBT is based on the following elements: Horticultural and body-awareness activities supplemented by individual therapeutic talks. The value of combining these elements is described by Corazon et al. [71]. The mindfulness or awareness activities aim to reduce the physiological effects of stress exposure and to re-establish healthy flexibility to the nervous system. Working with the psychological trauma when appropriate and implementing nature and mindfulness-based tools for coping with PTSD are considered to enhance the ability to handle challenging life situations.

The length of the NBT was ten weeks, with three hours of therapy three times a week. The duration of the weekly individual therapeutic conversations was one hour. It was part of a therapeutic approach to encourage the veterans to be aware of and respect their bodily sensations, and use this knowledge to choose activities matching their mental and bodily capacity. The intention was to build up the veterans' self-confidence and experience of success in the activities.

The intervention had a daily structure, the purpose of which was to create a recognizable and safe frame for the participants. The day started with a walk through the arboretum forest to the therapy garden. Upon arrival, a gathering around the fireplace was the first item of the day. Body awareness is considered as potentially beneficial for health [72]. Body-awareness exercises like 'body-scan', mindful awareness of breathing, and sounds and thoughts in the nature-setting were used. The aim was to reduce the high arousal level, and bring calmness into the nervous system. This was followed by horticultural activities and private time.

The horticultural activities involved a physical element, e.g., wood splitting and planting of trees that could benefit their needs for physical challenges [70], as well as more relaxing activities conducted alone, with staff members, or in the group.

2.4. Participants

Potential participants were recruited through advertisements in newspapers and on websites for soldiers and veterans. Those who had served abroad and were diagnosed with PTSD could apply for participation and could visit the therapy garden. The next step was a meeting with members of the staff. Eight male veterans, aged 26–47 years, were included in the project. Veterans with psychotic conditions were excluded.

With regard to the veterans included in the study, the time since they had first received their PTSD diagnosis ranged between nineteen months and two years, while the time until onset of symptoms after service ranged from a few months to more than eighteen years. The veterans had served in war zones for one to four periods (of six months) in the Balkans, Iraq, and Afghanistan. Seven of the included veterans used medicine for mental PTSD symptoms, such as anxiety, anger, and sleeplessness. Drugs (not prescribed by physicians) formed part of the self-medication for five of the participants. Three participants from the group were working part-time at the military barracks. The remaining five were on sick leave for a period between two to twelve years, and received unemployment benefits.

Dropouts: After three weeks, one of the participants developed psychotic symptoms and was therefore excluded from the study. One participant started an education two weeks before the NBT ended.

2.5. Data Collection and Analysis

Before the intervention, the first author conducted initial talks (pilot interviews) with veterans with PTSD (non-applicants). This resulted in a pre-understanding of the experiences and the physical and mental wounds that can arise during active service. This recognition was used to develop the interview guide and the appropriate approach during the data collection. Interview guides were created, with the aim to explore how veterans live with PTSD on a daily basis and their experiences of how NBT affected their lives.

Four individual, semi-structured, open-ended interviews were carried out with each participant. The first interview was conducted before the intervention, the second after five weeks, the third after ten weeks (at the end of intervention), and the last interview was conducted one year after the intervention. There were separate interview guides for all four interviews. The first interview focused on the veterans' previous relation to nature, their experiences with activities in nature, and how they perceived having PTSD, including bodily changes and sensations, their coping tools, and experiences when not being able to alleviate symptoms. The focus of interview two was on the veterans' experiences with the therapy garden and changes in symptoms and function during the therapy, and activities of special importance. In the third interview, the questions were once again about changes in wellbeing, but there was also a focus on cooperation and fellowship with the group and future relations to nature. The last interview, one year after the termination of therapy, was about the veterans' wellbeing, their continued relation to nature, and their evaluation of the effect of the therapy on their daily life. The interviews lasted between 46 and 94 min. In addition, one focus-group interview with all participants was conducted after ten weeks of treatment.

During the interviews, it was considered important to generate an atmosphere in which the participants felt physically and emotionally safe. This was achieved by, for example, letting the participants decide where the first interview should be conducted. Four of the participants chose their homes due to experiencing anxiety when venturing outside the home. Two interviews were held in the military barracks, and two at the interviewer's office.

The second interview was conducted in the therapy garden while walking on paths chosen by the participants. The third interview was conducted in the therapy garden near the bonfire area, while the fourth interview took place in the participants' homes or at the interviewer's office.

Due to dropouts, seven veterans participated in the first three interviews. By the end of the fourth interview one year later, five veterans participated.

Notes about the interview situation or the participants' physical reactions were taken during the interviews, in order to include the circumstances around the statements and body language that might reveal knowledge or improve the interviewer's opportunities to ask clarifying questions [73,74]. The notes were added to the transcriptions. All interviews were conducted, digitally recorded, and transcribed verbatim by the first author.

2.6. Data Analysis

Interpretative phenomenological analysis (IPA) was used to analyse the data. IPA has its roots in phenomenology, and the method aims to explore in detail the participants' life-world and their personal experiences and perception [75,76]. The method involves a dynamic process with the researcher playing an active role and, thus, acknowledges the influence of the researcher's personal conceptions and the interpretative activity involved [77]. The method is used increasingly within the psychological field, as well as in social research [78,79]. Data were analysed following the stepwise procedure of the IPA method: Repeated readings of each interview to gain an overall impression, notes on passages of special interest, followed by identification of initial themes that capture the essence of the interview [75]. This procedure was repeated with all interviews, and initial themes were identified. Following this, themes were clustered, common themes were identified across the interviews, and, finally, main themes were identified. This formed the basis for the narrative writing up. The first author conducted the first steps of the analysis process, including the first clustering of themes and identification of main themes, together with the third author, who is a qualitative researcher with experience in the IPA-method. The analysis process was discussed among all authors, and they all participated in the process of identifying the five main themes. Divergent views were discussed until agreement was reached.

3. Results

The analysis resulted in five superordinate themes: When the body speaks; relationships, imperative and unbearable; building a self; the future, dreams, fears and hopes; and lessons learned. These themes will be elaborated below.

3.1. When the Body Speaks

All the veterans reported that they had experienced bodily sensations before being diagnosed with PTSD. Some weeks or months after returning home, they noticed changes in their bodily reactions. They complained of headaches, memory impairment, sleep disturbances, and increased sensitivity to sounds that triggered memories of the war, for example the sound of a helicopter or an accelerating motor vehicle. They said that, at first, the bodily symptoms were confusing and they did not relate them to a possible PTSD diagnosis. Some described it as an experience of being out of touch with their bodies, and of feeling a need to escape physically by running away or mentally by sleeping:

> "I was like a volcano; I felt the pressure inside and out. Suddenly it says BOOM. Sometimes I felt like I had to run as fast as I could to get away from myself."

Most of the veterans said that they had sought help at a hospital for their symptoms, because they experienced the symptoms as being physical and in some cases even life-threatening, as if they were having a heart attack.

> "First there's a pressure on my chest, like a child pressing, then it tightens like a band round my trunk, and in the end, it's like an elephant planting a foot on my chest, pressing so hard I can't breathe."

The medical examinations did not lead to a physical explanation for their symptoms. Some began to consider whether there was a connection between their physical problems and their mental state and contacted the military health service. Others said that they continued to search for a physical diagnosis. A few described it as a struggle with large personal costs; it was no longer a question of getting a diagnosis, but of being respected as a person.

"I have struggled tremendously the last year to make them aware of my problems [. . .] It has been the most stressful thing in my whole life. I just hope that I will be treated as I deserve."

During the last five weeks of the intervention, all the veterans described changes in their bodily symptoms. These changes occurred at a different pace and did not always lead to a complete absence of symptoms. However, the veterans talked about how even a small change led to the realisation of how their symptoms had influenced their daily lives. In the third interview (toward the end of the intervention), one of the veterans mentioned that he had been able to sleep through the night for the first time in 18 years. Others talked about better quality of sleep, or about managing to let go of the anxiety connected with falling asleep and the nightmares the sleep might bring:

"My dreams . . . I have positive dreams now. I still have some of those dreams that are hard to handle, but I am more distanced from them. Like standing outside and looking down on it. It does not affect me in the same way. More relaxed, you can say."

The veterans said that the feelings of turmoil and of being in a state of constantly heightened alertness was reduced during the nature-based intervention. Most of the veterans experienced a peaceful feeling in their bodies during the nature-based activities. One said that it was as if breathing had become easier and this had led to reduced tension in his muscles. Another mentioned that this relaxed condition was a big motivator for doing some of the activities that he liked less:

"All that yoga and stuff, I do it because I am looking forward to lying down and listening [] . . . I love to be in that trance-like state . . . I'm almost counting down."

In the second interview (halfway through the intervention), all the veterans stressed that the breathing techniques had become a useful tool for coping with stressful situations, such as sitting close to other people on a bus or going shopping in a crowded supermarket. They also told that they used to be very sensitive to other people's emotions, but that this had changed during the intervention. One of the veterans described this change in the third interview:

"I feel like the body is relaxing more. . . . normally I feel like a radar for people's anger, even though it doesn't have anything to do with me. If I go down the street and see someone who is angry, my system is up high [..]. Now I can tell myself it has nothing to do with me."

This change in behavioural patterns made it possible for the veterans to participate in social activities.

3.2. Relationships, Imperative and Unbearable

Two types of relationships were described as being affected by the veterans' condition: Relationships with soldier comrades, and relationships with family and friends. The veterans described in detail the close relationships they had with comrades that had developed during service. They had felt a responsibility toward each other in their everyday lives, which had given them a sense of safety in spite of living with the constant threat of attack. The veterans described this fellowship with other soldiers in the first interview:

"Your comrades are the ones you would die for . . . and the ones who help you handle your problems."

When a comrade became wounded or died, the veterans experienced grief and guilt because they were alive. One of the veterans expressed it as follows:

"I feel guilty about being alive, and that I did not bring my comrade back home with me, even though I promised his mum I would."

This veteran said that he had taken on a personal responsibility and that he blamed himself for his friend's death. The fact that he had promised his friend's mother that he would bring his friend home made it even worse. Two of the participants were sent home for treatment before they had finished their posting and recounted how they felt ashamed about leaving their comrades behind.

Being on sick leave stimulated thoughts about what others might think of them, and made them feel that they were seen as cheats who had invented the symptoms themselves. Some felt it as if other people were talking badly about them behind their backs:

"That guy, is he really sick?"

In the first interview, most of the veterans described a feeling of loneliness after coming home, and some felt an urge to isolate themselves from their relatives and friends. They said that during service, they considered their comrades to be replacements for their families. When they first returned home, their families could not replace this relationship. The veterans described their relationships with their families as difficult and often contradictory; on the one hand, their families were the most important thing in the world to them, while on the other hand, they could not handle being together with them. All the veterans thought that they had changed and were different from how they had been before service, and they found it difficult to meet their families' needs for affection. One veteran, when talking about his girlfriend, who used to call him or send him messages every day, said the following:

"I haven't got the room inside me to be there for her every day . . . I can't . . . for me feelings are just not like before."

In the first interview, the veterans also emphasised how they had changed after they had served; they were now in a constant state of alertness and unable to refrain from observing people's behaviour when in a crowd. They said that they always felt the need to check for snipers and hide under tables when hearing the sound of airplanes. This behaviour frightened other people and was seen as being extreme. They felt that it had a significant effect on their ability to take part in social arrangements and it also led to unintended suspicion from their families. One veteran related the following episode about his wife coming home from work:

"I look at her . . . her hands, if she is carrying something, keys or . . . or if something looks different. If her hand is closed, I have to follow her movements until I have seen what she has got there."

All the veterans described how both physical contact and being able to sense affection were hard after coming home. One of them was unable to pick up his little son:

"It has been terrible. Especially for my son. He has his needs . . . [interviewer: And you can't give this to him?] "No, I can't take it [touching and skin-contact]."

They also said that they experienced difficulties sharing feelings and talking about how they felt, which made their emotional communication with their relatives difficult:

"It's hard for me to express how I'm feeling and maybe also hard for them to know what to say to me [...] Not even my family knows much about how I'm doing. It stays inside me, and it's very very hard to open up and talk about how I'm feeling and thinking."

In the interviews conducted midway through the intervention, the veterans emphasised some changes that had occurred in the way they perceived relationships. They all experienced a positive feeling of being part of the group of veterans during the NBT. Being surrounded by people with the same background, similar experiences, and challenges was considered more comforting than being with civilians.

"If I had started in another group, where people had PTSD but for civil reasons, I don't think it would have been the same . . . we have this mutual understanding [...] There are things we don't need to say . . . we know what it's like to serve abroad and be in a state of constant alertness."

This understanding resulted in an atmosphere in the group in which they felt free to put memories and reflections into words. They expressed the importance of being in an ambience of understanding where no explanations were needed.

In the same round of interviews as above, several of the veterans highlighted how the term 'acceptance' had become a cornerstone in their thinking about life. Gradually, the veterans expressed acceptance of what life might bring instead of fighting it. In addition, during the NBT, the veterans described different strategies they had developed to cope with stressful situations and quarrels with their families.

3.3. The Future, Dreams, Fears, and Hopes

In the first interview, all the veterans related a history of long-term treatment with medication and/or psychotherapy. Some of the treatments had provided small improvements, but had also shattered hopes and dreams when the improvements did not last or even failed to materialise. Even so, in the first interview, all the participants expressed positive expectations to the intervention. However, their expectations differed and reflected their present life situation. Some felt the need for specific tools to help them to regain control:

"I need an instrument to control the turmoil and nerves in my body because I hate it. I hate having it [. . .] it's a heavy burden."

Several of the veterans' statements reflected their hopes and fears regarding their PTSD symptoms. Being disappointed could affect their mood and reinforce anxiety. For the veterans, the alternative to not getting better was frightening. One veteran with a background as a social worker said in the second interview:

"You get anxious of this change [of oneself]. And where does it lead to? You see the weirdo on the street, and suddenly you imagine that's the way you're going."

Another participant was unable to see a future for himself. He expressed it like this in the second interview, giving an impression of the deep worry that the veterans face:

"Future? It's almost like it's just some letters on a piece of paper that I see. A mathematical formula on a white wall . . . "

However, at the end of the intervention, the veterans' thoughts about the future had changed. Anxiety was considered less dominant. Instead, the veterans accepted the slow pace of the improvements they experienced, and time became an important factor in their healing processes. They expressed an awareness that they should not put pressure on themselves.

"Before, I was so preoccupied with saying, in six months I will have got so far with my disease. But I've dropped everything to do with time horizons and that sort of thing. Things must come as they are, the more I hurry, the more I stress myself, and the less energy I have to handle things."

This expresses a growing insight into the condition among the veterans, and it acknowledges their own role in a recovery process. During the intervention and the year after the NBT, some of the veterans even experienced being able to handle their problems and imagine a future. A veteran expressed it like this in the final interview (one year after the intervention):

"Now I manage to do some of those things that I had completely avoided before [. . .] Yes I have a dream . . . being more independent [financially] through having a job. Sometimes I really wonder if I am that damaged that it's a utopia for me . . . but, then I think, if I really could make it, I would create a life together with my son."

3.4. Identity—Construction of a Self

The veterans described their identities as soldiers as strong and important parts of themselves in the first interview. Coming home, feeling different, and receiving a PTSD diagnosis had a huge impact on their lives. They said that being constrained and not being able to do the same things as before had resulted in their view of themselves as having changed, and this forced them to work on constructing another identity.

Almost all of the participants were young and had recently graduated when they were sent to war areas. They experienced how life as a soldier in a war zone often differed from their expectations, for example, that it was often difficult to distinguish enemies from civilians. The military rank system caused contrasting feelings: Some felt strengthened by rising up the ranks, while others felt the responsibility as a burden. There were also times when it was difficult to make situations fit into the rank system. One of the participants described a situation where he was accompanying a critically injured comrade into the helicopter to say goodbye. He felt this existential point between life and death where emotions exceeded the military rank within the group.

"Then my boss comes up to me and grabs me. I remember, I tried to get away, but then he gave me a hug. And then it starts! A tiny little spark . . . And then the priest comes over, and he's a fucking good priest. He's like a dad. He always blesses us when we go on patrol, and it might look silly on television, but it's bloody important when you're in a place like that."

All the veterans expressed in the first and second interviews that fellowship, the uniforms, the weapons, and the common language of the military were important factors which bonded them together and gave them a common identity. One of them expressed (15 years after leaving the military) how he still felt strongly connected to his weapon:

"Well it's a bit strange, but when I was in the military, I was walking in the night, it was much more comfortable if I had my rifle, although it was secured and only fired blanks . . . it was still my weapon, and it gave me some calmness and protection [. . .] and even when I walk around as a civilian, I miss it, walking at night."

Some veterans described that after returning home and experiencing the changes as a result of PTSD, their self-perception gradually turned into a feeling of alienation. One felt like he was just an observer of his own life instead of actually living it:

"I'm a stranger in the world, but also to my own body, and the only thing that ties me to the world is a sewing thread."

The NBT provided an insight into the participants' self-perception. During the first interview, one veteran described how he was no longer *"a master in his own house."* This can be interpreted as PTSD had taken over the control of his life. However, one year later, in the last interview, when asked the same question, he answered:

"I've found out that I don't even have the foundations of the house . . . you build up a little, and find out that it must be in another way because it doesn't work for me that way."

The participants said that when they were no longer able to serve as a soldier, finding a new occupation became an important task in constructing a new identity and being a respected member of society. When talking about his new job, one veteran said (interviewed one year after NBT):

"It's a place where I feel respected, and they talk to me as a human being and not just a worker, so I want to give more, and I can push myself more [. . .] I've got my professional pride back."

Being able to handle one's own situation is a huge step in gaining control over life in spite of having PTSD.

3.5. Lessons Learned, Reflections

During the therapy, the veterans experienced changes in their way of thinking and handling life situations presented in the four above themes. 'Lessons learned' can be seen as the veterans' own reflections on the whole process, from starting the NBT, to one year after it had ended.

The veterans expressed how the NBT helped them take more initiatives (for example, they became gradually more socialized) and find solutions (they could now use different tools) to the restrictions in their daily lives with PTSD.

"So I try to do different things . . . there's a dog's playground next to my place, and for a period, I sat on a bench nearby. Partly not to be too close, but on the other hand, I wanted to be so close that I got some human contact without being in focus."

One veteran reflected on how a better understanding and acceptance of himself could be a stepping stone to gaining more control of his life. However, it could also imply extra work:

"One might think about things in a totally different way now, and it [the PTSD symptoms] makes you rise to the challenge, but at the same time, you become more handicapped . . . or what you might say."

He used the word "handicapped", which is usually associated with a physical disability. However, the term expressed his feeling of being unable to function on equal terms with others.

Accepting one's needs and capacities was part of the NBT. It was a challenge for some of the participants to implement acceptance in their daily lives, as this was considered to be in opposition to structure and order as an expression of being in control. One veteran described how he had felt that untidiness and things being out of place was unacceptable before he took part in the NBT. However, now this was seen as a positive thing:

"I've found out that everything does not have to be exactly in order all the time, right? Before, it meant a great deal to me that everything was in the right place. I think it's because I found out that my head can't deal with it."

It takes time to implement some of the content from the NBT. During the third interview, one veteran talked about a frustrating episode in the garden: The horticultural therapist had asked all the veterans to hold hands in a circle and this was something he felt very uncomfortable doing. After a while, he spoke up and the therapist praised him for doing so:

"I was not the only one who felt that way,—but we are soldiers and follow orders [..]"

During the final interview, he mentioned the same episode again and said:

"I have changed now because I dare to say 'no', and it will be easier for me in my future life."

4. Discussion

First, a brief summary of the findings for each superordinate theme is presented. Then the results are discussed and related to the literature.

In general, the veterans experienced changes in their lives with PTSD from baseline to one year after the intervention. In the first interview, they described their bodily experiences from having PTSD as pain, sleep disturbances, high arousal, and flashbacks. For some, the changes occurred in the intervention period, while others described these changes in the last interview one year after the intervention. Not only had the symptoms decreased, the veterans also expressed a feeling of control in relation to distress.

The veterans described their relationships with their comrades during service as strong, and they felt guilty about leaving before completing their service or when comrades were killed. Being in a group of comrades that shared their experiences during the intervention helped them deal with the situation. Their relationships with family members were described as complex; the veterans wanted close relationships, but at the same time they were not always able to endure them. In the last interview, more veterans expressed how being in nature made them feel more calm, and how it was now less difficult to be with family and friends and to talk about their feelings.

All the veterans expressed a fear that the condition might worsen due to earlier experiences of highs and lows in relation to treatment. In the beginning of the intervention, the veterans expressed it as almost impossible to imagine the future. This changed during the intervention period. Through NBT, they seemed to gain more control over their lives, and it brought them to a state in which they dared to imagine a positive future.

The process of learning to accept the loss of their strong identity as a soldier and the creation of a new identity was described as demanding. For some veterans, being able to manage a job gave a feeling of being respected. During the intervention, the veterans improved their ability to find new solutions and strategies for handling challenges in their life in more appropriate ways.

When comparing the participants' bodily reactions, they were in line with frequently reported literature [5,18,80,81]. PTSD symptoms can be understood from a biological, physiological, or sociological perspective. Bosco et al. [82] reviewed three models for understanding PTSD and chronic pain. They mentioned how different models, the fear-avoidance model, the mutual maintenance model, and the shared vulnerability model, might contribute to the different aspects of understanding pain in this group. There is now a consensus that this type of pain related to PTSD does not have an external cause [83]. Ruden [84] found that the pain was often associated with somatosensory changes and comorbidity with mental diseases. He suggested that during the traumatic event an encoding occurred, where a sense of powerlessness and inability to take responsive action could lead to pain as an outcome of the event. He explained that emotions produced in a fearful situation might cause delayed pain after the event, activated by a subconscious stimulus from the memory of which the person is not necessarily aware. The NBT seemed to change the veterans' response to such situations and their reactions to their symptoms. The mindfulness exercises, where breathing exercises were used to maintain focus and bodily control [85], are believed to have had this impact. The stress-reducing effect of the intervention seems to have been useful. The NBT therapy garden was specifically designed to support people suffering from stress-related diseases [86,87].

The NBT offered the veterans an opportunity to join a group of fellow veterans. The veterans described how this fulfilled two of their needs: To be in a group representing the military culture with which they had lost connection, and to meet with people with similar experiences and PTSD symptoms.

The importance of relationships with comrades during service has also been identified in other studies [88,89], including studies of Danish soldiers [90] in which comrades were referred to as the 'military family'. The special culture that prevails in the military and the impact on young soldiers is well described in the literature [91,92]. In this culture, the individual is dedicated to the country and his fellow soldiers with binding commitment to his unit. The concept of honor is important and fundamental for the function of the military [93]. However, this also implies that seeking help could be seen as a sign of weakness, and it might even be seen as dangerous to have people in need of psychological help on a combat team [88,94]. The veterans in the present study expressed the feeling of failure and guilt when comrades died, and inadequacy due to not being able to finish their time of service. Having mental instead of visual physical wounds was considered problematic; one veteran even said that he felt that others thought he was a cheat.

All the veterans said that their families were very important parts of their lives, but at the same time the relationships were also a source of problems. During and after the NBT, the veterans handled their relationships with their families differently. Emotional numbing and the feeling of dissociation from their families were described as reasons for the complicated relationships. While numbness may be a useful emotion during war, it complicated the veterans' family relationships. Emotional numbness is listed as one of the PTSD symptoms that affects both the veterans and their families [5,26,94]. An important part of NBT is experiencing nature through the senses. Actions such as touching the bark of a tree, putting your hand in the stream and feeling the cold water, or listening to the birds activates positive memories and emotions. Establishing a relationship to nature can be a step toward establishing relationships to other human beings [95].

All the veterans who participated in the NBT wanted their lives to be less affected by PTSD. They asked for tools to help them reduce bodily stress and understand their bodily signals. This could be interpreted as an instrumental way of viewing the body as a 'thing' one must gain control over. This view may have its roots in the military system with discipline and bodily control [92,96], which has also been described by Foucault in his concept of "the docile bodies" [97]. However, through being in nature and doing therapeutic activities in nature, the participants learned some very concrete tools, such as breathing techniques, that facilitated a feeling of bodily control. Moreover, they also experienced a more spiritual awakening, for example, that seeking out nature can lead to an inner calmness. In addition, working with nature activities, such as producing bird boxes and hanging them on the trees in the garden, chopping firewood, or sowing seeds, was considered meaningful.

The design of the study made it possible to follow the effect of the NBT through the veterans' experiences. The theme "lessons learned" addressed the veterans' reflections regarding the effect. They mentioned acting more appropriately in difficult situations and using tools from the NBT as some of the positive effects of the therapy. NBT helped the veterans to develop dynamic strategies, which had a positive effect on their relationships, identity, and dreams for the future. Working with mindfulness activities seemed to give a deeper insight into themselves and their resources. The veterans described how working with 'acceptance' as part of the mindfulness activities gave them the opportunity to develop and deal with a new identity; maybe different from who they were before, but no longer an inferior version. Mindfulness conducted in a nature environment may have been tolerated better by the veterans, because many of the sounds like birdsong and running water are well known to the brain, and because no sudden noises, for example honking horns and people shouting, occur.

The NBT took place in nature and was an active contributor, both directly by simply being in nature, and indirectly through the horticultural activities. Kaplan [64] describes how soft fascination, which is stimulated by natural environments, has a restorative influence on individuals and helps reduce stress-related symptoms. Particularly the heightened arousal level that is part of PTSD symptoms seemed to be reduced by being in and sensing nature.

In the NBT, the therapeutic acceptance of the veterans' own experiences of their resources and support of their choice of activities (e.g., relaxing instead of being more active) built up the veterans' self-confidence. The veterans described how NBT influenced their ability to take the initiative and seek new solutions in their lives, and strengthened their capacity to construct a new identity. We do not necessarily see NBT as a treatment that is either a 'stand-alone' treatment or an 'add-on' therapy. The condition of the individual participant must be taken into account when determining the most beneficial treatment. Some of the veterans in this group had suffered from PTSD for just a few years, whereas as others had suffered from it for more than 18 years. Our results indicate that veterans who have been included in many 'vet programmes' or who have had bad experiences with medical treatment or who have felt that cognitive therapy was too provoking for their condition experienced the best results. This indicates that it is a suitable therapy for vulnerable veterans.

The study has some limitations. The participants were recruited through advertisements in newspapers and social media and webpages for soldiers and veterans. Therefore, our sample may have been comprised by a group of especially motivated veterans or veterans with especially mild or severe symptoms. In addition, only male veterans responded. However, the veterans in our study differed with regard to age and time since the onset of PTSD. In addition, they all represented rather well-known PTSD symptoms. Therefore, we think that our results are transferable to other male veterans. We cannot know if the results also apply to female veterans. As the study is qualitative, the question of generalisability cannot be answered. Nevertheless, the participants in our study experienced an effect of the intervention and the effect was sustained after one year. This means that the intervention is experienced as effectual by some male veterans.

5. Conclusions

The veterans of this study seemed to be split between two worlds. Living with the PTSD meant that at the beginning of the intervention, their awareness was in the military world; they had been enculturated to the military world with its extreme situations and they had lost the competences required to navigate in the civilian world. Their loyalty was also to the military world and was directed towards their comrades. They were locked emotionally in the traumatic situations they had experienced and brought their war identity home with them, where it did not fit in. They had to go through therapy to return home and adapt to a new civilian identity. The NBT helped them take on this new identity through a process where they, together with comrades, could gradually allow themselves to let go of their military identity. Even though they could not just take on their former identity again, the ability to relax again that they achieved through the experiences in nature helped them on their way to finding a new identity.

After the ten-week NBT programme in a therapy forest garden, the veterans diagnosed with PTSD reported that their bodily symptoms were less burdensome, and that being in a group with people with a similar military background and culture had been beneficial. Moreover, they noticed an improved ability to take part in social activities with their families. They had learnt to be more accepting of their condition and the slow pace of recovery, including the need for developing new identities. This opened a door to imagining a future again with an ability to work and improved self-esteem. The veterans' reflections on the NBT process at the follow-up revealed that tools from the therapy had enabled them to better handle potentially difficult situations and gain more control of their lives. This means that the results seem sustainable. In the last interview, all the veterans expressed that living with PTSD had become easier. Although the study is based on a small number of informants, the results seem promising and NBT should possibly be considered as a therapy complementary to the existing evidence-based therapies.

Author Contributions: D.V.P. and U.K.S. designed the study. D.V.P. collected data. Data analysis and interpretation was performed by D.V.P. and A.S.D. And D.V.P. and U.K.S. drafted the manuscript. All authors revised the manuscript and approved the final version of the manuscript.

Funding: The project was made possible with the financial support from the Soldiers' Foundation, University College Zealand, and University of Copenhagen.

Acknowledgments: The authors would like to thank the participants in the project, the horticultural therapists, and the therapists from Kalmia, the Center again stress.

References

1. Wise, J. *Digging for Victory: Horticultural Therapy with Veterans for Post-Traumatic Growth*; Routledge: Abingdon, UK, 2015.

2. Jones, E.; Wessely, S. Battle for the Mind: World War 1 and the Birth of Military Psychiatry. *Lancet* **2014**, *384*, 1708–1714. [CrossRef]

3. Chater, K. Exploring a Growing Field: Canadian Horticultural Therapy Organizations. Ph.D. Thesis, City University of Seattle, Seattle, MA, USA, 2015.

4. Reed, C.; Christopher. The Origins, Development and Perceived Effectiveness of Horticulture-Based Therapy in Victoria. Ph.D. Thesis, Deakin Univeristy, Victoria, Australia, 2015.

5. American Psychiatric Association. *Diagnostic and Statistical Manual of Mental Disorders*, 5th ed.; American Psychiatric Association: Washington, DC, USA, 2013.

6. Dursa, E.K.; Reinhard, M.J.; Barth, S.K.; Schneiderman, A.I. Prevalence of a Positive Screen for PTSD among OEF/OIF and OEF/OIF-Era Veterans in a Large Population-Based Cohort. *J. Trauma. Stress* **2014**, *27*, 542–549. [CrossRef] [PubMed]

7. McFarlane, A.; Hodson, S.E. *Mental Health in the Australian Defence Force: 2010 ADF Mental Health Prevalence and Wellbeing Study: Report*; Department of Defence: Washington, DC, USA, 2011.

8. Hoge, C.W.; Auchterlonie, J.L.; Milliken, C.S. Mental Health Problems, Use of Mental Health Services, and Attrition from Military Service after Returning from Deployment to Iraq or Afghanistan. *JAMA* **2006**, *295*, 1023–1032. [CrossRef] [PubMed]

9. Richardson, L.K.; Frueh, B.C.; Acierno, R. Prevalence Estimates of Combat-Related Post-Traumatic Stress Disorder: Critical Review. *Aust. N. Z. J. Psychiatry* **2010**, *44*, 4–19. [CrossRef] [PubMed]

10. Zamorski, M.A.; Bennett, R.E.; Rusu, C.; Weeks, M.; Boulos, D.; Garber, B.G. Prevalence of Past-Year Mental Disorders in the Canadian Armed Forces, 2002–2013. *Can. J. Psychiatry* **2016**, *61* (Suppl. 1), 26S–35S. [CrossRef] [PubMed]

11. Fulton, J.J.; Calhoun, P.S.; Wagner, H.R.; Schry, A.R.; Hair, L.P.; Feeling, N.; Elbogen, E.; Beckham, J.C. The Prevalence of Posttraumatic Stress Disorder in Operation Enduring Freedom/Operation Iraqi Freedom (OEF/OIF) Veterans: A Meta-Analysis. *J. Anxiety Disord.* **2015**, *31*, 98–107. [CrossRef] [PubMed]

12. Karstoft, K.-I.; Nielsen, A.B.S.; Andersen, S.B. *ISAF7—6,5 År Efter Hjemkomst*; Veterancentret: Copenhagen, Denmark, 2017.

13. Reisman, M. PTSD Treatment for Veterans: What's Working, What's New, and What's Next. *Pharm. Ther.* **2016**, *41*, 623–627, 632–634.

14. Andrews, B.; Brewin, C.R.; Philpott, R.; Stewart, L. Delayed-Onset Posttraumatic Stress Disorder: A Systematic Review of the Evidence. *Am. J. Psychiatry* **2007**, *164*, 1319–1326. [CrossRef] [PubMed]

15. Dobson, A.; Treloar, S.; Zheng, W.; Anderson, R.; Bredhauer, K.; Kanesarajah, J.; Loos, C.; Pasmore, K. *Census Study Report*; Centre for Military and Veterans Health, The University of Queensland: Brisbane, Australia, 2012.

16. The Mental Health of the UK Armed Forces. 2013. Available online: https://www.kcl.ac.uk/kcmhr/publications/Reports/Files/mentalhealthsummary.pdf (accessed on 1 June 2018).

17. Hoge, C.W.; Terhakopian, A.; Castro, C.A.; Messer, S.C.; Engel, C.C. Association of Posttraumatic Stress Disorder with Somatic Symptoms, Health Care Visits, and Absenteeism among Iraq War Veterans. *Am. J. Psychiatry* **2007**, *164*, 150–153. [CrossRef] [PubMed]

18. Lew, H.L.; Otis, J.D.; Tun, C.; Kerns, R.D.; Clark, M.E.; Cifu, D.X.; Otis, J.D.; Tun, C.; Kerns, R.D.; Clark, M.E.; et al. Prevalence of Chronic Pain, Posttraumatic Stress Disorder, and Persistent Postconcussive Symptoms in OIF/OEF Veterans: Polytrauma Clinical Triad. *J. Rehabil. Res. Dev.* **2009**, *46*, 697–702. [CrossRef] [PubMed]

19. Asnaani, A.; Reddy, M.K.; Shea, M.T. The Impact of PTSD Symptoms on Physical and Mental Health Functioning in Returning Veterans. *J. Anxiety Disord.* **2014**, *28*, 310–317. [CrossRef] [PubMed]

20. Norman, S.B.; Haller, M.; Hamblen, J.L.; Southwick, S.M.; Pietrzak, R.H. The Burden of Co-Occurring Alcohol Use Disorder and PTSD in U.S. Military Veterans: Comorbidities, Functioning, and Suicidality. *Psychol. Addict. Behav.* **2018**, *32*, 224–229. [CrossRef] [PubMed]

21. Keane, T.M.; Kaloupek, D.G. Comorbid Psychiatric Disorders in PTSD. *Ann. N. Y. Acad. Sci.* **1997**, *821*, 24–34. [CrossRef] [PubMed]

22. Milliken, C.S.; Auchterlonie, J.L.; Hoge, C.W. Longitudinal Assessment of Mental Health Problems among Active and Reserve Component Soldiers Returning from the Iraq War. *JAMA* **2007**, *298*, 2141–2148. [CrossRef] [PubMed]

23. Barrett, D.H.; Doebbeling, C.C.; Schwartz, D.A.; Voelker, M.D.; Falter, K.H.; Woolson, R.F.; Doebbeling, B.N. Posttraumatic Stress Disorder and Self-Reported Physical Health Status among US Military Personnel Serving during the Gulf War Period: A Population-Based Study. *Psychosomatics* **2002**, *43*, 195–205. [CrossRef] [PubMed]

24. Galovski, T.; Lyons, J.A. Psychological Sequelae of Combat Violence: A Review of the Impact of PTSD on the Veteran's Family and Possible Interventions. *Aggress. Violent Behav.* **2004**, *9*, 477–501. [CrossRef]

25. Vogt, D.; Smith, B.N.; Fox, A.B.; Amoroso, T.; Taverna, E.; Schnurr, P.P. Consequences of PTSD for the Work and Family Quality of Life of Female and Male U.S. Afghanistan and Iraq War Veterans. *Soc. Psychiatry Psychiatr. Epidemiol.* **2017**, *52*, 341–352. [CrossRef] [PubMed]

26. Ray, S.L.; Vanstone, M. The Impact of PTSD on Veterans' Family Relationships: An Interpretative Phenomenological Inquiry. *Int. J. Nurs. Stud.* **2009**, *46*, 838–847. [CrossRef] [PubMed]

27. RAND Corporation. 2008. Available online: http://www.rand.org/news/press/2008/04/17.html (accessed on 1 June 2018).

28. Tanielian, T.L.; Jaycox, L. *Invisible Wounds of War: Psychological and Cognitive Injuries, Their Consequences, and Services to Assist Recovery*; Rand Corporation: Santa Monica, CA, USA, 2008; Volume 1.

29. Puetz, T.W.; Youngstedt, S.D.; Herring, M.P. Effects of Pharmacotherapy on Combat-Related PTSD, Anxiety, and Depression: A Systematic Review and Meta-Regression Analysis. *PLoS ONE* **2015**, *10*, e0126529. [CrossRef] [PubMed]

30. Lipinska, G.; Baldwin, D.S.; Thomas, K.G.F. Pharmacology for Sleep Disturbance in PTSD. *Hum. Psychopharmacol. Clin. Exp.* **2016**, *31*, 156–163. [CrossRef] [PubMed]

31. Hoge, C.W.; Grossman, S.H.; Auchterlonie, J.L.; Riviere, L.A.; Milliken, C.S.; Wilk, J.E. PTSD Treatment for Soldiers after Combat Deployment: Low Utilization of Mental Health Care and Reasons for Dropout. *Psychiatr. Serv.* **2014**, *65*, 997–1004. [CrossRef] [PubMed]

32. Office of Evidence. *VA/DOD Clinical Practice Guideline for the Management of Posttraumatic Stress Disorder and Acute Stress Disorder the Management of Posttraumatic Stress Disorder Work Group the Office of Quality, Safety and Value*; Office of Evidence: Washington, DC, USA, 2017.

33. McLay, R.N.; Wood, D.P.; Webb-Murphy, J.A.; Spira, J.L.; Wiederhold, M.D.; Pyne, J.M.; Wiederhold, B.K. A Randomized, Controlled Trial of Virtual Reality-Graded Exposure Therapy for Post-Traumatic Stress Disorder in Active Duty Service Members with Combat-Related Post-Traumatic Stress Disorder. *Cyberpsychol. Behav. Soc. Netw.* **2011**, *14*, 223–229. [CrossRef] [PubMed]

34. Goodson, J.; Helstrom, A.; Halpern, J.M.; Ferenschak, M.P.; Gillihan, S.J.; Powers, M.B. Treatment of Posttraumatic Stress Disorder in US Combat Veterans: A Meta-Analytic Review 1. *Psychol. Rep.* **2011**, *109*, 573–599. [CrossRef] [PubMed]

35. Resick, P.A.; Wachen, J.S.; Mintz, J.; Young-McCaughan, S.; Roache, J.D.; Borah, A.M.; Borah, E.V.; Dondanville, K.A.; Hembree, E.A.; Litz, B.T.; et al. A Randomized Clinical Trial of Group Cognitive Processing Therapy Compared with Group Present-Centered Therapy for PTSD among Active Duty Military Personnel. *J. Consult. Clin. Psychol.* **2015**, *83*, 1058–1068. [CrossRef] [PubMed]

36. Forbes, D.; Lloyd, D.; Nixon, R.D.V.; Elliott, P.; Varker, T.; Perry, D.; Bryant, R.A.; Creamer, M. A Multisite Randomized Controlled Effectiveness Trial of Cognitive Processing Therapy for Military-Related Posttraumatic Stress Disorder. *J. Anxiety Disord.* **2012**, *26*, 442–452. [CrossRef] [PubMed]

37. Frost, N.D.; Laska, K.M.; Wampold, B.E. The Evidence for Present-Centered Therapy as a Treatment for Posttraumatic Stress Disorder. *J. Trauma. Stress* **2014**, *27*, 1–8. [CrossRef] [PubMed]

38. Lorber, H.L. The Use of Horticulture in the Treatment of Post-Traumatic Stress Disorder in a Private Practice Setting. *J. Ther. Hortic.* **2011**, *21*, 18–29.

39. Steenkamp, M.M.; Litz, B.T.; Hoge, C.W.; Marmar, C.R. Psychotherapy for Military-Related PTSD. *JAMA* **2015**, *314*, 489. [CrossRef] [PubMed]

40. Haagen, J.F.G.; Smid, G.E.; Knipscheer, J.W.; Kleber, R.J. The Efficacy of Recommended Treatments for Veterans with PTSD: A Metaregression Analysis. *Clin. Psychol. Rev.* **2015**, *40*, 184–194. [CrossRef] [PubMed]

41. Hopwood, T.L.; Schutte, N.S. A Meta-Analytic Investigation of the Impact of Mindfulness-Based Interventions on Post Traumatic Stress. *Clin. Psychol. Rev.* **2017**, *57*, 12–20. [CrossRef] [PubMed]

42. Polusny, M.A.; Erbes, C.R.; Thuras, P.; Moran, A.; Lamberty, G.J.; Collins, R.C.; Rodman, J.L.; Lim, K.O. Mindfulness-Based Stress Reduction for Posttraumatic Stress Disorder Among Veterans. *JAMA* **2015**, *314*, 456. [CrossRef] [PubMed]

43. O'Malley, P.G. In Veterans with PTSD, Mindfulness-Based Group Therapy Reduced Symptom Severity. *Ann. Intern. Med.* **2015**, *163*, 15–163. [CrossRef] [PubMed]

44. Serpa, J.G.; Taylor, S.L.; Tillisch, K. Mindfulness-Based Stress Reduction (MBSR) Reduces Anxiety, Depression, and Suicidal Ideation in Veterans. *Med. Care* **2014**, *52*, S19–S24. [CrossRef] [PubMed]

45. Niles, B.L.; Polizzi, C.P.; Voelkel, E.; Weinstein, E.S.; Smidt, K.; Fisher, L.M. *Initiation, Dropout, and Outcome from Evidence-Based Psychotherapies in a VA PTSD Outpatient Clinic*; American Psychological Association: Washington, DC, USA, 2017.

46. Imel, Z.E.; Laska, K.; Jakupcak, M.; Simpson, T.L. Meta-Analysis of Dropout in Treatments for Posttraumatic Stress Disorder. *J. Consult. Clin. Psychol.* **2013**, *81*, 394–404. [CrossRef] [PubMed]

47. Yehuda, R.; Hoge, C.W. The Meaning of Evidence-Based Treatments for Veterans with Posttraumatic Stress Disorder. *JAMA Psychiatry* **2016**, *73*, 433. [CrossRef] [PubMed]

48. Blais, R.K.; Renshaw, K.D. Stigma and Demographic Correlates of Help-Seeking Intentions in Returning Service Members. *J. Trauma. Stress* **2013**, *26*, 77–85. [CrossRef] [PubMed]

49. Miller, S.M.; Pedersen, E.R.; Marshall, G.N. Combat Experience and Problem Drinking in Veterans: Exploring the Roles of PTSD, Coping Motives, and Perceived Stigma. *Addict. Behav.* **2017**, *66*, 90–95. [CrossRef] [PubMed]

50. Bonfils, K.A.; Lysaker, P.H.; Yanos, P.T.; Siegel, A.; Leonhardt, B.L.; James, A.V.; Brustuen, B.; Luedtke, B.; Davis, L.W. Self-Stigma in PTSD: Prevalence and Correlates. *Psychiatry Res.* **2018**, *265*, 7–12. [CrossRef] [PubMed]

51. Yehuda, R.; Vermetten, E.; McFarlane, A.C.; Lehrner, A. PTSD in the Military: Special Considerations for Understanding Prevalence, Pathophysiology and Treatment Following Deployment. *Eur. J. Psychotraumatol.* **2014**, *5*, 25322. [CrossRef] [PubMed]

52. McMahan, E.A.; Estes, D. The Effect of Contact with Natural Environments on Positive and Negative Affect: A Meta-Analysis. *J. Posit. Psychol.* **2015**, *10*, 507–519. [CrossRef]

53. Hartig, T.; Mitchell, R.; de Vries, S.; Frumkin, H. Nature and Health. *Annu. Rev. Public Health* **2014**, *35*, 207–228. [CrossRef] [PubMed]

54. Han, K.-T. The Effect of Nature and Physical Activity on Emotions and Attention While Engaging in Green Exercise. *Urban For. Urban Green.* **2017**, *24*, 5–13. [CrossRef]

55. Sidenius, U.; Stigsdotter, U.K.; Dahl Refshauge, A. A Year in the Therapy Forest Garden Nacadia®-Participants' Use and Preferred Locations in the Garden during a Nature-Based Treatment Program. *Int. J. Sustain. Trop. Des. Res. Pract.* **2015**, *8*, 44–53.

56. Corazon, S.S.; Nyed, P.K.; Sidenius, U.; Poulsen, D.V.; Stigsdotter, U.K. A Long-Term Follow-up of the Efficacy of Nature-Based Therapy for Adults Suffering from Stress-Related Illnesses on Levels of Healthcare Consumption and Sick-Leave Absence: A Randomized Controlled Trial. *Int. J. Environ. Res. Public Health* **2018**, *15*, 137. [CrossRef] [PubMed]

57. Lee, I.; Choi, H.; Bang, K.-S.; Kim, S.; Song, M.; Lee, B. Effects of Forest Therapy on Depressive Symptoms among Adults: A Systematic Review. *Int. J. Environ. Res. Public Health* **2017**, *14*, 321. [CrossRef] [PubMed]

58. Grahn, P.; Pálsdóttir, A.M.; Ottosson, J.; Jonsdottir, I.H. Longer Nature-Based Rehabilitation May Contribute to a Faster Return to Work in Patients with Reactions to Severe Stress and/or Depression. *Int. J. Environ. Res. Public Health* **2017**, *14*, 1310. [CrossRef] [PubMed]

59. Lee, S.; Kim, M.S.; Suh, J.K. Effects of Horticultural Therapy of Self-Esteem and Depression of Battered Women at a Shelter in Korea. In Proceedings of the 8th International People-Plant Symposium Proceedings, Awaji, Japan, 4–6 June 2004; pp. 139–142.

60. Debeer, B.B.; Kimbrel, N.A.; Meyer, E.C.; Gulliver, S.B.; Morissette, S.B. Combined PTSD and Depressive Symptoms Interact with Post-Deployment Social Support to Predict Suicidal Ideation in Operation Enduring Freedom and Operation Iraqi Freedom Veterans. *Psychiatry Res.* **2014**, *216*, 357–362. [CrossRef] [PubMed]

61. Kimbrel, N.A.; Meyer, E.C.; DeBeer, B.B.; Gulliver, S.B.; Morissette, S.B. A 12-Month Prospective Study of the Effects of PTSD-Depression Comorbidity on Suicidal Behavior in Iraq/Afghanistan-Era Veterans. *Psychiatry Res.* **2016**, *243*, 97–99. [CrossRef] [PubMed]

62. Shoemaker, C.A. The Profession of Horticultural Therapy Compared with Other Allied Therapies. *J. Ther. Hortic.* **2002**, *13*, 74–81.

63. Hewson, M.L. *Horticulture as Therapy: A Practical Guide to Using Horticulture as a Therapeutic Tool*; Idyll Arbor: Enumclaw, WA, USA, 1994.

64. Kaplan, S. The Restorative Benefits of Nature: Toward an Integrative Framework. *J. Environ. Psychol.* **1995**, *15*, 169–182. [CrossRef]

65. Duvall, J.; Kaplan, R. Enhancing the Well-Being of Veterans Using Extended Group-Based Nature Recreation Experiences. *J. Rehabil. Res. Dev.* **2014**, *51*, 685–696. [CrossRef] [PubMed]

66. Hawkins, B.L.; Townsend, J.A.; Garst, B.A. Nature-Based Recreational Therapy for Military Service Members A Strengths Approach. *Ther. Recreat. J.* **2016**, *50*, 55–74. [CrossRef]

67. Duvall, J.; Kaplan, R. Exploring the Benefits of Outdoor Experiences on Veterans. *Ann. Arbor.* **2013**, *1001*, 48109–51041.

68. Kaplan, R.; Kaplan, S.; Ryan, R. *With People in Mind: Design and Management of Everyday Nature*; Island Press: Washington, DC, USA, 1998.

69. Harper, N.J.; Norris, J.; D'astous, M. Veterans and the Outward Bound Experience: An Evaluation of Impact and Meaning. *Ecopsychology* **2014**, *6*, 165–173.

70. Poulsen, D.V.; Stigsdotter, U.K.; Refshage, A.D. Whatever Happened to the Soldiers? Nature-Assisted Therapies for Veterans Diagnosed with Post-Traumatic Stress Disorder: A Literature Review. *Urban For. Urban Green.* **2015**, *14*, 438–445. [CrossRef]

71. Corazon, S.S.; Stigsdotter, U.K.; Jensen, A.G.C.; Nilsson, K. Development of the Nature-Based Therapy Concept for Patients with Stress-Related Illness at the Danish Healing Forest Garden Nacadia. *J. Ther. Hortic.* **2010**, *20*, 33–51.

72. Mehling, W.E.; Price, C.; Daubenmier, J.J.; Acree, M.; Bartmess, E.; Stewart, A. The Multidimensional Assessment of Interoceptive Awareness (MAIA). *PLoS ONE* **2012**, *7*, e48230. [CrossRef] [PubMed]

73. Hersen, M.; Thomas, J.C. *Handbook of Clinical Interviewing with Adults*; Sage Publications: Thousand Oaks, CA, USA, 2007.

74. Rubin, H.J.; Rubin, I. *Qualitative Interviewing: The Art of Hearing Data*, 3rd ed.; SAGE: Thousand Oaks, CA, USA, 2012.

75. Smith, J.; Flowers, P.; Larkin, M. *Interpretative Phoneomological Analysis: Theory, Method and Research*; Sage Publications: Thousand Oaks, CA, USA, 2009.

76. Smith, J.A. *Qualitative Psychology: A Practical Guide to Research Methods*; Sage Publications: Thousand Oaks, CA, USA, 2007.

77. Murray, S.J.; Holmes, D. Interpretive Phenomenological Analysis (IPA) and the Ethics of Body and Place: Critical Methodological Reflections. *Hum. Stud.* **2014**, *37*, 15–30. [CrossRef]

78. VanScoy, A.; Evenstad, S.B. Interpretative Phenomenological Analysis for LIS Research. *J. Doc.* **2015**, *71*, 338–357. [CrossRef]

79. Pietkiewicz, I.; Smith, J.A. A Practical Guide to Using Interpretative Phenomenological Analysis in Qualitative Research Psychology. *Psychol. J.* **2014**, *20*, 7–14.

80. Pacella, M.L.; Hruska, B.; Delahanty, D.L. The Physical Health Consequences of PTSD and PTSD Symptoms: A Meta-Analytic Review. *J. Anxiety Disord.* **2013**, *27*, 33–46. [CrossRef] [PubMed]

81. Gironda, R.J.; Clark, M.E.; Massengale, J.P.; Walker, R.L. Pain among Veterans of Operations Enduring Freedom and Iraqi Freedom. *Pain Med.* **2006**, *7*, 339–343. [CrossRef] [PubMed]

82. Bosco, M.A.; Gallinati, J.L.; Clark, M.E. Conceptualizing and Treating Comorbid Chronic Pain and PTSD. *Pain Res. Treat.* **2013**, *2013*, 174728. [CrossRef] [PubMed]

83. Woolf, C.J. Central Sensitization: Implications for the Diagnosis and Treatment of Pain. *Pain* **2011**, *152*, S2–S15. [CrossRef] [PubMed]

84. Ruden, R.A. Encoding States: A Model for the Origin and Treatment of Complex Psychogenic Pain. *Traumatol. Int. J.* **2008**, *14*, 119–126. [CrossRef]

85. Kabat-Zinn, J. *Full Catastrophe Living: How to Cope with Stress, Pain and Illness Using Mindfulness Meditation*, 2nd ed.; Bantam Books: New York, NY, USA, 2013.

86. Stigsdotter, U.K. Nacadia Healing Forest Garden, Hoersholm Arboretum, Copenhagen, Denmark. In *Therapeutic Landscapes: An Evidence-Based Approach to Designing Healing Gardens and Restorative Outdoor Spaces*; Marcus, C.C., Sachs, N.A., Eds.; John Wiley & Sons Ltd.: Hoboken, NJ, USA, 2013; pp. 198–205.

87. Stigsdotter, U.K.; Grahn, P. What Makes a Garden a Healing Garden. *J. Ther. Hortic.* **2002**, *13*, 60–69.

88. Coll, J.E.; Weiss, E.L.; Yarvis, J.S. No One Leaves Unchanged: Insights for Civilian Mental Health Care Professionals into the Military Experience and Culture. *Soc. Work Health Care* **2011**, *50*, 487–500. [CrossRef] [PubMed]

89. Demers, A. When Veterans Return: The Role of Community in Reintegration. *J. Loss Trauma* **2011**, *16*, 160–179. [CrossRef]

90. Andersen, S.B.; Madsen, T.; Karstoft, K.-I.; Elklit, A.; Nordentoft, M.; Bertelsen, M. *Efter Afghanistan-Rapport over Soldaters Psykiske Velbefindende to et Halvt År Efter Hjemkomst*; Veterancentret: Copenhagen, Denmark, 2013.

91. Green, G.; Emslie, C.; O'Neill, D.; Hunt, K.; Walker, S. Exploring the Ambiguities of Masculinity in Accounts of Emotional Distress in the Military among Young Ex-Servicemen. *Soc. Sci. Med.* **2010**, *71*, 1480–1488. [CrossRef] [PubMed]

92. Hall, L.K. The Importance of Understanding Military Culture. *Soc. Work Health Care* **2011**, *50*, 4–18. [CrossRef] [PubMed]

93. Reger, M.A.; Etherage, J.R.; Reger, G.M.; Gahm, G.A. Civilian Psychologists in an Army Culture: The Ethical Challenge of Cultural Competence. *Mil. Psychol.* **2008**, *20*, 21. [CrossRef]

94. Sayers, S.L.; Farrow, V.A.; Ross, J.; Oslin, D.W. Family Problems among Recently Returned Military Veterans Referred for a Mental Health Evaluation. *J. Clin. Psychiatry* **2009**, *70*, 163. [CrossRef] [PubMed]

95. Ottosson, J. The Importance of Nature in Coping with a Crisis: A Photographic Essay. *Landsc. Res.* **2001**, *26*, 165–172. [CrossRef]

96. Eichberg, H. Body Culture. *Phys. Cult. Sport Res.* **2009**, *46*, 79–98. [CrossRef]

97. Foucault, M. *Discipline and Punish Trans. The Birth of the Prison*; Vintage Books: New York, NY, USA, 1979.

15

Signs in People with Intellectual Disabilities: Interviews with Managers and Staff on the Identification Process of Dementia

Göran Holst [1] (iD), Maria Johansson [2] (iD) and Gerd Ahlström [2,*] (iD)

[1] The Swedish Red Cross University College, Box 1059, SE-141 21 Stockholm, Sweden; Goran.Holst@rkh.se
[2] Department of Health Sciences, Faculty of Medicine, Lund University, Box 157, SE-221 00 Lund, Sweden; maria.johansson@med.lu.se
*   Correspondence: gerd.ahlstrom@med.lu.se

Abstract: The life expectancy of people with intellectual disabilities (ID) has steadily increased, which has been accompanied by an increased risk of dementia. Staff and managers are key resources for safety diagnosis since they deliver information about people with ID behavior every day. The aim of the present study was to explore the identification process employed by staff and managers to detect signs of suspected dementia in people with an ID within intellectual disability services (ID-services). Twenty managers and 24 staff within an ID-service were interviewed and qualitative latent content analysis was applied. A model consisting of three themes on three levels of resources for the identification process of signs of suspected dementia emerged from the analysis. On the first level was the time and continuity in the care relationship, which is crucial for identifying and responding to changes in cognitive ability that indicate dementia. On the second level, the staff identify deficiencies in their own knowledge, seek support from colleagues and managers within their workplace and, on the third level, outside their workplace. Staff and managers expressed a need for early and continuous guidance and education from specialists in dementia and primary healthcare. This finding indicates an urgent need for intervention research and digital support for staff in dementia care.

Keywords: intellectual disability; mental retardation; learning disability; older people; dementia; signs of dementia; frailty; qualitative study; interview study; caregivers' experiences

1. Introduction

Aging people in the general population and dementia prevalence are increasing [1], as well as for people with an intellectual disability (ID). [1]. ID is typically a life-long condition with onsets occurring before the age of 18 years characterized by significant limitations in intellectual and cognitive functioning as expressed in reasoning, learning, problem solving, and behavior adaptive skills [2,3]. Aging people with an ID have a high incidence of dementia and, especially among people with Down's syndrome, dementia presents early [4,5]. When people with an ID are aging, many of them are cared for in community residential care [6]. The characteristics of developing dementia in a general population are mainly stated in the form of increasing memory difficulties, language difficulties, and, hence, difficulties in coping with many of the challenges of everyday life. Recognizing these changes in people with an ID is even more complex and implies several challenges [7,8] in the sense that they already have a cognitive impairment and linguistic difficulties. Even depression and anxiety, which are common in the early stages of dementia, are more difficult to detect in people with an ID [8]. Previous research about dementia among older people with ID comprised issues regarding epidemiology, assessments tools for diagnosis, and management in the form of pharmacological and non-pharmacological treatment [9]. However, assessment for early identification of dementia can be complicated due to a lack of well-established instruments adapted to people with ID, which also had comprehensive information about reliability and validity. The most instruments used to diagnose dementia are based on people who previously had intact cognitive functioning. Due to the pre-existing decreased cognitive abilities in the population with ID, the early detection of dementia is challenging. However, accurate screening for diagnosis of dementia is crucial in order to provide appropriate interventions, care, and support as early as possible [10–14].

People with an ID have the same right as others for an investigation based on the individual's needs and ability when they show signs of dementia [15]. However, a barrier to meeting this requirement in practice is the absence of a clear structure and methodological support for the implementation of a dementia investigation adapted to people with an ID. According to The British Psychological Society [16], there has been an awareness for several years about dementia mainly in the general population and a proliferation of strategies and standards documents have ensued. However, dementia among people with an ID has still received minimal focus. One possible reason for this is the diagnostic challenges due to the complexity involved in detecting the early signs of dementia in a person with an ID, which is mentioned above. However, Moran and colleagues [17] focus on an assessment in several steps conducted using national recommendations for the evaluation and management of dementia. This includes a medical examination, review of medications, baseline functioning, current functioning, and documentation of family and social history. Therefore, a family member or caregiver have, along with the medical specialist, a decisive role in such an investigation due to their knowledge about the history of the person with an ID [17].

Staff and managers are key resources for supporting dementia care in the early stages of screening and diagnosing dementia by delivering information about the person with an ID who lives and is cared for in residential care [8]. It is well known that people with an ID may have difficulty seeking care, according to their actual needs. One of the reasons may be the difficulty to express their wishes and needs in a manner that is understandable to others. Furthermore, because of their ID, they may show signs that may be similar to cognitive difficulties that develop in dementia patients, which may complicate the investigation and further planning for adapted care [8]. Based on findings from an explorative study conducted by Cleary and Doody [18], knowing the person well is a key element in providing a mode of care that supports and comforts the person with an ID or dementia, i.e., providing a mode of care according to actual needs. In a review of the literature by Cleary and Doody [19], it was found that a professional caregiver considered caring for people with an intellectual disability and dementia sometimes challenging, stressful, and time consuming and believed that professional caregivers required further knowledge and educational training concerning all stages of dementia. It was also found that the ability of staff to seek advice and support from multidisciplinary professionals and management appears to be determined based on successful coping and an ability to handle these challenges [19].

In addition, leaders greatly influence the quality of the services and care delivered to people with an ID. Studies have shown the importance of leaders in organizations and their indirect influence on outcomes [20] through their leadership of the staff [21]. The development and the support of staff need to focus on the service users´ quality of life, how and when support is delivered, and the organization of meaningful activities for the service users [21]. Taking into consideration the important role of staff and managers for the person with an ID in the early stages of dementia, their experience should, therefore, be explored and can thus provide a source of knowledge about how signs of dementia can manifest in everyday life. This knowledge may lead to continued development of a person-centered care aimed at persons with an ID and dementia. Therefore, the aim of the present study was to explore the identification process employed by staff and managers to detect signs of suspected dementia in people with an ID within intellectual disability services.

2. Materials and Methods

The design of the study was an explorative qualitative semi-structured interview study with staff and managers within the intellectual disability service for people with an ID.

2.1. Study Setting

The Swedish welfare system is mainly public, largely funded by taxes, and designed to provide everyone with equal access to health care, elderly care, and disability and social services based on each person's need for services, support, and care. The responsibility is shared between 21 county councils (primary health care and specialist health care) and 290 municipalities (elderly care, disability, and social services). Since 1994, there is an entitlement law in Sweden named the *LSS* (Act Concerning Support and Service for People with Certain Functional Impairments), which is based on the Human Rights Convention [22,23] and for people with extensive and permanent functional impairment. This Act guarantees that people with comprehensive disabilities have the right to the same living conditions as the general population, which ensures support in daily living and the capacity to influence the received support. A person who fulfill the criteria of the LSS Act can apply for support, personally or with support from someone else, and any decision on a measure under the LSS can be appealed at the County Administrative Court [15]. The eight support services for adult persons with an ID, according to LSS, are: Residence with special services for adults or other specially adapted housing, daily activities, counseling and other personal support, personal assistance, companion service, contact person, relief service in the home, and a short stay away from home [22].

The current Swedish policy for people with a disability as well as for older people in the general population is "aging in place", which means enabling people to continue to live in their own homes for as long as possible and providing assistance in accordance with their needs [24]. A group home is a private-residence located in a block of flats or a house in ordinary housing areas with special services or specially adapted accommodation for people with an ID [15]. Residents have their own small flat and share common areas such as a dining room and a large kitchen. Each group home houses 6 to 8 people from 18 years of age or older with different levels of ID. They receive the support needed in daily living from the staff at the group home who are available 24 hours a day. The residents pay a plausible fee for accommodation, recreation, and cultural activities but must be left with a sufficient amount of money for personal use.

People with ID have a right to participate in daily activity centers up to five days a week from the age of 18 to the age of 67. Activities at the daily activity centers give people with ID who are not working in the labor market nor studying some interesting and meaningful, day-to-day structured activities. The daily activity centers provide various types of activities from more open social cohesion to more structured employment adapted to the needs of each individual. It is mandatory for the municipalities to provide intellectual disability services (ID-service) in Sweden in accordance with the *LSS act* [15,22].

2.2. Sampling and Participants

2.2.1. The Selection of Managers

The study included staff and managers working in an ID-service in a Southern city in Sweden. The inclusion criterion for managers to participate in the study was that they have had experience leading a group home or daily activity center where older residents 55 years of age and above live or have lived. The inclusion criteria for staff attending the study were at least one year of experience in working in one of these organizations and experience in providing support to older persons with IDs aged 55 or above. The first-line managers in the municipality were in general responsible for two to three group homes or daily activity centers while the second-line managers were responsible for all first-line managers within their designated area of the town.

All 12 second-line managers in the current city were contacted by e-mail with an informative letter about the study and a request to participate in the study if they fulfilled the inclusion criteria. The second-line managers then contacted the first-line managers within the relevant responsibility area with information letters and a request to participate in the study. There were four second-line managers and 16 first-line managers who judged that they met the criteria and accepted to participate in the study. These managers were included in this study. Fifteen of the 20 managers worked in group homes and five worked in daily activity centers. Five were men and 15 were women. To avoid the risk of revealing the four second-line managers' identities, no more background data were collected about the participating managers.

2.2.2. The Selection of Staff

The 16 first-line managers were given an information letter to hand to the staff in the group homes or the daily activity centers where they work as managers and asked whether they were interested in participating in the study. Twenty-seven staff wanted to participate in the study. Two of them were dropouts because of long sick-leave and one for unknown reasons. Thus, 24 staff were included in this study. Seventeen of the 24 staff worked in group homes and seven worked at daily activity centers. Four were men and 20 were women. The age of the staff ranged from 24 to 65 years of age with a mean age of 48 years (SD 10.4). They had between 2 and 41 years of experience working in a group home or a daily activity center and 75% of them had more than nine years of experience. Four of them had a university level education, six had a post-secondary education (post-gymnasium), 13 had two or three years of secondary education (gymnasium), and one person had elementary education.

Thus, the total study group was comprised of 44 participants.

2.3. Data Collection

The interviewer (MJ) contacted the managers and staff and asked about the willingness to participate after given information about the study and a time for the interview was decided. Just before the interview, the information about the study was repeated orally and the participants were given the opportunity to ask questions before signing a written informed consent. All interviews took place at the workplace of the managers and staff outside of the place in which people with IDs have their activities.

A semi-structured interview guide was used in the 44 interviews, which had two main questions: What does aging mean for a person with an ID? and How do you perceive the need for support, service, and care in aging people with an ID? Follow-up questions were asked depending on how comprehensively the interviewee had answered the main open questions. The interviews were taped digitally and transcribed verbatim including pauses and emotional expressions. In the interviews emerged rich narratives that revealed that aging with ID for managers and staff meant having concern about providing service to persons who they believed had dementia. Thus, this became the focus of this study.

2.4. Analysis

The analysis was a qualitative latent content analysis [25,26], which was followed by an inductive approach in which codes abstracted into themes were made. The analysis was provided in the structure of Preparation, Organizing, and Reporting [25]. The Preparation phase started with reading the transcribed interviews several times to obtain a sense of the wholeness of the content. Then the units of meaning about changes in the everyday life of the person with an ID were selected from the interviews, which included signs of dementia and descriptions of the strategies of staff and managers in understanding and acting to provide care based on actual needs. In the next step, Organizing, these units of meaning were condensed, i.e., the text units that describe, in different ways, the possible signs of dementia and/or strategies for care and support. The condensed units of meaning from staff and managers were then labeled with codes, which describe the content of the text. The units of meaning, the condensed units of meaning, and the codes with similar content were read several times and, from patterns of core content, the themes were developed. The Organizing phase ended with thorough discussions by all the authors together in several meetings about the result of the analysis and the themes were refined. Reporting means to describe the results of the analysis process by illustrating a conceptual map [25] with three themes and with illustrated quotations.

2.5. Ethics Approval and Consent to Participate

Before starting the study, the responsible health care and social welfare manager in the current city as well as the Regional Ethics Review Board in Lund, Sweden (reference number: 2013/83) approved the study. The research was guided by the research ethical principles in the Declaration of Helsinki and the participants gave their oral and written informed consent before the interviews. To respect the participants' autonomy, all the participants were informed that they had the right to withdraw from the study at any time without any consequences. To maintain the principle of non-maleficence, the participants were guaranteed confidentiality, which was taken into account in data collection by coding the interviews and presenting the data on the group level.

3. Results

Three themes emerged from the data and these constitute three levels of the identification process of signs when dementia is suspected in a person with an ID. The three themes are known as: A close caring relationship provides reflection and understanding, a team relationship provides a basis for knowledge, support and continued action, and external relations support examination and more adapted care (Figure 1). Each theme was generated from patterns of core content (see Table 1).

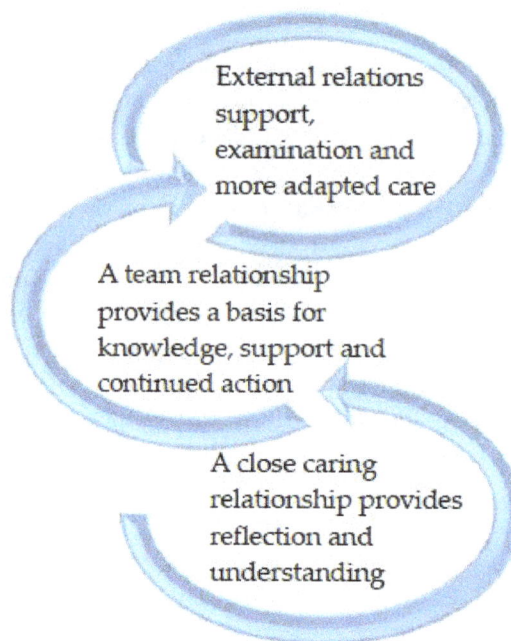

Figure 1. A model of the three levels of resources for the identification process of signs of people with an ID and suspected dementia.

Table 1. Actors and patterns of core content in the three levels in the model (Figure 1) of resources for the identification process of signs among people with an ID and suspected dementia.

Level: Themes	Actors and Patterns of Core Content
First level: A close caring relationship provides reflection and understanding	Actors in this part of the caring process consist of the person with an ID and staff. • Time and continuity in the care relationship are crucial to identify and respond to signs of a change in cognitive ability and thus indicate dementia. • Staff must strive to understand the person's changed expression and observed behaviors. • Internal reflection, seeking to understand what the changes lead to, and how treatment and care can best be adapted.
Second level: A team relationship provides a basis for knowledge, support and continued action	Actors in this second part of the caring process consist of staff and managers in their own workplace. • Necessary to obtain support from colleagues. • Transfer experiences and reflections from the long-standing and ongoing process together with the person with an ID to colleagues and managers in recurring meetings. • Staff express how managers have a responsibility and an opportunity to provide support based on their knowledge and experience.
Third level: External relations support examination and more adapted care	Actors on this third level consist of, beside the staff and managers in the ID-service, external staff from other municipal units, primary health care, and specialist care. • Managers pave the way for contact with external resources and initiate an investigation for suspected dementia. • Staff who know the older person with an ID accompany them to the office of the physician. • In cases when the staff needs more knowledge about dementia and specialist support, dementia nurses are consulted.

3.1. A Close Caring Relationship Provides Reflection and Understanding

The described actors in this part of the caring process consist of the person with an ID and staff (Figure 1, Table 1). Under this theme, the staff clearly describe how time and continuity in the care relationship are crucial to being able to identify and respond to the often-subtle changes in behaviors, which can indicate signs of a change in cognitive ability and thus indicate dementia.

"I can't say how many years ago it was. His behavior just changed completely and we didn't understand a thing. He'd been the nicest man in the world and then he just changed completely." (Member of staff, group home, female)

A care relationship based on good conditions provides guidance on how treatment and support need to be adapted, according to changes in needs and new circumstances, since time and continuity allow staff to detect changes. The participants described a long-term caring relationship and how changes that mark possible dementia usually requires staff who strive to understand the person's changed expression and observed behaviors.

"A person's memory gets worse. But if you know what it's been like over time, you can see that there's a new situation." (Member of staff, daily activity center, female)

The transition from a caring relationship, without signs of dementia, to a relationship where such signs are detected will affect both parties. Everyday life and its activities are affected. It can be forgetfulness that makes it harder for the person with an ID to orientate in time and finish a meal. For the staff who should provide the support, the change requires an understanding of what is happening and, based on this, the insight that efforts need to be adapted and how to adapt. The staff expressed a compassion and concerns over changes in the behavior and everyday habits of the person. Based on this sympathy, they needed an internal reflection by seeking to understand what the changes lead to and how treatment and care can best be adapted. They express how it is a challenge to see signs of dementia since it manifests in behaviors like irritation, aggressiveness, forgetfulness, and confusion rather than being spoken in linguistic terms.

> "There are two whose behavior indicates dementia, though not quite in the same way. The fact that they don't talk makes things a bit more difficult, of course. But you do notice changes in behavior especially in the case of one of them. For instance, you'll suddenly find him standing in the shower at four in the afternoon, which hasn't happened before. He has a shower in the morning and he's always been careful to keep to that routine." (Member of staff, group home, female)

This imposes other demands on the staff's responsiveness compared to when someone expresses their forgetfulness in words. The staff emphasize how continuity in contact is an important part of being able to "feel needs that are expressed as behaviors" among persons with IDs. It also appears that staff are uncertain about how a changed behavior of the person with an ID should be interpreted as signs of dementia, signs of normal aging for people with IDs, or signs of symptoms of other bodily disorders such as an infection or pain. Necessary knowledge about normal and abnormal aging is, therefore, needed.

> "But you have the same problem with people with dementia who don't talk. A person can hit themselves and it can be a sign that they're in pain. And I think, I really do think, that we all need to know what happens when we get older." (Member of staff, group home, female)

3.2. A Team Relationship Provides a Basis for Knowledge, Support, and Continued Action

The described actors in this second part of the three-step level consist of staff and managers in their own workplace (Figure 1, Table 1). According to staff, it is necessary in many cases to obtain support from colleagues, which can lead to a proper investigation of the changes they discover in the person with an ID. This indicates either an onset of dementia or the expression of a challenging behavior, which is difficult to master. The staff explains how to transfer their experiences and reflections from the long-standing and ongoing process together with the person with an ID to colleagues and managers in recurring meetings. By doing so, they can gain understanding and relief as well as confirmation of their interpretation of a strange act of suspected dementia or insights that can lead to an understanding of how to respond differently.

> "You've got to take the situation as it comes, so to speak. And then, of course, we talk a lot about it in the staff group, so that everybody's alert to the fact that something's happened with regard to the person. As when one person went around picking up this, that and the other—collecting little things. She hadn't done that before." (Member of staff, daily activity centre, female)

The staff emphasizes the importance of having this forum and how it enables a changed action in care, which may be the best available to the person with an ID. The staff expresses how managers have a responsibility and an opportunity to provide support based on their knowledge and experience. The managers, in turn, received descriptions from the staff of situations in which changes in behavior have occurred and they try to find possible internal support methods.

> "Well, what made the staff start to suspect dementia was that the person became confused and couldn't find the way home and . . . " (Manager, group home, male)

The person with an ID may, because of a cognitive impairment and possible dementia, develop a radically changed need for support in his everyday life. The changed behavior affects the individual himself but also his surroundings in the form of other residents and staff. An experienced problem was when other persons living at the group home could not handle the changed behavior associated with dementia. For managers, it is common to think about a change of housing and/or the adaptation of the workplace. They express a willingness to let, as far as possible, the person with an ID stay in their current residence and compensate with more customized support to make this possible. There were different opinions among managers and staff and between managers as to whether it was better for the older person with dementia to stay at the group home or to move to an ordinary group home for older persons with dementia. If the person had lived at the group home for a long time and felt secure and comfortable there, the main opinion was that it was better for him/her to stay and adapt to the environment.

"I mean, it's where they live, and if they feel a sense of security there, you mustn't make them move just because they're older and you can't make somebody move because they suffer from dementia." (Member of staff, daily activity center, female)

Another opinion was that it could be better to move the person with ID to an ordinary group home for older people with dementia when the staff have not had enough experience and do not have sufficient knowledge about dementia care. A leader gave an example of a group home for older people with dementia, but it did not turn out well for organizational reasons. From the interviewees, it appears that there is no optimal housing that suits those with ID and dementia.

"Is it dementia that should determine where he's going to live or is it quality of life? It's maybe more important that he's here where he knows the staff and his neighbors and the environment and the area. Yes, that's maybe more important." (Member of staff, group home, female)

There is, however, a desire of managers for staff to have better education regarding dementia in the ordinary group home instead of adapted housing, so that future demands of the growing group of older persons with an ID who are developing dementia can be met.

"I don't think the person would have been better off in an ordinary home for people with dementia. On the other hand, the staff at the group home do need greater competence concerning dementia." (Manager, group home, female)

3.3. External Relations Support Examination and More Adapted Care

The described actors on this third level consist of the staff and managers in the ID-service, external staff from other municipal units, and primary health care and specialist care (Figure 1, Table 1). Managers pave the way for contact with external resources in the form of support from, for example, nurses specially trained in dementia care for educational efforts and skills development, but they can also assist in finding ways to employ external actors from municipal, primary health care, or specialist care. Specialists, outside their own group, can support examinations and education.

"In connection with a person being diagnosed as having Alzheimer's, this wonderful nurse came here one morning and talked to us all. Very committed. She's attached to the primary healthcare center where the person with Alzheimer's is registered. She's fantastic and so is the doctor." (Member of staff, daily activity center, female)

In cases where the primary healthcare nurse who is connected to the group home found that the staff needed more knowledge about dementia and specialist support, a dementia nurse was consulted. If there occurred difficulties in the care of the person with an ID and dementia at the end of life such as anxiety and screaming, the staff could experience frustration and problems in handling the situation.

"It felt as if nothing we did was right, but then the dementia nurse was an enormous help, simply by being able to put it into words and showing it was normal. She said there was nothing more we could do." (Manager, daily activity center, male)

However, the availability of consultation with dementia nurses varied in different areas of the actual city. There could have been a dementia nurse previously available but not at the moment. The dementia nurses were employed in the community and not especially in the ID-service, which means their knowledge about people with IDs was limited. Support from external specialists was important at the end of a dementia progress especially in the phase with palliative care, which could be tough on the staff. Other than support from the staff group and manager, the staff could get support from nurses and physicians from the primary healthcare field on how to care for the older person at the end of life.

> *"Our nurses from this part of town were brought in and her own general practitioner made regular calls towards the end. We worked together in the palliative care when the person was dying. This gave me a firm sense of security."* (Member of staff, group home, male)

The managers' outline the importance of an environment that is well adapted to the changing abilities and needs of the person with an ID, which can, for example, include the support of an occupational therapist. The advice could be to consider using colors and lights.

> *"When we furnish a flat in co-operation with the person, what do we have to think about? No dark mats on a light-coloured floor, for instance . . . You don't want to feel as if you're falling into a hole! And the curtains mustn't be made of a material that reflects the light . . . You don't want a situation where the person can't really see whether there's someone standing outside the window or not, or where, when it's dark, the artificial light is reflected. These are things you don't think about until they're pointed out to you."* (Member of staff, group home, female)

For the most part, the staff as well as the managers experience a lack of support in diagnosing the condition in accordance with the guidelines and rights relevant to dementia. Managers expressed that there were difficulties in conducting an investigation into suspected dementia. This was mainly due to five factors: (1) the physicians at primary healthcare and other outside specialists did not have enough knowledge concerning dementia in persons with an ID; (2) a lack of developed methods to measure changes in people who already had dysfunctions; (3) a lack of knowledge in the ID-service of supportive intervention in dementia care is directed to a person with an ID; (4) a negative attitude from healthcare staff to an ID; and (5) an ethical and legal question of subjecting persons to examinations that they did not understand or want. One suggestion to facilitate the investigation was to do it at the person's home instead of at the primary healthcare center. There was also a major issue of what benefit the person with an ID received from an investigation and dementia diagnosis. The changes in, or loss of, abilities would, nonetheless, be compensated and treated by more support from the staff.

> *"What can you ask of them and how important is it? It differs from one person to another. The staff must always adjust to the person's individual needs; find what aid or appliance the person requires at the particular time."* (Manager, group home, female)

It appeared that physicians in primary health care centers had difficulties in establishing a dementia diagnosis for people with an ID and it was important that staff who knew the older person with an ID well accompanied them to the office of the physicians. The staff could describe the changes in the behavior and deliver information about the older persons' normal skills and capacities that he or she had a year ago.

> *"Of course, the person needs to be accompanied by a member of staff that works closely with them. If the person goes unaccompanied to a healthcare center, the examination can be just who knows what because the dementia isn't visible. All you see is the intellectual impairment. It needs to be made clear how the person functioned until a year ago before we started thinking that something was not as it should be."* (Manager, daily activity center, female)

4. Discussion

The interviews with staff and managers revealed that dementia is a main concern in aging for people with an ID, which, in this study, is expressed in a model of three themes on three levels of resources for the identification process of suspected dementia signs. The first theme illustrates a level where caregivers, through their everyday contact, can get information about early signs of possible dementia. In the next step, this knowledge is discussed with colleagues and managers and, lastly, managers can consult external resources to further investigate their suspicion of dementia and consider the need of staff for education and support. The study points to the need for skills development of staff who work close to the person with an ID and the shortcomings in methods, forms, and procedures for the implementation of an adequate dementia investigation for persons with an ID. Additionally, the study points to the difficulty in deciding on an accommodation and environment that is optimally adapted to the target group, i.e., aging in place with the continual development and adaptation of the staff's skills and the environment or the being moved to adapted accommodation.

The time and continuity of the relationship between the person with an ID and staff as well as knowledge support from colleagues and managers were considered as important prerequisites for the detection of possible signs of dementia and the adaptation of the caring process in the interviews. Northway [27] argues that staff who are close to the person with ID have a unique knowledge of changes in health conditions and, therefore, points to the importance of respecting the knowledge that staff have access to. Llewellyn [28] indicates that the unique knowledge of staff represents a crucial prerequisite for starting a care process designed to discover dementia and adapt support based on changing needs. Additionally, Cleary and Doody [18] point to the fact that knowing the person with an ID and dementia is key to providing care based on individual needs and they point to proactive planning that supports the carers and, as an effect, also the person with an ID. This is also in line with, for example, Moran et al. [17] who state that a standard diagnostic workup in the evaluation and management of dementia for a person with an ID includes a detailed history that is presented by someone who is well-acquainted with the individual such as, for example, a family member or caregiver. Staff who participated in this study demonstrated a high level of commitment and motivation for their work, but they also expressed the desire for more knowledge and education as a prerequisite for continued support in line with the progression of dementia and increased need for care. The managers and staff working in an intellectual disability service generally have a social or pedagogic education, which means that they may have the same level of knowledge about dementia as the population in general regardless of any experiences they get through their work. A previous interview study from the UK shows that people in general expressed uncertainty about the illness trajectory, boundaries between age-related memory decline, cognitive impairment, and dementia [29].

Janicki [30] argues that constructive staff education and training are crucial components for the quality care of people with IDs and dementia. Thus, personalized training for staff and a proactive approach from managers where education is planned and adapted to the changing needs of caregivers is important. Managers have a key role [8] in organizing work so that space is provided for a continuous dialogue between staff in which they can discuss individual cases and problems with the inclusion of collegial support or supervision from an expert, i.e., a nurse specialized in dementia care. This form of support is presented as very important to better understanding, for example, a changed behavior but is also found to have an emotional relief function through the confirmation from colleagues [31]. However, staff does not always have knowledge about the changes that are relevant for the development of dementia or the effectiveness of any treatment and they, therefore, have difficulty participating in dialogue with other professionals. Furthermore, educational interventions may improve the awareness of mental health problems such as depression and anxiety. Costello and colleagues [32] and Tsiantis and colleagues [33] found a significant improvement in the knowledge and attitudes of staff working with persons with IDs and thus better prepared them to differentiate better various mental health problems after receiving the educational intervention.

The findings from the study also show that further support is needed and emphasize the manager's responsibility to consult external resources when early signs of dementia can be a suspected diagnosis and the need for support increases. Actors outside of the workplace of the managers and staff such as general practitioners, occupational therapists, and registered nurses specialized in dementia care, are important resources as dementia progresses over time, but other means may also be considered. Research showing promising results using a digital diary method such as the Experience Sampling Method (ESM), which was described by Knippenberg et al. [34] to assess caregiver functioning, has emerged. The method is mainly designed for spousal caregivers to persons with dementia, but, since the relationship between professional caregivers and individuals with IDs and dementia is often long-term, it should be possible to develop similar digital methods that are refined and adapted to this caring relationship. This type of a digital diary method may provide an opportunity to better understand the everyday life of both caregivers and persons with dementia and it offers possibilities for adapting support based on the needs of the person.

The findings also indicates an opinion of staff as well as managers that the person with an ID should be offered a specialized assessment and investigation of possible dementia. However, sometimes the experts due to the experiences of staff and managers in the present study had a lack of knowledge about methods of dementia investigation and support targeted at a person with an ID and sometimes they also reflected a somewhat negative attitude towards the value and significance of special dementia investigation for this group of older people. It is well known that the diagnosis of dementia is complex in adults with ID due to their intellectual, psychosocial deficits and, most often, atypical presentation [7]. However, in recent years, several instruments have been developed, which are available or under development. For example, international experiences from special memory clinics for persons with IDs and possible dementia [4] in which a system using informant-based tools as well as objective-based tools for measuring possible dementia and evaluating the dementia process is proposed. The so-called Dementia Care Mapping (DCM) is widely used in general dementia care and may benefit care workers as well as people living with dementia in care settings [35]. DCM has been designed to improve the quality and effectiveness of person-centered care and it can be used either as an assessment of residents' well-being and quality of life or as an outcome measure of intervention [35,36]. Schaap and colleagues [37] recently evaluated a modified form of DCM for use in ID-care and found it to be an appropriate and valuable method to support staff in their work with aging people. There are interesting examples to consider and it is a challenge for healthcare to implement any of these systems to make care more equal even for people with an ID. However, these instruments are not tested with regard to their validity and reliability and there is a need for psychometric studies in further research.

The findings of the study also deal with the question of the rights of people with IDs and dementia with respect to the choice between aging in place or moving to an adapted accommodation for dementia in general [15,22]. The staff and managers stress several possible benefits of staying in the environment where the person feels at home and the environment and treatment are adjusted as far as possible based on changing needs. Wilkinson and colleagues [38] argue that support for the staff in terms of strategic deployment of staff, i.e., extra staff in cases of disturbing behavior, is important and thus organizational flexibility is also important. This requires a good dialogue between staff and managers, which would allow many situations and problems to be solved within the staff team and the well-being of the person with an ID as well as the caregiver to be supported. However, besides dementia, this is also applicable in the case of multi-morbidities such as epilepsy, depression, vision impairments, and hearing impairments [8,39–41]. This means that, in addition to the increased needs arising from dementia, the staff must also handle problems related to multi-morbidity and the connected polypharmacy [42,43], which creates a great demand for knowledge and support concerning how to handle such problems when a decision has been made to let the person age in place. The development and evaluation of adapted housing to meet future demands as the group of persons with IDs and severe dementia increase is apparently an important area for further research.

The interviewees experience a diagnosis of dementia in people with IDs as problematic and as a question of the necessity for persons who do not understand or ask for the investigation. One of the ethical issues in clinical care, according to WHO [44], is "What criteria should be used to assess whether a patient has the capacity to make his or her own decisions about treatment." It is an important ethical issue concerning, on the one hand, the same rights of health and healthcare as the general population with access to treatment and, on the other hand, the right to self-determination. The ethical principles of beneficence and non-maleficence [44] seem to be opposed. A way for managers and staff to handle this problem seemed to be to accept the situation and adapt to the older persons' changed behavior and needs. However, the risk is that differential diagnoses such as depression, a brain tumor or hearing, and vision impairments are missed because of a diagnostic overshadowing [8]. If people with an ID are not diagnosed, there is a risk that the staff will not receive support and guidance from the healthcare, i.e., memory clinics, which they need. Staff in the disability service need support, guidance, and education because very few have health education and/or previous experience in the care of people with ID and dementia.

It would be desirable to get people with an ID to express their thoughts and wishes by themselves, which would illuminate the process from the first appearance of signs of dementia. However, since this implies methodological difficulties, staff and managers in this study can, in light of their several years of experience in working with older people with IDs, be considered their representatives. Descriptions in the interviews of staff and managers who together have extensive experience may possibly give a somewhat idealized picture of the situation given their knowledge about dementia and other common health problems in aged people with an ID. This needs to be taken into consideration when reading the results. However, extensive narrations as a basis for the analysis in this study and the overall experience of the interviewees counts as validity. Dementia among people with an ID was not the main question in the interview guides, but it became the clear concern that needed to be raised. If dementia had been the main focus of the interview, more aspects of dementia could have appeared. However, there were important experiences in the data provided in this study, which will hopefully contribute to the field of knowledge about people with an ID and dementia, but further research about the whole care pathway is needed.

The context of group homes and daily activity centers is organized in similar ways and, based upon a strong entitlement law known as the LSS act, it is based on the core values of autonomy, influence, and participation [22]. The culture in these two organizations, therefore, do not differ to any larger extent in Sweden, which means that the result is perceived to have transferability to the Swedish context and also to the Norwegian context due to a similar law. However, the transferability to other countries need to be considered carefully from the following perspectives: the organization of intellectual disability services, laws, and disability policy as well as the competence of managers and staff in each country. The similarities between most of the world's countries is the implementation of human rights that protect the rights of vulnerable groups in societies [23].

5. Conclusions

This study presents results expressed as a model based on three themes about resources for the identification process of signs of suspected dementia. The importance of a caregiver relationship based on time and continuity is the basic resource for collegial and manager support as well as the consultation of specialists outside the intellectual disability service. Only when these resources are used will it be possible for staff to identify, and react to, dementia symptoms in a safe and knowledge-based way, initiate examination, design well-adapted care, and, if necessary, consider moving the person to adapted housing. A close collaboration with specialists within dementia care may contribute to a good working environment for staff with skilled guidance and support, continuous education, and the initiation of intervention research concerning the best accommodation form and digital support for people with an ID and staff.

The results are important for policy making in their ambition to improve the care for this vulnerable group. More focus needs to put on teaching staff about dementia among older people with ID since this important area is insufficient in medical and nursing education today. Further qualitative research may include those with ID and family members' experiences of early signs as well as the staff's experiences, which means that they acquire deeper knowledge of detecting and distinguishing signs of dementia over time and exploring the type of living standards and the environment, i.e. stay in place or specialized environment. Knowledge from these studies needs to be translated into interventions of integrated care for people with ID and dementia based on the complexity that this type of intervention implies.

Author Contributions: G.H. conceptualized the study in collaboration with G.A. and M.J. M.J. performed all the interviews. The qualitative analysis was made by G.H. and M.J. G.H. and G.A. wrote the first draft of the manuscript. Comments on the results of the analysis and improvements of the manuscript draft were made by M.J. All authors (G.H., M.J. and G.A.) approved the final version of the manuscript. G.A. and M.J. were responsible for funding acquisition.

Funding: The study is supported by a grant from the Lundström's Memory Foundation and the Vårdal Foundation.

Acknowledgments: We would also like to acknowledge the support from the research group Health Promoting Complex Interventions, Department of Health Sciences, Faculty of Medicine, Lund University and support from the Swedish Red Cross University College in Sweden.

References

1.   World Health Organization. *Towards a Dementia Plan: A Who Guide*; World Health Organization: Geneva, Switzerland, 2018; pp. 6–8.

2.   American Psychiatric Association. *Diagnostic and Statistical Manual of Mental Disorders*, 5th ed.; American Psychiatric Association: Washington, DC, USA, 2013.

3.   Schalock, R.L.; Borthwick-Duffy, S.A.; Bradley, V.J.; Buntinx, W.H.E.; Coulter, D.L.; Craig, E.M.; Gomez, S.C.; Lachapelle, Y.; Luckasson, R.; Reeve, A.; et al. *Intellectual Disability: Definition, Classification, and Systems of Supports*, 11th ed.; American Association on Intellectual and Developmental Disabilities: Washington, DC, USA, 2010.

4.   McCarron, M.; McCallion, P.; Reilly, E.; Dunne, P.; Carroll, R.; Mulryan, N. A prospective 20-year longitudinal follow-up of dementia in persons with down syndrome. *J. Intellect. Disabil. Res.* **2017**, *61*, 843–852. [CrossRef] [PubMed]

5.   Strydom, A.; Chan, T.; King, M.; Hassiotis, A.; Livingston, G. Incidence of dementia in older adults with intellectual disabilities. *Res. Dev. Disabil.* **2013**, *34*, 1881–1885. [CrossRef] [PubMed]

6.   Kelly, C.; O'Donohoe, A. *Hrb Statistics Series 24 Annual Report of the National Intellectual Disability Database Committee 2013*; Health Research Board: Dublin, Ireland, 2014.

7.   Nagdee, M. Dementia in intellectual disability: A review of diagnostic challenges. *Afr. J. Psychiatry* **2011**, *14*, 194–199. [CrossRef]

8.   Strydom, A.; Al-Janabi, T.; Houston, M.; Ridley, J. Best practice in caring for adults with dementia and learning disabilities. *Nurs. Stand.* **2016**, *31*, 42–51. [CrossRef] [PubMed]

9.   Sheehan, R.; Ali, A.; Hassiotis, A. Dementia in intellectual disability. *Curr. Opin. Psychiatry* **2014**, *27*, 143–148. [CrossRef] [PubMed]

10.   McCarron, M.; McCallion, P.; Coppus, A.; Fortea, J.; Stemp, S.; Janicki, M.; Wtachman, K. Supporting advanced dementia in people with down syndrome and other intellectual disability: Consensus statement of the international summit on intellectual disability and dementia. *J. Intellect. Disabil. Res.* **2018**, *62*, 617–624. [CrossRef] [PubMed]

11.   McKenzie, K.; Metcalfe, D.; Murray, G. A review of measures used in the screening, assessment and diagnosis of dementia in people with an intellectual disability. *J. Appl. Res. Intellect. Disabil.* **2018**, *31*, 725–742. [CrossRef] [PubMed]

12. Elliott-King, J.; Shaw, S.; Bandelow, S.; Devshi, R.; Kassam, S.; Hogervorst, E. A critical literature review of the effectiveness of various instruments in the diagnosis of dementia in adults with intellectual disabilities. *Alzheimer's Dement Diagn. Assess. Dis. Monit.* **2016**, *4*, 126–148. [CrossRef] [PubMed]

13. Froggatt, K.; Payne, S.; Morbey, H.; Edwards, M.; Finne-Soveri, H.; Gambassi, G.; Pasman, H.R.; Szczerbinska, K.; Van den Block, L. Palliative care development in european care homes and nursing homes: Application of a typology of implementation. *J. Am. Med. Dir. Assoc.* **2017**, *18*, 550.e7–550.e14. [CrossRef] [PubMed]

14. Zeilinger, E.L.; Stiehl, K.A.; Weber, G. A systematic review on assessment instruments for dementia in persons with intellectual disabilities. *Res. Dev. Disabil.* **2013**, *34*, 3962–3977. [CrossRef] [PubMed]

15. The National Board of Health and Welfare. *Swedish Disability Policy—Service and Care for People with Functional Impairments; Measures under the Act Concerning Support and Service for Persons with Certain Functional Impairments*; The National Board of Health and Welfare: Stockholm, Sweden, 2009; pp. 126–188.

16. The British Psychological Society; Royal College of Psychiatrists; Division of Clinical Psychology. *Dementia and People with Intellectual Disabilities: Guidance on the Assessment, Diagnosis, Interventions and Support of People with Intellectual Disabilities Who Develop Dementia*; The British Psychological Society: Leicester, UK, 2015.

17. Moran, J.A.; Rafii, M.S.; Keller, S.M.; Singh, B.K.; Janicki, M.P. The national task group on intellectual disabilities and dementia practices consensus recommendations for the evaluation and management of dementia in adults with intellectual disabilities. *Mayo Clin. Proc.* **2013**, *88*, 831–840. [CrossRef] [PubMed]

18. Cleary, J.; Doody, O. Nurses' experience of caring for people with intellectual disability and dementia. *J. Clin. Nurs.* **2017**, *26*, 620–631. [CrossRef] [PubMed]

19. Cleary, J.; Doody, O. Professional carers' experiences of caring for individuals with intellectual disability and dementia. *J. Intellect. Disabil.* **2017**, *21*, 68–86. [CrossRef] [PubMed]

20. Clement, T.; Bigby, C. Competencies of front-line managers in supported accommodation: Issues for practice and future research. *J. Intellect. Dev. Disabil.* **2012**, *37*, 131–140. [CrossRef] [PubMed]

21. Beadle-Brown, J.; Mansell, J.; Ashman, B.; Ockenden, J.; Iles, R.; Whelton, B. Practice leadership and active support in residential services for people with intellectual disabilities: An exploratory study. *J. Intellect. Disabil. Res.* **2014**, *58*, 838–850. [CrossRef] [PubMed]

22. Swedish Parliament. *Act Concerning Support and Service for Persons with Certain Functional Impairments*; Independent Living Institute: Stockholm, Sweden, 1993.

23. The United Nations. *Convention on the Rights of Persons with Disabilities (CRPD)*. 2006. Available online: http://www.un.org/disabilities/documents/convention/convoptprot-e.pdf (accessed on 4 August 2018).

24. Wiles, J.L.; Leibing, A.; Guberman, N.; Reeve, J.; Allen, R.E.S. The meaning of "aging in place" to older people. *Gerontologist* **2012**, *52*, 357–366. [CrossRef] [PubMed]

25. Elo, S.; Kyngas, H. The qualitative content analysis process. *J. Adv. Nurs.* **2008**, *62*, 107–115. [CrossRef] [PubMed]

26. Vaismoradi, M.; Turunen, H.; Bondas, T. Content analysis and thematic analysis: Implications for conducting a qualitative descriptive study. *Nurs. Health Sci.* **2013**, *15*, 398–405. [CrossRef] [PubMed]

27. Northway, R.; Holland-Hart, D.; Jenkins, R. Meeting the health needs of older people with intellectual disabilities: Exploring the experiences of residential social care staff. *Health Soc. Care Community* **2017**, *25*, 923–931. [CrossRef] [PubMed]

28. Llewellyn, P. The needs of people with learning disabilities who develop dementia: A literature review. *Dementia* **2011**, *10*, 235–247. [CrossRef]

29. Robinson, L.; Dickinson, C.; Magklara, E.; Newton, L.; Prato, L.; Bamford, C. Proactive approaches to identifying dementia and dementia risk: A qualitative study of public attitudes and preferences. *BMJ Open* **2018**, *8*, e018677. [CrossRef] [PubMed]

30. Janicki, M.P. Quality outcomes in group home dementia care for adults with intellectual disabilities. *J. Intellect. Disabil. Res.* **2011**, *55*, 763–776. [CrossRef] [PubMed]

31. McCarron, M.; Reilly, E. *Supporting Persons with Intellectual Disability and Dementia: Quality Dementia Care Standards. A Guide to Practice*; Daughters of Charity Service: San Antonio, TX, USA, 2010.

32. Costello, H.; Bouras, N.; Davis, H. The role of training in improving community care staff awareness of mental health problems in people with intellectual disabilities. *J. Appl. Res. Intellect. Disabil.* **2007**, *20*, 228–235. [CrossRef]

33. Tsiantis, J.; Diareme, S.; Dimitrakaki, C.; Kolaitis, G.; Flios, A.; Christogiorgos, S.; Weber, G.; Salvador-Carulla, L.; Hillery, J.; Costello, H. Care staff awareness training on mental health needs of adults with learning disabilities: Results from a greek sample. *J. Learn. Disabili.* **2004**, *8*, 221–234. [CrossRef]

34. Van Knippenberg, R.J.M.; De Vugt, M.E.; Ponds, R.W.; Myin-Germeys, I.; Van Twillert, B.; Verhey, F.R.J. Dealing with daily challenges in dementia (deal-id study): An experience sampling study to assess caregiver functioning in the flow of daily life. *Int. J. Geriatr. Psychiatry* **2017**, *32*, 949–958. [CrossRef] [PubMed]

35. Barbosa, A.; Lord, K.; Blighe, A.; Mountain, G. Dementia care mapping in long-term care settings: A systematic review of the evidence. *Int. Psychogeriatr.* **2017**, *29*, 1609–1618. [CrossRef] [PubMed]

36. Kitwood, T.; Bredin, K. Towards a theory of dementia care: Personhood and well-being. *Ageing Soc.* **1992**, *12*, 269–287. [CrossRef] [PubMed]

37. Schaap, F.D.; Dijkstra, G.J.; Finnema, E.J.; Reijneveld, S.A. The first use of dementia care mapping in the care for older people with intellectual disability: A process analysis according to the re-aim framework. *Aging Ment. Health* **2017**. [CrossRef] [PubMed]

38. Wilkinson, H.; Kerr, D.; Cunningham, C. Equipping staff to support people with an intellectual disability and dementia in care home settings. *Dementia* **2005**, *4*, 387–400. [CrossRef]

39. Sandberg, M.; Ahlstrom, G.; Kristensson, J. Patterns of somatic diagnoses in older people with intellectual disability: A swedish eleven year case-control study of inpatient data. *J. Appl. Res. Intellect. Disabil.* **2017**, *30*, 157–171. [CrossRef] [PubMed]

40. Axmon, A.; Bjorne, P.; Nylander, L.; Ahlstrom, G. Psychiatric diagnoses in older people with intellectual disability in comparison with the general population: A register study. *Epidemiol. Psychiatr. Sci.* **2017**. [CrossRef] [PubMed]

41. McCarron, M.; McCallion, P.; Reilly, E.; Mulryan, N. A prospective 14-year longitudinal follow-up of dementia in persons with down syndrome. *J. Intellect. Disabil. Res.* **2014**, *58*, 61–70. [CrossRef] [PubMed]

42. Axmon, A.; Kristensson, J.; Ahlstrom, G.; Midlov, P. Use of antipsychotics, benzodiazepine derivatives, and dementia medication among older people with intellectual disability and/or autism spectrum disorder and dementia. *Res. Dev. Disabil.* **2017**, *62*, 50–57. [CrossRef] [PubMed]

43. Axmon, A.; Sandberg, M.; Ahlstrom, G.; Midlov, P. Prescription of potentially inappropriate medications among older people with intellectual disability: A register study. *BMC Pharmacol. Toxicol.* **2017**, *18*, 68. [CrossRef] [PubMed]

44. WHO. Global Health Ethics; Key Issues; Global Network of Who Collaborating Centres for Bioethics. Available online: http://apps.who.int/iris/bitstream/handle/10665/164576/9789240694033_eng.pdf; jsessionid=4835FE3B07E6988565CE7C3FAE67E83C?sequence=1 (accessed on 14 July 2018).

16

Oral Health in Pregnant Chinese Women in Singapore: A Call to Go beyond the Traditional Clinical Care

Preethi Balan [1], Hong-Gu He [2], Fengchunzhi Cao [2], Mun Loke Wong [1], Yap-Seng Chong [3,4], Violeta Lopez [2], Shu-E. Soh [3,5] and Chaminda Jayampath Seneviratne [1,*

[1] Discipline of Oral Sciences, Faculty of Dentistry, National University of Singapore, Singapore 119083, Singapore; p.preethidr@gmail.com (P.B.); denwml@nus.edu.sg (M.L.W.)
[2] Alice Lee Centre for Nursing Studies, Yong Loo Lin School of Medicine, National University of Singapore, Singapore 117597, Singapore; nurhhg@nus.edu.sg (H.G.H.); caofengchunzhi@gmail.com (F.C.); nurvl@nus.edu.sg (V.L.)
[3] Singapore Institute for Clinical Sciences, Agency for Science, Technology and Research, Singapore 117549, Singapore; obgcys@nus.edu.sg (Y.-S.C.); paesse@nus.edu.sg (S.-E.S.)
[4] Department of Obstetrics and Gynaecology, Yong Loo Lin School of Medicine, National University of Singapore, Singapore 119074, Singapore
[5] Department of Paediatrics, Yong Loo Lin School of Medicine, National University of Singapore, Singapore 119228, Singapore
* Correspondence: jaya@nus.edu.sg

Abstract: Objective: To examine the correlations among oral health knowledge, attitude, practices and oral disease among pregnant Chinese women in Singapore. **Methods**: A descriptive correlational study was conducted in pregnant Chinese women in Singapore. A questionnaire was used to collect data of oral health knowledge, attitude and practices. Plaque index scores were used to assess the oral health of subjects. **Results**: A total of 82 pregnant women participated in the study, out of whom 38% showed adequate oral health knowledge, nearly half of them achieved adequate and oral health attitude and practice scores while 34% had good Plaque index scores. The lower income group had higher experience of self-reported dental problems during pregnancy than those in the higher income group (p = 0.03). There were significant positive correlations between scores of oral health practice, attitude and oral health knowledge levels. The plaque index scores negatively correlated with the oral health practice scores (p = 0.02). **Conclusions**: Our findings provided evidence that oral health knowledge, attitude and practices among Chinese pregnant women were not optimal which implies the importance of promoting their oral health during pregnancy through the improvement of knowledge and attitudes. This would facilitate formulation and implementation of appropriate oral health promotion policies.

Keywords: attitudes; Chinese; knowledge; oral health; practice; pregnant women

1. Introduction

Pregnancy brings about progressive physical and psychological changes in women along with hormonal changes. The increased physical and emotional demands during pregnancy might contribute to the neglect in oral hygiene leading to poor oral health. Inadequate oral hygiene and hormonal changes increase the risk of developing oral health problems such as gingivitis and periodontitis [1]. Gingivitis is the most commonly reported oral problem during pregnancy, with a prevalence of 60 to 75% [2]. Women with pre-existing gingivitis may also show significant exacerbation of the condition during pregnancy [3]. In the first trimester, women commonly experience morning sickness, which leads to increased acidity in the oral cavity and this high acidity erodes the tooth enamel [4]. In the second trimester, pregnancy granuloma has been commonly documented, which frequently occurs in areas of inflamed gingivitis and other recurrent irritation areas. A systematic review has concluded that oral disease especially periodontitis is a contributing factor in pre-term low birth weight babies due to the elevation of inflammatory markers and transmission of oral bacteria into the feto-placental unit [5]. Therefore, a critical step in preventing oral diseases and its complications during pregnancy is to practice good oral hygiene habits.

The literature suggests that the common factors for poor oral health during pregnancy include low oral health literacy [6,7], stress in pregnancy [8], high cost of dental services [9,10], failure of prioritizing oral care [11,12] and poor social economic status [13]. Despite good tooth brushing habits, usage of adjuvant dental products such as dental floss, interdental brush, and mouth rinse is low [14,15]. Further, with the generally lower education levels, this group of women has a poor understanding of the information gathered which ultimately contributes to poor oral health practices [16].

Singapore with its unique blend of ethnicities and traditions brings a different perspective to knowledge on oral health, child bearing practices and confinement period where general health practices may be modified [16]. This is especially significant in Chinese population, where dietary habits incorporate the "hot and cold" elements [17]. These cultural beliefs and practices can at times facilitate or act as barriers to oral health maintenance and access to health care services. Hence, in this study, we have taken oral health knowledge, attitude, practices and plaque index scores as oral health determinants to gain insights into the oral health of pregnant Chinese women in Singapore. A better understanding of oral health as influenced by knowledge, attitudes and practices will be useful in formulating appropriate oral health promotion interventions.

The aims of the study were to investigate various oral health determinants (oral health knowledge, attitude, practices and plaque index scores) in pregnant Chinese women in Singapore and their correlations. Moreover, the association of oral health status during pregnancy with the oral health determinants and the social demographic factors was also explored.

2. Materials and Methods

2.1. Study Design, Setting and Participants

This study adopted a cross-sectional, descriptive and correlational research design to investigate the current oral health related knowledge, attitudes and practices in Singapore Chinese pregnant women. Participants were recruited from the Obstetrics clinic of National University Hospital, a public tertiary hospital in Singapore, from October 2015 to April 2016. The study recruited 82 women who met the following selection criteria:

Inclusion criteria: (a) Singaporean or permanent residents of Chinese ethnicity; (b) Aged 21–50 years; and (c) Pregnant at less than 24 weeks' gestation.

Exclusion criteria: Women with any systemic health conditions such as diabetes, cardiovascular diseases or blood dyscrasias were excluded from the study to ensure there was no influence of these factors on the oral health.

The sample size was calculated through power analysis for Pearson product-moment correlation coefficient. As there were no similar studies examining the correlation among the three dependent variables, we anticipated a conventional medium effect size of 0.25, and hence a minimum of 82 participants were needed to achieve a 80% power at 0.05 (two-sided) significance level [18].

2.2. Outcomes and Measurements

A structured self-administered questionnaire was used to explore the demographic background, oral health knowledge, attitude and practices of the participants. The questionnaire was self-developed based on the Pregnancy Risk Assessment Monitoring System (PRAMS) [19], Rustvold Oral Health

Knowledge Inventory (ROHKI), and Oral Health Attitudes Questionnaire (OHAQ) [19,20] and experts' opinion. The questionnaire consisted of five parts. Part one included socio-demographic characteristics including age, number of pregnancies, monthly household income, highest educational level attained, and smoking history. In Part two, oral health knowledge was assessed with questions on diet and the etiology of oral disease, safety of dental treatment and use of dental X-rays during pregnancy, association of poor oral health and adverse pregnancy outcomes and need for care regimes when oral diseases develop during pregnancy. Part three consisted of oral health attitude questions and participants were asked about their opinions about dental visits and importance of oral health during pregnancy and general health. A five-point Likert scale with responses ranging from 1 (Strongly Disagree) to 5 (Strongly Agree) was used to assess each item in the oral health knowledge and attitude sections. The knowledge on association between adverse pregnancy outcome and maternal dental health was assessed with a three point Likert scale with "Agree", "Unsure" and "Disagree" as the responses. Part four assessed their oral health practices with closed-ended questions on tooth brushing techniques, frequency of brushing and dental visits. Self-rated oral health status was assessed on a five-point rating scale with responses ranging from 1 (very poor) to 5 (very good). In Part five, the participants were asked if they were experiencing any oral health problems during pregnancy with responses as "yes" or "no" and if they did, details of the problem were noted.

The plaque index was graded by a single trained examiner on a scale from 1 to 3, where 1 = "One third or less than one third of all teeth present have dental plaque/calculus deposits", 2 = "More than one third of the teeth but less than half of all teeth present have dental plaque/calculus deposits" and 3 = "Half or more than half of all teeth present have dental plaque/calculus".

Oral health knowledge, attitude and practice and plaque index scores, were considered as the determinants of oral health. The oral health status of participants during pregnancy was determined by self-reported presence of oral problems and was considered the dependent variable.

An overall score was generated for oral health knowledge, attitude and practices by summing the response codes from the questionnaire items. The cut-off for scores of oral health determinant variables were set at the median. Placing the cut-off at the median is a commonly used method to set the cut-off score in health knowledge tests [21]. Accordingly, participants scoring more than the median score were identified as having good performance while participants scoring less than or equal to the median score were considered to have poor performance with respect to oral health attitude, knowledge and practice. The reverse relation was considered for the plaque index score.

2.3. Data Collection Procedure

The researchers recruited Chinese women who were currently undergoing prenatal care in the study clinic. Potential participants were given an information sheet explaining the study's aims, procedures, their responsibility, possible risks and side effects, possible benefits, alternatives to participation, confidentiality of data and voluntary participation. Those who were willing to participate, provided signed consent to take part in the study. Following this, they were given a self-administered questionnaire, which took about 20–30 min to complete. Thereafter, Plaque Index Score was evaluated by examining all the teeth. This was conducted in a private room to ensure privacy. A token of appreciation was given to each participant after they had completed the questionnaire and dental examination.

2.4. Ethical Considerations

The study was approved by the Institutional Review Board of the study hospital (NHG DSRB Ref: 2014/00979). Signed informed consent was obtained from all participants upon recruitment. Voluntary participation and confidentiality of the data collection were ensured. Participants could choose to terminate participation at any time.

2.5. Statistical Analysis

Data were entered into SPSS® version 22 (IBM SPSS Statistics for Windows, Version 22.0. IBM Corp, Armonk, NY, USA) and analysed. Descriptive statistics were computed to compile data for the demographics and other key variables of interest. As the data were not normally distributed, non-parametric tests were used. Prior to analysis, some of the knowledge and attitude questions were reverse-coded to facilitate an appropriate scoring system for oral health knowledge and attitudes. The responses for income level and educational level were collapsed to form a three levelled response for data analysis. In addition, response for self-perception of oral health status was also categorised for data analysis. As there were many tied ranks in the sample, Kendall's tau-b (τb) was used to evaluate the statistical significance and correlations between oral health determinants. The association of oral health determinant and sociodemographic factors on the oral health status during pregnancy was analyzed using chi-square or Fisher's exact. The level of statistical significance was set at $p \leq 0.05$.

3. Results

3.1. Socio-Demographics and Self-Reported Clinical Characteristics of Participants

A total of 82 pregnant Chinese women attending their antenatal care in a public tertiary hospital were recruited. The age of the participants ranged from 21 to 43 years (Mean $\pm$ SD = 31.8 $\pm$ 4.5 years). The majority of participants (98.8%) were married and their mean gestational age was 12.1 weeks (SD = 5.2). The educational levels of the participants ranged from primary school education to Doctor of Philosophy with a preponderance of participants with secondary school/general equivalency diploma (46.3%) and bachelor's degree (41.4%). All participants were reported to be non-smokers. The majority of the participants (81.7%) intended to go through post-partum confinement practice. Out of the 82 participants, 24.4% reported dental problems since the start of pregnancy. Of the participants who had dental problems during pregnancy, 75% reported bleeding gums. However, only 6.7% visited dentist for treatment of bleeding gums, even though 73.2% of them perceived their oral health status as moderate or poor. More than half of the participants (56.1%) were unsure that there could be a potential association between maternal dental problems and risk of having adverse pregnancy outcomes (Table 1).

Table 1. Sociodemographic and oral health characteristics (N = 82).

Sociodemographic and Oral Health Characteristics	Mean $\pm$ SD	N (%)
Sociodemographic characteristics		
Age in years	31.8 ($\pm$ 4.5)	
Gestational age	12.1 ($\pm$ 5.2)	
Marital status		
Married		84 (98.8%)
Single		1 (1.2%)
Highest educational level		
Secondary school/diploma		38 (46.3%)
Graduate		34 (41.4%)
Masters/PhD		10 (12.2%)
Monthly household income		
Low ($\leq$2999$)		23 (28.1%)
Medium (3000 to 4999$)		19 (23.2%)
High ($\geq$5000$)		40 (48.8%)
Smoking status		
Yes		0 (0.0%)
No		82 (100%)
Intentions of practicing confinement		
Yes		70 (81.7%)
No		15 (18.3%)

Table 1. *Cont.*

Sociodemographic and Oral Health Characteristics	Mean ± SD	N (%)
Oral health characteristics		
Dental problems during pregnancy (Self-reported)		
Yes		20 (24.4%)
No		62 (75.6%)
Self-reported dental complaints		
Tooth decay		2 (2.4%)
Bleeding gums		15 (18.3%)
Gum boil		0 (0.0%)
Tooth-ache		5 (6.1%)
Tooth injury		1 (1.2%)
Bleeding gums within participants with dental problems during pregnancy		
Yes		15 (75.5%)
No		5 (25.5%)
Participants who visited dentist for bleeding gums during pregnancy		
Yes		1 (6.7%)
No		14 (93.9%)
Self-perception of oral health status		
Good		22 (26.8%)
Poor/moderate		60 (73.2%)
Association between adverse pregnancy outcomes and oral health		
Agree		31(37.8%)
Disagree		5 (6.1%)
Unsure		46 (56.1%)

3.2. Levels of Oral Health Determinants among Participants

Table 2 shows the mean scores for oral health knowledge, attitude and practices and dental plaque. The cut-off for oral health determinant's score was set at the median [21]. Accordingly, 38% of the participants displayed adequate oral health knowledge at cut-off 28. Nearly half of the participants had satisfactory oral health attitude (50%) and practice (46%) scores as defined by the cut-off scores of 28 and 4 respectively. Plaque index scores were good in 34% of participants at cut-off 1 (Figure 1).

Table 2. Levels of oral health determinant factors (N = 82).

Score	Mean ± SD	Median	Minimum	Maximum
Oral health knowledge	27.5 ± 3.2	28	16.00	37.00
Oral health attitude	27.7 ± 2.9	28	22.00	34.00
Oral health practice	4.4 ± 1.8	4	0.00	9.00
Plaque index	1.4 ± 0.6	1	1.00	3.00

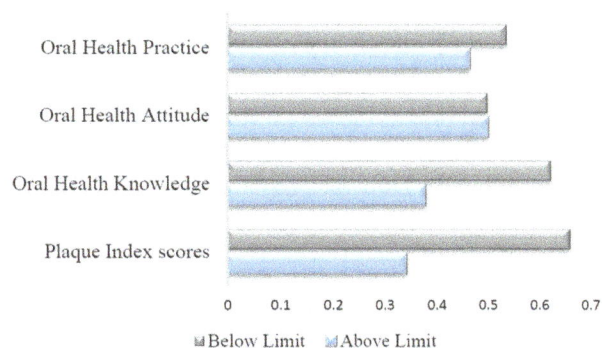

Figure 1. Distribution of scores of oral health determinant factors based on cut-off value.

3.3. Association of Oral Health Status during Pregnancy with the Oral Health Determinant Factors and the Social Demographic Factors

Oral health knowledge scores were higher in respondents not experiencing any dental problems during pregnancy than those who had problems (Table 3). Similarly, the oral health attitude and practice scores were also higher in participants in whom dental problems were absent, although the results were not statistically significant. Furthermore, the plaque index scores were better in participants without dental problems than those who had problems.

Table 3. Association of oral health status with oral health determinant factors and social demographic factors (N = 85).

	Oral Health Status during Pregnancy		
	Problem present N = 20 (24.4%)	Problem absent N = 62 (75.6%)	*p*-value
Oral health determinants			
Oral health knowledge score (Mean) [a]	38.9	42.3	0.572
Oral health attitude score (Mean) [a]	39.3	42.1	0.640
Oral health practice score (Mean) [a]	40.0	41.9	0.747
Plaque index (Mean) [a]	44.4	40.5	0.462
Social demographic factors			
Age (Mean) [a]	34.3	43.8	0.121
Income status (N, %) [b]			
High (5000$–>10,000$)	5 (12.5)	35 (87.5)	0.03
Medium (3000$–4999$)	7 (36.8)	12 (63.2)	0.890
Low (<1000$–2999$)	8 (34.8)	15 (65.2)	
Educational level (N, %) [b]			
Masters/PhD	1 (10.0)	9 (90.0)	0.172
Graduate	7 (20.6)	27 (79.4)	0.291
Secondary school/Diploma	12 (31.6)	26 (68.4)	

[a] Mann-Whitney test; [b] Chi-square test.

Participants who reported having dental problems were older than those who did not report having any dental problems. There was an income-related gradient in the dental problem experience among the respondents. Those who were in the lower income group had a statistically higher experience of dental problems during pregnancy than those in the higher income groups ($p = 0.03$). A similar trend in relation to dental problems was also reported with the educational level, as non-graduate participants appeared to be at higher risk of having dental problems during pregnancy than the more highly educated participants. However, the difference was not statistically significant. This information proves instrumental in identifying the target population which needs auxiliary dental care during pregnancy.

3.4. Correlations among Oral Health Determinants

Kendall tau b test provided support for the correlations between the scores for oral health determinants. The plaque index scores negatively correlated with the oral health practice scores ($r = -0.2$, $p = 0.02$). The scores for oral health practice were shown to be significantly and positively correlated with the levels of oral health attitude ($r = 0.2$, $p = 0.01$). Furthermore, oral health attitude correlated positively with the oral health knowledge ($r = 0.3$, $p < 0.001$) (Table 4).

Table 4. Correlations among oral health determinant factors (N = 82).

		1	2	3	4
1.	Oral health knowledge score	1.000			
2.	Oral health attitude score	0.300 **	1.000		
3.	Oral health practice score	0.056	0.215 *	1.000	
4.	Plaque index score	−0.108	−0.081	−0.200 *	1.000

$* p < 0.05; ** p < 0.01.$

4. Discussion

To our knowledge, this is the first study which has explored the oral health behavior and outcomes in the pregnant population in Singapore. Pregnant Chinese women were the focus of this study as the vast majority of Singapore's population is made up of Chinese (74.3%) [22]. The mean age of the mothers in this study was 31.8 year (SD ± 4.5), which was consistent with the fertility age of Singaporean women (30–34 years) [23]. The majority of the participants (81.7%) intended to go through postpartum confinement practice.

This study indicated bleeding gums as the major dental complaint experienced during pregnancy in 75% of the participants who reported having dental problems. This is consistent with the report on the increase in the prevalence and severity of gingival inflammation occurring during pregnancy [2]. These gingival changes could be the result of hormonal fluctuations or alteration in immune responses during pregnancy [24]. There is an exacerbated inflammatory response to dental plaques leading to swollen gingivae which tend to bleed on provocation. Management of pregnancy gingivitis involves regular dental visits for professional cleaning and monitoring. In addition, educating women about the etiology and prevention of the condition is also essential [25]. However, in this study only 6.7% of the participants with bleeding gums visited the dentist for treatment. This figure is meagre as compared to other countries like Australia, where Thomas et al. reported that 30% of the women accessed dental care during pregnancy [26] and in the US, where 22.7–34% of the pregnant women utilized dental services during pregnancy [27]. A possible consequence of such oral hygiene neglect could be an increased risk for adverse pregnancy outcomes such as pre-term deliveries, low birthweight babies, and preeclampsia, especially in the light of mounting evidence of association between the oral health and birth outcomes [28]. The periodontal health status has been associated with adverse pregnancy outcomes, especially in pregnant women older than 40 years of age [29]. In this study, more than half of the respondents were unsure of such associations while approximately 6% disagreed with this. However, numerous studies have also indicated that most women were unaware of the association between poor oral health and the well-being of the fetus [7,10,30]. This indicates that there is an imperative need to educate pregnant women regarding maintaining their oral health during pregnancy.

Oral health knowledge regarding safety of dental treatment or X-ray examination during pregnancy, causes or presentation of dental caries, care for bleeding gums experienced during pregnancy was found to be poor amongst the participants in the study. Poor knowledge about oral health among pregnant women could be attributed to the prevalence of misconceptions that poor oral health is normal and accepted during pregnancy or that dental treatment can be harmful to the fetus [31]. Confusion over safety of dental treatment has been found to be the most important factor limiting access to dental care among mothers in Greece [32]. Moreover, most pregnant women do not receive enough information about oral health and the importance of dental care prior to and during pregnancy [11,33]. The common consensus is that prevention, diagnosis and treatment of dental conditions including use of dental X-rays (with shielding of abdomen and thyroid) is safe during pregnancy [34]. Dental health professionals must update their knowledge on pregnancy related conditions and their proper management without imposing any adverse impact on the patient and fetus [35]. Referral and consultation to patient's gynecologist's or physician should be considered, whenever required.

The oral health attitudes were also observed to be low with half of the participants falling below the cut-off value for desirable attitude. This could perhaps be due to the fact that the most of the women did not consider it important to have a dental check-up during pregnancy and chose to defer it until after pregnancy [33,36]. These misperceptions and erroneous beliefs about oral health care may contribute to the low utilization rate of dental services [37]. This was evident in this study where only 6.7% of participants sought treatment after developing bleeding gums during pregnancy.

This study also showed low practice levels in more than half of the participants (54%). Moreover, the plaque index scores, which is an indicator of oral hygiene and a proxy for gingival health [38], was also high in about 66% of participants, suggesting a low level of oral hygiene among the pregnant women. This finding was in line with results from a study by Bressane et al., 2011; reporting inadequate oral health behaviors during pregnancy [39]. Figure 2 summarizes the correlation between these oral health determinant factors. This study also suggested that, while 73.2% of the participants perceived their oral health status to be poor or moderate, they did not consider oral health care as an urgent need and preferred delaying the dental visit until after delivery.

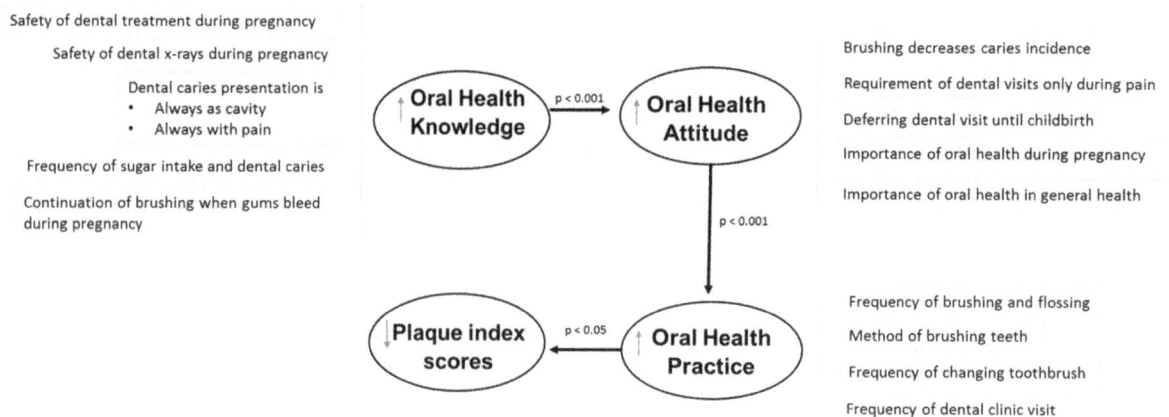

Figure 2. Correlation between the oral health determinant factors.

In this study, the oral health status during pregnancy (with or without dental problem) was associated with oral health-determining factors and sociodemographic factors. Although the results were not significant, it was found that the oral health knowledge, attitude and practice scores were lower in the participants who were experiencing oral health problems during pregnancy as compared to those who did not. Similarly, the plaque scores were also higher in participants with dental problems during pregnancy. As the inflammatory response to dental plaque is increased during pregnancy, it is crucial that women take additional effort in oral care to avoid having dental problems during gestation [25]. Oral health, especially the prevention of gingivitis and accumulation of plaque, is very much dependent on the adherence to oral hygiene behaviors and regular dental visits [40]. Pregnancy being a stressful period, with the increased physical and emotional demands, could potentially contribute to stress-related neglect on oral hygiene as was shown by Amin and ElSalhy [30], where almost half of the pregnant women surveyed had instances of forgetting to brush their teeth during pregnancy. The findings also showed that people of low socioeconomic status were significantly more likely to have dental problems during pregnancy than those of higher socioeconomic status

(p = 0.03).The high cost of dental services is a strong deterrent for dental visits [9,10]. Women with higher household income have the financial capability for regular dental visits and are more likely to seek dental treatments, both preventive and curative, as compared to women with lesser household income [10]. Oral health services are often cited as one of the more expensive services. For example, in a national survey of 801 pregnant women conducted by Cigna Corporation a, only half of the women were observed to have dental insurance. Furthermore, those with dental insurance were twice as likely to visit the dentist [41]. Hence, having dental insurance coverage has been identified as an enabling factor that promotes dental visits [15,30] to potentially bridge the gap.

To add to the aforementioned information, our findings also showed significant positive correlations between oral health knowledge and attitude (r = 0.3), and oral health attitude and practice (r = 0.2). This is consistent with previous findings showing similar correlational strengths [42]. Given that poor oral hygiene practices can result in build-up of dental plaque, oral health practices had significant negative correlations with plaque index scores (r = −0.210). These findings concur with findings from existing literature [43].

As this study was a self-reported survey it may have inherent weaknesses and biases. Our cohort included participants with a gestational age of less than 24 weeks. As oral finding tend to increase with progressing gestational age, assessing oral health at a fixed time point would have helped better correlation of time specific oral findings prevalent during pregnancy with the oral health determining factors. Nevertheless, to our knowledge, this is the first empirical study that has examined oral health determining factors in the Chinese population in Singapore. From this study, it appears that oral health knowledge is lacking in pregnant Chinese women in Singapore. This could possibly result in the adoption of negative attitudes and a lack of emphasis on oral health care. The existence of interactions between culture-related factors such as normative beliefs, knowledge, and behaviors with economic and social factors structure one's health chances and choices [44]. Unless an individual's adopted system of assumptions is challenged and revolutionized, it is not possible to bring change to their healthcare behavior patterns. All these pregnancy-related oral health problems could be mitigated with good oral hygiene practices, highlights the importance of oral care during pregnancy [45]. In addition, researches have indicated that oral health knowledge and attitudes do influence the oral health practices, such as tooth brushing habits, use of adjunct dental products and frequency of dental visits. This signals an imperative need to impart oral health education to pregnant women, with the greatest need in the lower socio-economic strata.

Pregnancy is among the best time for information seeking and a good opportunity for improving health knowledge, and pregnant women are generally more motivated to make behavior change for the well-being of the baby [46]. Improving health knowledge and practices will require the support of oral healthcare and prenatal care providers. Communication by health care providers should address the myths and misconceptions many women have about oral health during pregnancy and increase their awareness.

5. Conclusions

Maternal periodontal disease has been associated with preterm birth, development of preeclampsia, and delivery of a small-for-gestational age infant. Evidence also suggests that infants and young children acquire caries-causing bacteria from their mothers. Given the considerable effect of oral diseases on pregnant women as well as a child's downstream oral health, the following future recommendations are proposed based on the findings of the study; firstly, conducting continuous oral health education programmes to heighten awareness of the oral–systemic health and clarifying myths regarding the safety of dental treatment during pregnancy; secondly, check-ups and oral healthcare should be encouraged during the perinatal visits by the healthcare professionals; and lastly, the availability of subsidized oral healthcare services for pregnant women who need such assistance. Equipped with more knowledge, women will have more self-efficacy and motivation for self-monitoring of brushing and flossing habits and subsequently better oral health outcomes.

Author Contributions: Y.-S.C., V.L., H.G.H. and S.-E.S. provided advice and contributed to the recruitment of the participants; C.F., H.G.H., V.L., W.M.L. and, C.J.S. devised the questionnaire. P.B. and C.F. recruited the participants; P.B., H.G.H. and C.F. performed data analysis; P.B., H.G.H., W.M.L. and, C.J.S. wrote the manuscript.

Funding: This study was supported by the Oral Health Seed Grant (R-221-000-076-733), Faculty of Dentistry, to CJS.

Acknowledgments: We thank the study participants, study coordinators and the nursing staff in the Obstetrical and Gynecology clinics of National University Health System, Singapore (NUHS).

Appendix A

List of abbreviations

SPSS	Statistical Package for the Social Sciences
PRAMS	Pregnancy Risk Assessment Monitoring System
ROHKI	Rustvold Oral Health Knowledge Inventory
OHAQ	Oral Health Attitudes Questionnaire
NHG DSRB	National Healthcare Group Domain Specific Review Boards
NUHS	National University Health System

References

1. La Marca-Ghaemmaghami, P.; Ehlert, U. Stress during Pregnancy. *Eur. Psychol.* **2015**, *20*, 102–119. [CrossRef]
2. Silk, H.; Douglass, A.B.; Douglass, J.M.; Silk, L. Oral health during pregnancy. *Am. Fam. Phys.* **2008**, *77*, 1139–1144.
3. Hey-Hadavi, J. Women's oral health issues: Sex differences and clinical implications. *Women's Health Prim. Care Clin.* **2002**, *5*, 189–199.
4. Sherman, P.W.; Flaxman, S.M. Nausea and vomiting of pregnancy in an evolutionary perspective. *Am. J. Obs. Gynecol.* **2002**, *186*, S190–S197. [CrossRef]
5. Shanthi, V.; Vanka, A.; Bhambal, A.; Saxena, V.; Saxena, S.; Kumar, S.S. Association of pregnant women periodontal status to preterm and low-birth weight babies: A systematic and evidence-based review. *Dent. Res. J.* **2012**, *9*, 368–380.
6. Hom, J.M.; Lee, J.Y.; Divaris, K.; Diane Baker, A.; Vann, W.F. Oral health literacy and knowledge among patients who are pregnant for the first time. *J. Am. Dent. Assoc.* **2012**, *143*, 972–980. [CrossRef] [PubMed]
7. Wu, Y.M.; Ren, F.; Chen, L.L.; Sun, W.L.; Liu, J.; Lei, L.H.; Zhang, J.; Cao, Z. Possible socioeconomic and oral hygiene behavioural risk factors for self-reported periodontal diseases in women of childbearing age in a Chinese population. *Oral Health Prev. Dent.* **2014**, *12*, 171–181. [CrossRef] [PubMed]
8. Le, M.; Riedy, C.; Weinstein, P.; Milgrom, P. Barriers to utilization of dental services during pregnancy: A qualitative analysis. *J. Dent. Child.* **2009**, *76*, 46–52.
9. Buerlein, J.K.; Horowitz, A.M.; Child, W.L. Perspectives of Maryland women regarding oral health during pregnancy and early childhood. *J. Publ. Health Dent.* **2011**, *71*, 131–135. [CrossRef]
10. George, A.; Johnson, M.; Blinkhorn, A.; Ajwani, S.; Bhole, S.; Yeo, A.E.; Ellis, S. The oral health status, practices and knowledge of pregnant women in south-western Sydney. *Aust. Dent. J.* **2013**, *58*, 26–33. [CrossRef] [PubMed]
11. Detman, L.A.; Cottrell, B.H.; Denis-Luque, M.F. Exploring dental care misconceptions and barriers in pregnancy. *Birth* **2010**, *37*, 318–324. [CrossRef] [PubMed]
12. Marchi, K.S.; Fisher-Owen, S.A.; Weintraub, J.A.; Yu, Z.; Braveman, P.A. Most pregnant women in California do not receive dental care: Findings from a population-based study. *Publ. Health Rep.* **2010**, *125*, 831–842. [CrossRef] [PubMed]
13. Gilbert, G.H. Racial and socioeconomic disparities in health from population-based research to practice-based research: The example of oral health. *J. Dent. Educ.* **2005**, *69*, 1003–1014. [PubMed]
14. Hunter, L.P.; Yount, S.M. Oral health and oral health care practices among low-income pregnant women. *J. Midwifery Women's Health* **2011**, *56*, 103–109. [CrossRef] [PubMed]

15. Thompson, T.A.; Cheng, D.; Strobino, D. Dental cleaning before and during pregnancy among Maryland mothers. *Matern. Child Health J.* **2013**, *17*, 110–118. [CrossRef] [PubMed]

16. Chen, L.W.; Low, Y.L.; Fok, D.; Han, W.M.; Chong, Y.S.; Gluckman, P.; Godfrey, K.; Kwek, K.; Saw, S.M.; Soh, S.E.; et al. Dietary changes during pregnancy and the postpartum period in Singaporean Chinese, Malay and Indian women: The GUSTO birth cohort study. *Public Health Nutr.* **2014**, *17*, 1930–1938. [CrossRef] [PubMed]

17. Naser, E.; Mackey, S.; Arthur, D.; Klainin-Yobas, P.; Chen, H.; Creedy, D.K. An exploratory study of traditional birthing practices of Chinese, Malay and Indian women in Singapore. *Midwifery* **2012**, *28*, e865–e871. [CrossRef] [PubMed]

18. Cohen, J. A power primer. *Psychol. Bull.* **1992**, *112*, 155–159. [CrossRef] [PubMed]

19. *Pregnancy Risk Assessment Monitoring System (PRAMS) Questionnaires*; Division of Reproductive Health, National Center for Chronic Disease Prevention and Health Promotion; Centers for Disease Control and Prevention: Atlanta, GA, USA, 2004–2008.

20. Rustvold, S.R. Oral Health Knowledge, Attitudes, and Behaviors: Investigation of an Educational Intervention Strategy with at-Risk Females. Doctoral Thesis, Portland State University, Portland, ON, USA, 2012.

21. Yuen, H.K.; Wolf, B.J.; Bandyopadhyay, D.; Magruder, K.M.; Salinas, C.F.; London, S.D. Oral health knowledge and behavior among adults with diabetes. *Diabetes Res. Clin.Pract.* **2009**, *86*, 239–246. [CrossRef] [PubMed]

22. Singapore Department of Statistics. *Population Trends*; Singapore Department of Statistics, Ministry of Trade & Industry: Singapore, 2016; p. 5, ISSN 1793–2424.

23. Singapore Department of Statistics. *Population Trends*; Singapore Department of Statistics: Singapore, 2016; p. 30.

24. Wu, M.; Chen, S.W.; Jiang, S.Y. Relationship between gingival inflammation and pregnancy. *Med. Inflamm.* **2015**, *2015*. [CrossRef] [PubMed]

25. Pirie, M.; Cooke, I.; Linden, G.; Irwin, C. Dental manifestations of pregnancy. *Obs. Gynaecol.* **2007**, *9*, 21–26. [CrossRef]

26. Thomas, N.J.; Middleton, P.F.; Crowther, C.A. Oral and dental health care practices in pregnant women in Australia: A postnatal survey. *BMC Pregnancy Childbirth* **2008**, *8*, 13. [CrossRef] [PubMed]

27. Gaffield, M.L.; Gilbert, B.J.; Malvitz, D.M.; Romaguera, R. Oral health during pregnancy: An analysis of information collected by the pregnancy risk assessment monitoring system. *J. Am. Dent. Assoc.* **2001**, *132*, 1009–1016. [CrossRef] [PubMed]

28. Baskaradoss, J.K.; Geevarghese, A.; Al Dosari, A.A.F. Causes of Adverse Pregnancy Outcomes and the Role of Maternal Periodontal Status—A Review of the Literature. *Open Dent. J.* **2012**, *6*, 79–84. [CrossRef] [PubMed]

29. Capasso, F.; Vozza, I.; Capuccio, V.; Vestri, A.R.; Polimeni, A.; Ottolenghi, L. Correlation among periodontal health status, maternal age and pre-term low birth weight. *Am. J. Dent.* **2016**, *29*, 197–200. [PubMed]

30. Amin, M.; ElSalhy, M. Factors affecting utilization of dental services during pregnancy. *J. Periodontol.* **2014**, *85*, 1712–1721. [CrossRef] [PubMed]

31. George, A.; Johnson, M.; Duff, M.; Ajwani, S.; Bhole, S.; Blinkhorn, A.; Ellis, S. Midwives and oral health care during pregnancy: Perceptions of pregnant women in south-western Sydney, Australia. *J. Clin. Nurs.* **2012**, *21*, 1087–1096. [CrossRef] [PubMed]

32. Hullah, E.; Turok, Y.; Nauta, M.; Yoong, W. Self-reported oral hygiene habits, dental attendance and attitudes to dentistry during pregnancy in a sample of immigrant women in North London. *Arch. Gynecol. Obs.* **2008**, *277*, 405–409. [CrossRef] [PubMed]

33. Al Habashneh, R.; Guthmiller, J.M.; Levy, S.; Johnson, G.K.; Squier, C.; Dawson, D.V.; Fang, Q. Factors related to utilization of dental services during pregnancy. *J. Clin. Periodontol.* **2005**, *32*, 815–821. [CrossRef] [PubMed]

34. Committee on Health Care for Underserved Women. Oral health care during pregnancy and through the lifespan. *Obs. Gynecol.* **2013**, *122*, 417–422. [CrossRef]

35. Naseem, M.; Khurshid, Z.; Khan, H.A.; Niazi, F.; Zohaib, S.; Zafar, M.S. Oral health challenges in pregnant women: Recommendations for dental care professionals. *Saudi J. Dent. Res.* **2016**, *7*, 138–146. [CrossRef]

36. Chacko, V.; Shenoy, R.; Prasy, H.E.; Agarwal, S. Self-reported awareness of oral health and infant oral health among pregnant women in Mangalore, India—A prenatal survey. *Int. J. Health Rehabilit. Sci.* **2013**, *2*, 109–115.

37. Saddki, N.; Yusoff, A.; Hwang, Y.L. Factors associated with dental visit and barriers to utilisation of oral health care services in a sample of antenatal mothers in Hospital Universiti Sains Malaysia. *BMC Public Health* **2010**, *10*, 75. [CrossRef] [PubMed]

38. Al-Sufyani, G.A.; Al-Maweri, S.A.; Al-Ghashm, A.A.; Al-Soneidar, W.A. Oral hygiene and gingival health status of children with Down syndrome in Yemen: A cross-sectional study. *J. Int. Soc. Prev. Commun. Dent.* **2014**, *4*, 82–86. [CrossRef]

39. Bressane, L.B.; Costa, L.N.B.D.S.; Vieira, J.M.R.; Rebelo, M.A.B. Oral health conditions among pregnant women attended to at a health care center in Manaus, Amazonas, Brazil. *Rev. Odonto Cienc.* **2011**, *26*, 291–296. [CrossRef]

40. Deinzer, R.; Granrath, N.; Spahl, M.; Linz, S.; Waschul, B.; Herforth, A. Stress, oral health behaviour and clinical outcome. *Br. J. Health Psychol.* **2005**, *10*, 269–283. [CrossRef] [PubMed]

41. Cigna Corporation. 2015 Cigna Corporation Healthy Smiles for Mom and Baby: Insights into Expecting and New Mothers' Oral Health Habits. 2015. Available online: https://www.cigna.com/assets/docs/newsroom/cigna-study-healthy-smiles-for-mom-and-baby-2015.pdf (accessed on 3 July 2018).

42. Tang, Y.; Zhu, Y.Q.; Wang, Y.; He, Y. A survey about knowledge, attitude, practice of oral health in pregnant women of one hospital in Shanghai municipality. *Shanghai J. Stomatol.* **2011**, *20*, 531–534.

43. Ifesanya, J.U.; Ifesanya, A.O.; Asuzu, M.C.; Oke, G.A. Determinants of good oral hygiene among pregnant women in Ibadan, south-western Nigeria. *Ann. Ib. Postgrad. Med.* **2010**, *8*, 95–100. [CrossRef] [PubMed]

44. Beegle, D. Overcoming the Silence of Generational Poverty: Invisible Literacies. 2003. Available online: http://www.combarriers.com/TP0151Overcoming.pdf (accessed on 10 February 2017).

45. Steinberg, B.J.; Hilton, I.V.; Iida, H.; Samelson, R. Oral health and dental care during pregnancy. *Dent. Clin. North Am.* **2013**, *57*, 195–210. [CrossRef] [PubMed]

46. Jackson, J.T.; Quinonez, R.B.; Kerns, A.K.; Chuang, A.; Eidson, R.S.; Boggess, K.A.; Weintraub, J.A. Implementing a prenatal oral health program through interprofessional collaboration. *J. Dent. Educ.* **2015**, *79*, 241–248. [PubMed]

17

Precision Medicine: The Role of the MSIDS Model in Defining, Diagnosing, and Treating Chronic Lyme Disease/Post Treatment Lyme Disease Syndrome and Other Chronic Illness: Part 2

Richard I. Horowitz [1,2,*]🆔 and Phyllis R. Freeman [2]🆔

1   HHS Tickborne Disease Working Group, Washington, DC 20201, USA
2   Hudson Valley Healing Arts Center, New York, NY 12538, USA; freemanp63@gmail.com
*   Correspondence: medical@hvhac.com

Abstract: We present a precision medical perspective to assist in the definition, diagnosis, and management of Post Treatment Lyme Disease Syndrome (PTLDS)/chronic Lyme disease. PTLDS represents a small subset of patients treated for an erythema migrans (EM) rash with persistent or recurrent symptoms and functional decline. The larger population with chronic Lyme disease is less understood and well defined. Multiple Systemic Infectious Disease Syndrome (MSIDS) is a multifactorial model for treating chronic disease(s), which identifies up to 16 overlapping sources of inflammation and their downstream effects. A patient symptom survey and a retrospective chart review of 200 patients was therefore performed on those patients with chronic Lyme disease/PTLDS to identify those variables on the MSIDS model with the greatest potential effect on regaining health. Results indicate that dapsone combination therapy decreased the severity of eight major Lyme symptoms, and multiple sources of inflammation (other infections, immune dysfunction, autoimmunity, food allergies/sensitivities, leaky gut, mineral deficiencies, environmental toxins with detoxification problems, and sleep disorders) along with downstream effects of inflammation may all affect chronic symptomatology. In part two of our observational study and review paper, we postulate that the use of this model can represent an important and needed paradigm shift in the diagnosis and treatment of chronic disease.

Keywords: Chronic Lyme disease; Post Treatment Lyme Disease Syndrome (PTLDS); dapsone; Multiple Systemic Infectious Disease Syndrome (MSIDS); persister bacteria; precision medicine; Chronic Variable Immune Deficiency (CVID); Postural Orthostatic Tachycardia Syndrome (POTS)

1. Introduction

Lyme disease is rapidly spreading and there has been a 320% increase in the number of US counties affected with Lyme disease within the past 20 years [1], with another recent threefold increase in the number of vector-borne disease cases [2]. Among the almost 650,000 vector-borne reported cases during a 12-year period, over 491,000 were tick-borne and over 150,000 were mosquito-borne [3]. According to prior National Institutes of Health (NIH) studies, those patients with symptoms of chronic Lyme disease, both diagnosed and undiagnosed, are extremely ill [4] and many are disabled and unable to work [5].

Nearly one out of two adults in the United States during the past decade have been found to suffer from at least one chronic condition [6], with estimates of US disability rates ranging from 13–19% [7]. Some of these disabling symptoms include arthritis, pain, fatigue, and cognitive difficulties. These are hallmark symptoms of Lyme disease and associated co-infections. Since the present Lyme disease diagnostic two-tiered testing strategy used for surveillance purposes [8] is known to have a sensitivity/specificity averaging around 56% [9], and as per the Centers for Disease Control and Prevention (CDC), the surveillance case definitions "are not intended to be used by health care providers for making a clinical diagnosis … " [10], approximately half of the individuals with Lyme disease may go undiagnosed. Some individuals suffering from "medically unexplained symptoms" (MUS) may therefore have contracted a tick-borne illness. Inadequate diagnostic testing for Lyme disease and associated *Borrelia* species may also be contributing to this diagnostic dilemma, as discussed in detail in Precision Medicine: Retrospective Chart Review and Data Analysis of 200 Patients on Dapsone Combination Therapy for Chronic Lyme Disease/PTLDS: Part 1. There has been an expansion of other *Borrelia sensu lato* species across the United States in the past decade [11], and many of these borrelia species, including Relapsing Fever *Borrelia* spp. and *Borrelia miyamotoi* as well as *Borrelia bissetti*, will not be found on standard two-tiered testing strategies for Lyme disease, yet they can lead to unexplained chronic illness [12–15].

The true healthcare burden for tick-borne illness may also be unappreciated due to Lyme disease and coinfections mimicking other chronic illnesses. Five percent of the US population suffers from Chronic Fatigue Syndrome (CFS)/Myalgic Encephalomyelitis and Fibromyalgia [16], which share the same symptoms as Lyme disease. The diagnostic criteria for these two diseases are based on symptomatology and establishing a differential diagnosis, not on specific laboratory testing. The true number of individuals with borreliosis and co-infections resulting in these chronic fatiguing, musculoskeletal illnesses with cognitive difficulties is therefore unknown. Prior reports on the role of *Bartonella* species indicate, for example, that this class of bacteria can cause a broad range of rheumatologic and neurologic symptoms resembling CFS/fibromyalgia [17–19].

Spirochetes have also been reported to be found in the brains of individuals suffering from dementia, and in the biofilms of patients suffering from Alzheimer's disease [20,21]. Multiple scientific peer-reviewed journal articles in the past two decades have implicated a possible association between bacterial and viral infections [22] along with environmental toxins in neurodegenerative conditions, with recent healthcare estimates approximating that 46 million Americans presently suffer from pre-clinical dementia [23]. Environmental toxins and spirochetes have both been associated with cognitive difficulties, as well as autoimmune illness, which presently affects tens of millions of Americans [24]. The necessity of effective prevention, diagnostic, and treatment strategies for Lyme disease and associated co-infections, and the need to evaluate their role in these disorders is urgently needed based on the above statistics. Just as important, however, is the need to determine the role of overlapping infections, environmental toxins, and other etiologies increasing inflammation, resulting in diverse chronic disease manifestations. If we are to improve public health and control rising health care costs, a new paradigm to account for the rising burden of chronic illness is needed.

The etiology and treatment of chronic Lyme disease/Post Treatment Lyme Disease Syndrome (PTLDS) has been a hotly debated topic in the medical literature for the past three decades. This problem exists in part because of a lack of clear definitions. PTLDS is defined as a syndrome in patients who have been treated for an erythema migrans rash (EM) with appropriate antibiotic treatment who have "persistent or recurrent patient-reported symptoms of fatigue, musculoskeletal pain, and/or cognitive complaints with associated functional decline, and this syndrome represents a defined subset of the larger patient population with the diagnosis of chronic Lyme disease, which is less understood and well defined" [25,26]. Theories of why patients remain ill generally range from autoimmune reactions post infection to tissue damage and/or persistent infection of the spirochete and/or its parts. No one model, however, has been sufficient to explain ongoing symptomatology after standard courses of antibiotics. The prevailing medical model used to describe and explain most chronic infectious disease is the "one microorganism/one disease" model based on Koch's postulates taught in medical school. This theory was established in the late 1800s. Scientific advances since that time include significant improvements in diagnostics as well as identifying expanding tick populations with a better understanding of the tick microbiome and associated coinfections, along with identifying the role of borrelia, other intracellular bacteria (i.e., *Bartonella* spp. and *Mycoplasma* spp.), the gastrointestinal (G.I). microbiome, and environmental toxin exposures in autoimmune illness. The role of nutritional deficiencies, food allergies/sensitivities, leaky gut [27], and/or sleep disorders, which can contribute to free radical/oxidative stress and further increase inflammation and symptomatology [28–39], have also been identified in the recent medical literature as potential etiological causes of chronic symptoms.

All these factors can have deleterious downstream effects on the body, including, but not limited to, mitochondrial and liver dysfunction; Hypothalamic-Pituitary-Adrenal (HPA) axis and autonomic nervous system dysfunction; as well as the ability to increase neuropsychiatric symptoms and pain syndromes [40,41]. The establishment of a new paradigm to account for all these factors and their roles in causing disabling symptoms after standard treatment for chronic Lyme disease/PTLDS is of vital importance based on the significant numbers of individuals contracting vector borne diseases. A data mining approach in a large cohort of symptomatic Lyme disease patients was undertaken to be able to better define the role of these multiple variables in those suffering from resistant symptoms of chronic Lyme disease/PTLDS.

In 2012, Horowitz described a multifactorial model for chronic disease known as MSIDS, or Multiple Systemic Infectious Disease Syndrome [39]. The individual patient's risks are evaluated during the initial evaluation as the model recognizes that a "one size fits all" approach using general medical guidelines may not account for individual differences and risk factors. The 16-point MSIDS model can efficiently screen through multifactorial etiologies contributing to chronic illness and focus on prevention (epigenetics), thus personalizing treatment. It represents a potential paradigm shift in the diagnostic and treatment approaches for chronic disease, as no one factor is assumed in advance to play a predominant role in the patient's symptomatology. It is only after taking a detailed history, evaluating chief complaints, reviewing family, social, and environmental histories, checking a review of systems, and performing a physical examination that medical hypotheses are formed, leading to focused laboratory testing.

Factors on the 16-point MSIDS model [42], which are then evaluated based on the history and physical examination, and can contribute to chronic disease include:

(1) **Infections**: Four types of infections are assessed. Some are tickborne and others may be mosquito borne, and/or transmitted by other vectors (including fleas, lice, mites, biting flies, and spider bites) or due to human to human transmission:

(a) Bacteria: i.e., *Borrelia burgdorferi* [Lyme disease]; other *Borrelia* species, such as *Borrelia sensu lato* species [43] and Relapsing Fever; *Ehrlichia, Anaplasma, Bartonella* species; *Mycoplasma* and *Chlamydia* species; *Rickettsia* species [*Rickettsia rickettsia* (Rocky Mountain spotted fever), *Coxiella burnetii* (Q fever), *Rickettsia typhi* (typhus)]; *Francisella tularensis* [tularemia]; and *Brucella* spp. [Brucellosis].

(b) Parasites: *B. microti* and *B. duncani* [Babesiosis], other piroplasms, *Toxoplasma gondii* (toxoplasmosis), intestinal parasites.

(c) Viruses: Herpes simplex virus 1 (HSV1), Herpes simplex virus 2 (HSV2), Human Herpes Virus 6 (HHV-6), Epstein Barr Virus [EBV], Cytomegalovirus [CMV], Coxsackie virus, Parvovirus, West Nile virus (WNV).

(d) Candida and other fungi.

(2) **Immune dysfunction**: *Borrelia burgdorferi* as well as European strains, including *Borrelia garinii*, have been associated with autoimmune phenomena [44,45]. Autoimmune markers, including antinuclear antibodies (ANA) and rheumatoid factors (RF), were assessed, as well as Human Leukocyte Antigen (HLA) markers (DR2, DR4) and immunoglobulin deficiencies and/or subclass deficiencies [46].

(3) **Inflammation**: Inflammatory chemokines and cytokines are produced during infection [47–49]. Erythrocyte Sedimentation Rate (ESR), C-Reactive Protein (CRP, an indirect marker of IL-6), Human Transforming Growth Factor beta 1 (TGFB1), Complement component 3a (C3a), Complement component 4a (C4a), and Vascular Endothelial Growth Factor (VEGF), an indirect marker of *Bartonella* infection [30]) were gauged as markers of inflammation.

(4) **Toxicity**: The burden of heavy metals, including mercury, lead, arsenic, cadmium, and aluminum, were recorded [50–52] as well as levels of mold toxins, including aflatoxins, trichothecenes, ochratoxins, and gliotoxins. Neurotoxins, such as quinolinic acid, may also be produced during infection [53,54]. Patients with a history of multiple chemical sensitivity (MCS) and/or Parkinson's disease were evaluated for the presence of pesticides, as well as a clinical response to intravenous and oral glutathione, which is known to play a role in chemical detoxification [55].

(5) **Allergies/Sensitivities**: Foods [56,57], medications, and environmental allergies were recorded. Inflammatory cytokine production, similar to those produced during a Lyme infection, may be found in those with allergic reactions. Markers, including total IgE antibody levels, IgE food allergies, evidence of gluten sensitivity or celiac disease (antigliadin antibodies, tissue transglutaminase (TTG)), and histamine levels were recorded if pruritis and/or symptoms of Mast Cell Activation Disorder were present [58].

(6) **Nutritional and enzyme deficiencies/functional medicine abnormalities in biochemical pathways** [59,60]: Patients with poor nutritional intake were tested for amino acid and/or fatty acid deficiencies. All patients were checked for methylenetetrahydrofolate reductase (MTHFR) gene mutations as well as mineral deficiencies, including iodine, copper, zinc, and magnesium. These minerals are essential cofactors in the biochemical pathways responsible for controlling free radical/oxidative stress, inflammation, hormone production, and detoxification.

(7) **Mitochondrial dysfunction [61–63]**: The mitochondria are essential for energy production in the muscles, nerves, brain, liver, kidney, and heart. Mitochondrial dysfunction was defined as those who had positive responses to the following mitochondrial support supplements: NT Factors, i.e., glycosylated phospholipids, CoQ10, acetyl-l-carnitine, and d-ribose.

(8) **Psychological disorders**: Neuropsychiatric symptoms may result from and/or worsen when Lyme disease and associated coinfections, such as *Bartonella* spp. and *Babesia* spp., are present [64,65]. Common manifestations, including depression, anxiety, Obsessive Compulsive Disorder (OCD), and Post Traumatic Stress Disorder (PTSD), were recorded [66].

(9) **Neurological dysfunction**: An infection with *Borrelia burgdorferi* and associated coinfections, including, but not limited to, other *Borrelia* species, *Babesia* spp., *Bartonella* spp., *Rickettsia* spp., and *Mycoplasma* spp., may increase neurological dysfunction [20,47,67]. We evaluated patients using our online symptom survey for evidence of neurological symptoms (headaches, cognitive dysfunction, as well as neuropathy). Proof of neuropathy with or without Chronic Inflammatory Demyelinating Polyneuropathy (CIDP) were also determined by direct chart review of physical examination/electromyogram (EMG)/small fiber biopsies.

(10) **Endocrine disorders [68–70]**: Hypothalamic-Pituitary-Axis (HPA) axis dysfunction may result from an infectious process. Evidence of thyroid, adrenal, and sex hormone dysfunction were recorded. Adrenal function was measured by blood, urine, and saliva testing [71]. Vitamin D levels (whose ratios can be an indirect marker for the presence of intracellular infections), as well as precursors of hormones, including Dehydroepiandrosterone sulfate (DHEA-S) and pregnenolone, were also noted.

(11) **Sleep disorders** [72,73]: Lyme disease is known to result in circadian rhythm disorders [74], including delayed sleep phase syndrome (DSPS) [75], where patients have a challenging time falling asleep and/or staying asleep. Hypersomnolence due to inflammatory cytokine production is also a known clinical manifestation [76–78]. Individuals were evaluated for evidence of any sleep related disorders, including obstructive sleep apnea (OSA), restless leg syndrome (RLS), hormone imbalance (menopause, elevated adrenal function at night), benign prostatic hypertrophy (BPH), and/or medication induced sleep problems.

(12) **Autonomic nervous system (ANS) dysfunction and Postural Orthostatic Tachycardia Syndrome (POTS)** [79–84]: Postural orthostatic tachycardia syndrome following Lyme disease has been reported [85], and four principal types of neuropathy can affect the nervous system in the patient infected with *Borrelia burgdorferi*. Autonomic neuropathy is a form of polyneuropathy that affects elements of the central nervous system (brain/hypothalamus and spinal cord), peripheral nervous

system with its sensory motor branches, and the enteric nervous system made up of nerve fibers that go to the bladder and gastrointestinal tract (including the pancreas and gallbladder). Problems with the autonomic nervous system can result in symptoms of resistant fatigue, dizziness, low blood pressure and fainting, anxiety, palpitations, cognitive difficulties, absent or excessive sweating, problems with temperature dysregulation [86], and problems with gastroparesis (nausea, vomiting) with or without constipation and/or bladder dysfunction. POTS is often diagnosed by a Head-up Tilt Table Test (HUT), but if such testing is not available, POTS can be diagnosed with bedside measurements of heart rate and blood pressure taken in the supine (laying down) and standing up position [87]. In our study, we performed sitting and standing blood pressures with corresponding pulse rates at time 0 (sitting for several minutes), 3, 6, and 9 min were recorded. Mild POTS was defined as a 1–10 mm Hg drop in blood pressure (BP), and/or 1–10-point increase in heart rate after standing for 9 min; moderate POTS was defined as a 11–29 mm drop in BP, and/or 11–29-point increase in heart rate after standing for 9 min; severe POTS was defined as a 30+ increase in heart rate standing and/or drop in systolic or diastolic blood pressure by 30 mm Hg or greater, standing for 9 min. More detailed tests to evaluate the autonomic nervous system [86], such as the Quantitative Sudomotor Axon Reflex Test (QSART), Heart Rate Response to deep breathing (HRDB), Valsalva maneuver (VM), Thermoregulatory Sweat Test (TST), Quantitative sensory testing (QST), skin biopsies evaluating the small fiber nerves, and gastric motility studies were performed in a small subset of patients with symptoms of severe autonomic neuropathy.

(13) **Gastrointestinal (G.I.) disorders** [27,88]: Certain G.I. disorders may result in increased inflammation, so patients were evaluated for one or more of the following gastrointestinal complaints: Gluten sensitivity, celiac disease, colitis, Candidiasis, leaky gut, parasites, *Helicobacter pylori* exposure, gastroesophageal reflux disease (GERD), and/or a history of *Clostridium difficile* while on dapsone combination therapy (DDS CT). Microbiome analysis and evaluation of beneficial short chain fatty acids (SCFA), inflammation, pancreatic enzymes, and fat malabsorption was done through Genova/Metametrix when clinically indicated.

(14) **Elevated liver function testing (LFT's)**: Elevated liver functions have been associated with inflammatory cytokine production [89], and may result from Lyme disease and associated tickborne infections, including, but not limited to, anaplasmosis, ehrlichiosis, Rocky Mountain spotted fever, babesiosis, and relapsing fever (*Borrelia miyamotoi*). Other causes of elevated liver functions include alpha-1 antitrypsin deficiency, Wilson's disease, hemochromatosis, viral and autoimmune hepatitis, gallstones, inflammatory bowel disease, connective tissue disease, congestive heart failure (right-sided), hepatic steatosis (Non Alcoholic Steatohepatitis, i.e., NASH), acute and chronic pulmonary disease, endocrine disorders, chemical and drug exposure, as well as cancer [90–92]. Evidence of elevated Aspartate Aminotransferase (AST), Alanine Aminotransferase (ALT), alkaline phosphatase, and total bilirubin were recorded. Patients were tested for the above liver pathologies if liver function abnormalities persisted.

(15) **Pain syndromes**: Muscular, arthritic, and neuropathic pain syndromes [93–96] (often migratory nature, which is one of the hallmarks of Lyme disease [96]) along with headaches/migraines can be seen with tick-borne disorders. Evidence of these syndromes were noted. Some patients were on compounded medications for pain and inflammation, including low dose naltrexone (LDN) and glutathione.

(16) **Physical Therapy (PT)/deconditioning** [97–99]: Many patients are deconditioned due to long-standing chronic illness. The need for physical therapy and reconditioning programs was evaluated along with their efficacy with improving fatigue, muscle strength, and coordination.

These numerous factors on the 16-point MSIDS model can be arranged into two categories (multiple causes of inflammation and the downstream effects of inflammation), which can account for persistent symptoms in tickborne and other chronic disease. The causes of inflammation include multiple infections, immune dysfunction, genetic causes of autoimmunity, imbalances of the microbiome of the gut, food allergies/sensitivities, leaky gut, mineral deficiencies and sleep disorders.

There are also factors which have adverse downstream effects at both the cellular and organ systems levels, leading to resistant fatigue, pain, and neurocognitive symptoms. These would include potential downstream effects of inflammation leading to endocrine disorders (low testosterone, estradiol, and progesterone with low libido; low adrenal function; hypothyroidism), neurological and psychological dysfunction, POTS/dysautonomia, mitochondrial dysfunction, pain syndromes, liver dysfunction, and autoimmune phenomenon. Any of these chronic disease manifestations may be worsened and/or due to one or multiple factors. This is the case with autoimmune reactions, which the scientific literature has shown can be affected by exposure to borrelia and other infections [100] (including, but not limited to, *Bartonella* and *Mycoplasma* species) [30,32,33], environmental toxin exposure (i.e., mercury, bisphenol A, asbestos, and/or small particle pollution) [50,51,101,102], imbalances in the microbiome of the gut, and/or from a genetic predisposition [103]. We therefore collected data from an online survey, which evaluated the efficacy of dapsone combined with other antibiotics and agents that disrupt biofilm for the treatment of chronic Lyme disease/PTLDS, along with information data mined directly from 200 patient records detailing abnormalities on the MSIDS model.

In part one, we evaluated the efficacy of newer "persister" drug regimens, like dapsone combination therapy, and found this protocol decreased the severity of eight major Lyme symptoms and improved treatment outcome. We also found multiple species of intracellular bacteria, including *Rickettsia*, *Bartonella*, *Mycoplasma*, *Chlamydia*, *F. tularensis*, and *Brucella*, contributing to the burden of illness, as well as a high prevalence of *Babesia* complicating management, with probable geographic spread of *Babesia WA1/duncani* to the Northeast. Occasional reactivation of viral infections, including HHV-6, in immunocompromised individuals was also seen in a small percentage of patients.

In part two, we seek to understand how Lyme disease can affect different body systems, how abnormalities on the MSIDS model can affect chronic symptoms in those with Lyme disease and associated coinfections, as well as which combination of factors might contribute to the burden of chronic illness leading to resistant symptomatology.

2. Materials and Methods

2.1. Participants

Participants included in this project were 200 adults recruited from a specialized Lyme disease medical practice using email and telephone contacts. Although situated in the Northeastern United States, the medical practice attracts patients from all over the world. Of 200 participants, 67 (33.5) were male, and 133 (66.5%) were female. Age ranged from 18–84 (M = 52.04, SD = 16.66). Out of 200 participants, 4 (2%) were Asian (Non-Hispanic), while the rest were all White (Non-Hispanic). Participants were mostly from the United States (N = 193), which was divided into demographic regions: West Coast (N = 1), Midwest (N = 16), East Coast (North) (N = 155), East Coast (South) (N = 20), and Other (Hawaii) (N = 1). Potential participants were sent an email invitation containing a link to the online symptom survey reported in Precision Medicine: Part 1.

2.2. Methodology

We conducted a retrospective chart review of a convenience sample of patients who agreed to have their medical charts reviewed. These charts (N = 657) were from the 200 patients who served as participants in our dapsone trial (reported in Part 1) and who had given informed consent to examine their medical records for MSIDS variables. Most of these patients had multiple charts documenting their treatment over the course of many years. Patients had enrolled in the preliminary dapsone trial based on the drug's action on "persister" bacteria [104–107]. Each participant received detailed instructions that outlined the need for blood testing every three weeks, dietary guidelines, and the name and phone number of the medical center's head nurse if anyone had questions or medical issues. Surveys were given in office, online, and via telephone to gather patient information.

Inclusion criteria: All 200 patients in our study met the criteria for a clinical diagnosis of Lyme disease supported by a physician documented erythema migrans (EM) rash and/or positive laboratory testing, including a positive ELISA/Enzyme Immunoassay (EIA), and/or C6 ELISA, Immunofluorescent Antibody (IFA), CDC positive IgM and/or IgG Western Blot, Polymerase Chain Reaction (PCR), *Borrelia* specific bands (23, 31, 34, 39, 83/93) on a Western blot [108] and/or positive ELISPOT (Lymphocyte Transformation Test, i.e., LTT). These patients had either failed or had an inadequate response to prior antibiotic therapy, and/or relapsed with persistent symptoms after stopping anti-infective therapy.

Exclusion criteria: Patients under the age of 18, patients having a known allergy to dapsone or any medication used in the trial, and/or having significant laboratory abnormalities, including a pre-trial anemia, were excluded from our study.

2.3. Data Mining Procedure

After we identified and operationally defined the MSIDS study variables we wished to explore, we provided those conducting the chart review with a list of these variables and their definitions, and provided them with a set of procedures to follow, including inclusion and exclusion criteria for each variable. Following the training of our data "miners" and a pilot test of the procedures, we provided them with oversight and closely monitored the procedure for consistency. All data mining was conducted via laptop computers using a standardized set of operationally defined variables recorded on duplicate Excel data sheets. Each research assistant on our team used his or her own Excel sheet and worked in pairs (one member entering data while the one member identified the variables in the chart). Excel sheet data were then combined/merged for data analysis. All data entry was from de-identified participants, and their PHI (personal health information) was entered via a research code assigned at random. Participant names and other identifiers were only known to the first author of this paper and the head nurse, who, with the first author, provided oversight to the procedures. All of those involved in data mining the charts and data analysis were HIPPA trained, had backgrounds and education in scientific data collection, and signed additional confidentiality agreements with our medical center. The first author was directly involved in data mining and data entry, and the second author provided oversight and team coordination. Data analysis of the Excel data was via SPSS software (version 25.0 from IBM SPSS Statistics, Armonk, NY, USA).

2.4. Laboratory Testing

Analysis of MSIDS variables were conducted using blood testing from several national reference laboratories (Quest Diagnostics, Secaucus, NJ, USA; LabCorp, Burlington, NC, USA; BioReference, Elmwood Park, NJ, USA; Pacific Toxicology Laboratories, Chatsworth, CA, USA), local state laboratories (i.e., Sunrise Medical Laboratories, Hicksville, NY, USA; NorDx, Scarborough, ME, USA; Affiliated Laboratory Inc., Rutland, VT, USA, AccuReference Medical Lab, Wappingers Falls, NY, USA), specialty laboratories for tick-borne diseases (Imugen, Norwood, MA, IgeneX, Palo Alto, CA, USA; Medical Diagnostic Laboratory, Hamilton Township, NJ, USA; Stony Brook Lyme Disease Laboratory, Stony Brook, NY, USA; Milford Molecular Diagnostics, Milford, CT, USA; Galaxy diagnostics, Morrisville, NC, USA; Immunosciences Lab, Inc, Los Angeles, CA, USA), and functional medicine laboratories (Aeron Lifecycles Clinical Laboratory, San Leandro, CA, USA; Labrix Clinical Laboratory, Clackamas, OR, USA; Genova Diagnostics, Asheville, NC, USA; Great Plains, Lenexa, KS, USA; Diagnos-Tech, Kent, WA, USA; Doctor's Data, St Charles, IL, RealTime Laboratory, Carrollton, TX, USA). More than one laboratory was used for each patient depending on laboratory capability, patient insurance, and availability in their home state (Galaxy diagnostics were not available in N.Y.). Measurement of environmental toxins was done by both blood and urine testing. A urine DMSA challenge through Doctor's Data was used to evaluate heavy metals (not just blood testing), since metals can leave the bloodstream and accumulate in tissues where they are no longer measurable, compartmentalizing in body tissues. DMSA effectively competes with tissue binding sites, releasing metals from sequestered sites, which then redistribute into the blood as a stable complex, and are then eliminated in the urine where they can be measured [109]. Patients were not tested with a DMSA challenge if there was evidence of significant sulfa sensitivity. Pesticide levels were measured by both blood (LabCorp) and urine analysis (PacTox Laboratories), and mold testing was done by urine analysis through the RealTime Laboratory in Texas, using liposomal glutathione (2 g) and sauna therapy prior to measurements [110]. G.I. evaluations included an upper endoscopy and colonoscopy if there was a history of GERD and/or colitis; H. pylori analysis was done by blood (and occasionally breath test, endoscopy); stool and microbiome analysis (bacteria, parasites, fungi) were done through both local laboratories and Genova/Metametrix. Liver function testing was done through local and national laboratories, with ultrasonography if NASH was suspected. Testing for Mast Cell Activation Disorder (MCAD) and food allergies included serum histamine, tryptase, chromogranin A, and IgE blood tests, respectively, (occasionally IgG4 delayed food allergy hypersensitivity testing was performed), when clinically indicated (MCAD can also be associated with POTS) [86]. Tilt table testing with or without small fiber biopsies and autonomic/electrodiagnostic testing (EMG) were done through private neurology and hospital settings (i.e., New York University). Sleep testing by polysomnography was done through Accusom (Novasom) home sleep testing (GlenBurnie, MD, USA) and in hospital settings with board certified pulmonary physicians (diplomates of the American Board of Sleep Medicine, Darien, IL, USA). A brief description of the tests and methods of evaluation for the 16 MSIDS variables appears on Table 1.

Table 1. MSIDS variables: Tests/method of evaluation.

1. Infections	Laboratory tests for the presence of *Borrelia* spp., *Babesia* spp., *Bartonella* spp., *Rickettsia* spp., etc.
2. Immune Dysfunction	Laboratory tests for autoimmune markers (ANA, RF), HLA status, immunoglobulin levels, and subclasses
3. Inflammation	Laboratory tests for markers of inflammation, i.e., ESR, CRP, TGFB1, C3a, C4a, and/or VEGF
4. Toxicity	Laboratory tests for heavy metals, mold toxins, pesticides, etc.
5. Allergies	Laboratory tests for IgE levels, food and environmental allergies, histamine, etc.
6. Nutritional and Enzyme Deficiencies	Laboratory tests for amino acids, fatty acids, mineral levels (serum, plasma, red blood cell)
7. Mitochondrial Dysfunction	Clinical evaluation of response to mitochondrial support (NT Factors, CoQ10, L-carnitine), evaluation of mtDNA mutations, etc.
8. Psychological Dysfunction	Clinical evaluation for evidence of depression, anxiety, OCD, PTSD, etc.
9. Neurological Dysfunction	Clinical examination, EMG, Small fiber biopsy, MRI brain, etc.
10. Endocrine Abnormalities	Laboratory evaluation of hormone levels (thyroid, adrenal, sex hormones, Vitamin D) and hormone precursors (DHEA-S, pregnenolone)
11. Sleep Disorders	Clinical evaluation (diet, medication), sleep studies, laboratory evaluation of hormone levels, etc.
12. Autonomic Nervous System Dysfunction	Tilt table testing with or without small fiber biopsies and autonomic/electrodiagnostic testing (EMG), clinical evaluation sitting/standing BP/heart rate
13. Gastrointestinal Dysfunction	Endoscopy, colonoscopy, clinical/laboratory evaluation (celiac markers, H. pylori), Comprehensive Digestive Stool Analysis (CDSA) for bacteria (*C. difficile*), ova and parasites, Candida, etc.
14. Elevated Liver Enzymes	Laboratory evaluation of AST, ALT, Alkaline phosphatase, total bilirubin, etc.
15. Pain Syndromes	Clinical evaluation, EMG, small fiber biopsy, laboratory markers for autoimmune disease (anti-myelin antibodies), etc.
16. Deconditioning	Clinical evaluation and need for physical therapy

3. Results

3.1. MSIDS (Data Mining)

The 16-point Multiple Systemic Infectious Disease Syndrome (MSIDS) is "a symptom complex of Lyme disease and multiple associated tick-borne coinfections which encompasses not only infections with *B. burgdorferi*, the etiologic agent of Lyme disease, but also encompasses other bacterial, viral, parasitic, and fungal infections. This symptom complex also includes issues with immune dysfunction, inflammation, environmental toxicity, allergies, nutritional and enzyme deficiencies with functional medical abnormalities in biochemical pathways, mitochondrial dysfunction, neuropsychological issues, autonomic nervous system dysfunction, endocrine abnormalities, sleep disorders, GI abnormalities, with abnormalities of liver function, and issues with pain, drug use, and physical deconditioning" [111]. These abnormalities on the MSIDS model can be found in both those with Lyme disease, i.e., "Lyme-MSIDS", and those with "non-Lyme MSIDS", i.e., those individuals without tick-borne disease, where MSIDS variables may be contributing to the burden of chronic illness.

Since the MSIDS model posits that patients may remain ill with persistent Lyme symptoms not only because of ongoing infection(s), but also because of a complex of other overlapping medical problems, we closely examined each patient's chart for evidence of these conditions and abnormalities. We found extensive evidence that patients did not have just Lyme disease alone. Figure 1 provides an overview of the percentage of patients experiencing each of the 16 points from the MSIDS map, data mined directly from the patient charts for the 200 participants in the study.

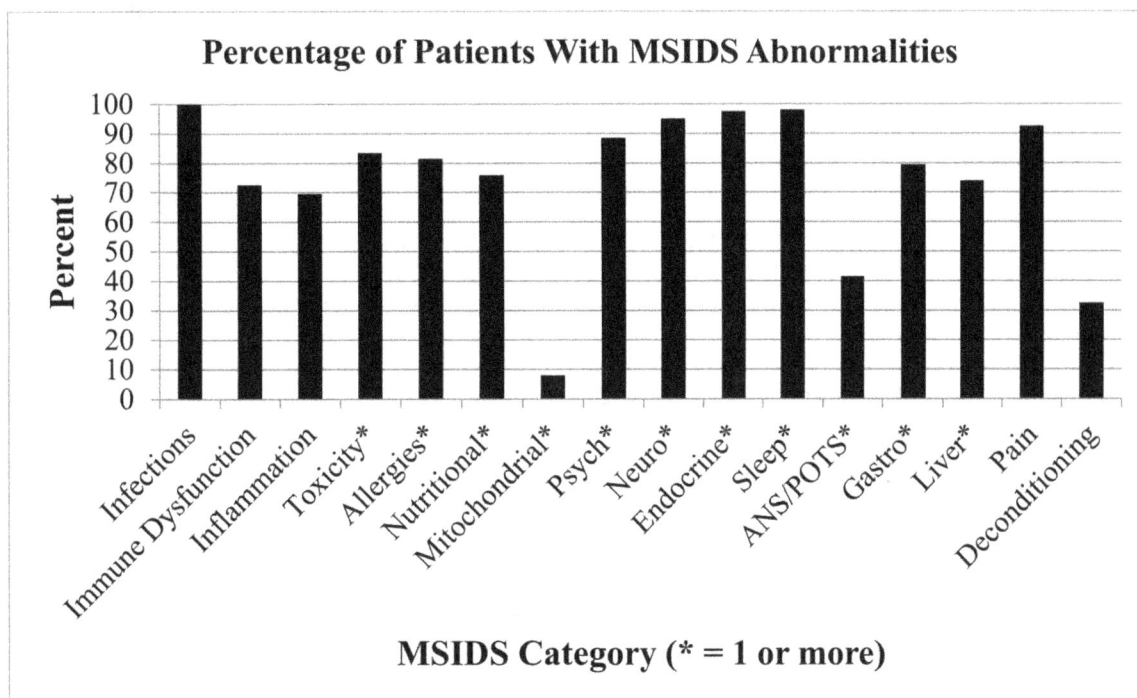

Figure 1. Percentage of patients with MSIDS abnormalities. Multiple overlapping abnormalities on the MSIDS map were associated with Lyme disease, contributing to ongoing symptomatology.

3.2. Patients Have More Than Lyme Disease: MSIDS Multifactorial Analysis

All our patients (100%) had evidence of exposure to one or more infections—all were being treated for Lyme disease as well as a range of coinfections (see Precision Medicine: Part 1). Babesiosis (*B. microti* and *B. duncani*) and *Bartonella* spp. (*B. henselae*) were the most commonly found coinfections. Among the 52% of patients with evidence of babesiosis by antibody titer and/or PCR/FISH, a significant percentage of *B. duncani* cases tested (28%) were found in the eastern seaboard. A small percentage of patients (2.5%) were found to have antibody titers for other *Bartonella* species, including *Bartonella quintana*.

Almost three quarters of patients (72.5%) had immune dysfunction (as measured by a positive ANA, RF with or without evidence of genetic HLA DR2, and DR4 markers with 85% having combined IgG subclass deficiencies). Several patients also had evidence of immune dysfunction based on the lack of increased antibody production in response to a pneumococcal vaccination. More than 69% of patients had evidence of inflammation (e.g., elevated ESR, CRP, TGFB1, C3a, C4a, and/or VEGF). Approximately 85% had positive tests for heavy metals, including elevated levels of lead, mercury, arsenic, cadmium, and aluminum (see Figure 2), with smaller numbers showing evidence of pesticide and mold exposure (not all patients were tested).

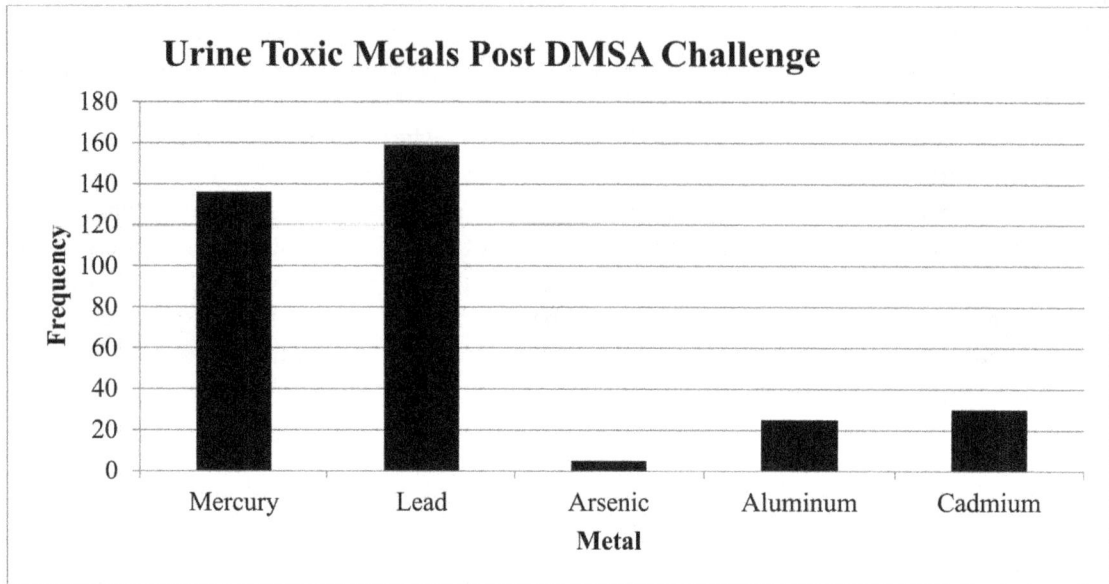

Figure 2. Urine toxic metals post dimercaptosuccinic acid (DMSA) challenge in 185 patients showed a high frequency of exposure to mercury and lead. Toxic metals were reported as micrograms/gram of creatinine to account for urine dilution variation. Ranges reported were within the reference range, elevated, and very elevated in comparison to a healthy population under non-challenge or non-provoked conditions.

Large numbers of patients (81%) had positive allergy testing (food allergies [45%] and drug allergies [56%]), with more than three quarters (76%) having one or more nutritional and enzyme deficiencies (MTHFR mutations were present in more than half of the patients [52.5%]). We also found that most individuals suffered from sleep disorders (98%), endocrine abnormalities (97.5%), neurological dysfunction (95%), pain syndromes (92.5%), psychological issues (88.5%), and some form of gastrointestinal and liver dysfunction (79.5% and 74% respectively), with less than half of the individuals having evidence of varying degrees of POTS/dysautonomia (41.5%), deconditioning (32%), and mitochondrial dysfunction (7.5%). In addition to coinfection testing, which was positive in our patients (see Precision Medicine: Part 1), the following is a detailed analysis of the number of individuals with multiple overlapping factors on the MSIDS map associated with their illness:

- Immune Dysfunction (positive ANA, RF, HLADR2, HLADR4: 145 (72.5%) participants had immune dysfunction, 13.5% had elevated IgM antibodies, and up to 85% had some form of immune deficiency:

  ○ 20.6% had total IgG deficiency;
  ○ 19.3% had IgM deficiency; and
  ○ 15.9% had IgA deficiency.

85.5% had combined IgG subclass deficiencies 1–4 (see Table 2).

Table 2. Frequencies and percentages of low, normal, and high immunoglobulin levels.

	N *	Low		Normal		High	
		Frequency	*Percent*	*Frequency*	*Percent*	*Frequency*	*Percent*
IgA	170	27	15.88	139	81.76	4	2.35
IgM	171	33	19.30	115	67.25	23	13.45
IgG	175	36	20.57	131	74.86	8	4.57
SubClass1	163	45	27.61	115	70.55	3	1.84
SubClass2	164	30	18.29	126	76.83	8	4.88
SubClass3	164	51	31.10	112	68.29	1	0.61
SubClass4	164	14	8.54	142	86.59	8	4.88

Frequencies and percentages of low, normal, and high immunoglobulin levels. A sizeable number of patients demonstrated immunoglobulin deficiencies and/or subclass deficiencies. Ranges for low, normal, and high values were determined by the reference laboratory. * Not every patient was tested for immunoglobulin and/or subclass deficiencies.

- Inflammation (Elevated ESR, CRP, TGFB1, C3a, C4a, TNF, VEGF): 139 (69.5%) participants had markers of inflammation.
- Toxicity: See Figure 2.

  ○ Heavy Metals: 169/185 (84.5%) had one or more elevated heavy metals using a 6-h urine DMSA challenge:

    ▪ 159 (79.5%) had elevated lead levels (N = 73 were elevated, and N = 59 were very elevated);
    ▪ 136 (68%) had elevated mercury levels (N = 77 were elevated, and N = 59 were very elevated);
    ▪ 5 (2.5%) had elevated arsenic levels (N = 3 were elevated, and N = 2 were very elevated);
    ▪ 25 (12.5%) had elevated aluminum levels (N = 25 were elevated); and
    ▪ 30 (15%) had elevated cadmium levels (N = 26 were elevated, and N = 4 were very elevated).

  ○ Mold: 30/42 (71.4%) had one or more elevated mold levels:

    ▪ 13/25 (52%) had elevated aflatoxins;
    ▪ 18/26 (69%) had elevated ochratoxins;
    ▪ 20/26 (76.9%) had elevated trichothecenes;
    ▪ 17/17 (100%) had elevated gliotoxins; and
    ▪ 7/18 (38.9%) had other elevated mold (Stachybotrys exposure).

  ○ Pesticides: 5 (2.5%) tested positive for pesticides*.

*Not all patients were tested for mold or pesticides: Only those with a history of significant mold exposure and/or pesticide exposure were checked, especially if there was evidence of significant chemical sensitivity and/or Parkinson's symptoms.

- Allergies: 163 (81.5%) of participants had allergies:

  ○ 90 (45%) had food allergies;
  ○ 43 (21.5%) had environmental allergies (e.g., seasonal allergies, allergy to animals, etc.);
  ○ 7 (3.5%) had high IgE levels;
  ○ 3 (1.5%) had high histamine levels (not all patients were tested for histamine sensitivity or Mast Cell Activation Disorder [MCAD]);
  ○ 112 (56%) had drug allergies; and
  ○ 12 (6%) had allergies categorized as "other".

- Nutritional and Enzyme Deficiencies: 152 (76%) participants had one or more of these deficiencies. All patients were tested for mineral deficiencies, but only patients with poor nutritional intake were tested for amino acid and/or fatty acid deficiencies:

  - 5 (2.5%) had amino acid deficiencies;
  - 2 (1%) had fatty acid deficiencies;
  - 36 (18%) had iodine deficiencies;
  - 14 (7%) had copper deficiencies;

    - 3 (1.5%) had deficiencies in serum copper;
    - 6 (3%) had deficiencies in red blood cell [RBC] copper;
    - 5 (2.5%) had deficiencies in plasma copper;

  - 31 (16%) had magnesium deficiencies;

    - 6 (3%) had deficiencies in serum magnesium;
    - 26 (13%) had deficiencies in RBC magnesium;

  - 36 (18%) had zinc deficiencies;

    - 22 (11%) had deficiencies in serum zinc;
    - 7 (3.5%) had deficiencies in RBC zinc;
    - 7 (3.5%) had deficiencies in plasma zinc; and

  - 105 (52.5%) had MTHFR mutations.

- Mitochondrial Dysfunction (defined by those who had positive responses to the following mitochondrial support supplements: ATP fuel (NT Factors, i.e., glycosylated phospholipids), Coenzyme Q10 (CoQ10), acetyl-l-carnitine, d-ribose): 15 (7.5%) had mitochondrial dysfunction.

- Psychological issues: 177 (88.5%) participants self-reported having at least one psychological problem:

  - 154 (77%) had depression;
  - 134 (67%) had anxiety;
  - 4 (2%) had Obsessive Compulsive Disorder (OCD);
  - 11 (5.5%) had Post Traumatic Stress Disorder (PTSD); and
  - 9 (4.5%) had other psychological issues.

- Neurological Dysfunction: 190 (95%) had at least one of the following Neurological symptoms/disorders:

  - 188 (94%) had neuropathy;
  - 5 (2.5%) had Chronic Inflammatory Demyelinating Polyneuropathy (CIDP);
  - 3 (1.5%) had Multiple Sclerosis;
  - 2 (1%) had seizures; and
  - 2 (1%) had other neurological issues (e.g., Parkinson's symptoms).

- Endocrine Abnormalities: 195 (97.5%) had at least one of the following endocrine abnormalities:

  - 121 (60.5%) had thyroid abnormalities;
  - 144 (72%) had adrenal abnormalities;
  - 82 (41%) had sex hormone abnormalities;
  - 136 (68%) had vitamin D deficiencies;
  - 3 (1.5%) had pregnenolone deficiencies; and
  - 74 (37%) had DHEA abnormalities.

- Sleep Disorders: 196 (98%) had at least one of the following sleep disorders:

    o   23 (11.5%) had Obstructive Sleep Apnea (OSA);
    o   1 (0.5%) had Restless Leg Syndrome (RLS);
    o   7 (3.5%) had Benign Prostatic Hyperplasia (BPH);
    o   4 (2%) were in menopause;
    o   2 (1%) had high adrenals;
    o   1 (0.5%) had medication induced sleep problems; and
    o   189 (94.5%) had other sleep problems, i.e., difficulties with insomnias, hypersomnias, circadian rhythm disorders (secondary to Lyme and tick-borne diseases).

- Autonomic Nervous System (ANS) Dysfunction/POTS: 83 (41.5%) had ANS dysfunction and/or POTS:

    o   23 (11.5%) had mild POTS (1–10 mm Hg drop in BP, and/or 1–10-point increase in heart rate after standing);
    o   41 (20.5%) had moderate POTS (11–29 mm drop in BP, and/or 11–29-point increase in heart rate after standing);
    o   9 (4.5%) had severe POTS (30+ increase in heart rate standing);
    o   19 (9.5%) had dysautonomia (e.g., gastroparesis, chronic constipation, bladder dysfunction, or dysfunction in temperature regulation); and
    o   2 (1%) had 'other' (tremors and/or discoloration hands/feet).

- Gastrointestinal Dysfunction: 159 (79.5%) had one or more of the following gastrointestinal disorders:

    o   10 (5%) had gluten sensitivity;
    o   10 (5%) had celiac disease;
    o   2 (1%) had colitis;
    o   43 (21.5%) had Candidiasis;
    o   15 (7.5%) had leaky gut;
    o   35 (17.5%) had parasites;
    o   17 (8.5%) had *H. Pylori* exposure;
    o   37 (18.5%) had gastroesophageal reflux disease (GERD);
    o   0% had a history of *C. Difficile* during treatment with dapsone; and
    o   83 (41.5%) had 'other' gastrointestinal dysfunction (Irritable Bowel Syndrome [IBS]).

- Elevated Liver Function Tests (LFTs): 148 (74%) had one or more of the following transient elevation in LFTs at some point during treatment

    o   90 (45%) had elevated AST;
    o   104 (52%) had elevated ALT;
    o   36 (18%) had alkaline phosphatase;
    o   47 (23.5%) had elevated T. Bilirubin; and
    o   5 (2.5%) had 'other' (low albumin).

- Pain Syndromes: 185 (92.5%) had migratory pain, which other research has demonstrated is one of the hallmark symptoms of active Lyme disease [39].
- Deconditioning: 64 (32%) were disabled and/or in physical therapy (PT).

4. Discussion

Results from Precision Medicine: Part 1 support and extend the findings of our published shorter term dapsone study in 100 patients on a dapsone protocol [106] for longer than three months. For the symptoms of Fatigue/Tiredness, Joint and/or Muscle Pain, Headache, Tingling/Numbness/Burning of the Extremities, Sleep Problems, Forgetfulness or Brain fog, Difficulty with Speech or Writing, and Day Sweats/Night Sweats/Flushing, 164 out of 200 patients (82%) had a statistically significant decrease of severity ratings of each symptom after treatment. Findings that differed from the 2016 study [106] include a significant decrease of symptom severity of headaches—this was not found previously. Although neuropathy (tingling/numbness/burning sensations) is a known potential side effect of dapsone [112], our study showed statistical improvement in this symptom when used in our three-drug antibiotic combination therapy.

4.1. Numerous Health Issues Confound Full Recovery

Apart from noting the incidence of coinfections outlined in Precision Medicine: Part 1, markedly different from the Horowitz and Freeman 2016 [106] study was the inclusion of a medical chart review of all 200 participants for evidence of abnormalities on the 16-point MSIDS map. The MSIDS information notably suggests that these patients, all of whom had persistent ongoing symptomatology (prior to DDS combination therapy), remained symptomatic because apart from documented evidence of Lyme disease, they had numerous other health issues likely interfering with a full recovery. Some of the most important medical problems which needed to be addressed on the MSIDS model to ensure clinical improvement included adequate treatment of babesiosis and bartonellosis, decreasing inflammation (avoiding allergic/sensitive foods, getting adequate sleep), assisting detoxification pathways for severe Herxheimer reactions, addressing immune dysfunction and/or immune deficiency, treating POTS/dysautonomia, as well as addressing any associated hormonal and psychological dysfunction. These multi-faceted health challenges made these patients' symptoms more difficult to treat. Chart review was also able to identify several effective combinations of antibiotics, as patients were frequently rotated through different combinations while on dapsone, as well as identify how multiple factors on the MSIDS map affected treatment outcomes.

In the three prior National Institutes of Health (NIH) randomized controlled trials for the treatment of Lyme disease [4,113,114], none of the above factors on the MSIDS map were considered. An analysis by Delong et al. [115] concluded that prior NIH double-blind treatment trials for Lyme disease produced mixed results. Although two of the three clinical NIH trials did show improvement in symptomatology, i.e., the Krupp trial showed improvements in fatigue, and the Fallon study showed improvement in encephalopathy with improved cognitive functioning, sustained clinical improvement was lacking. This is commonly observed in clinical practice once patients with chronic Lyme symptoms stop anti-infective therapy.

Several explanations as to why the NIH studies did not find consistent clinical improvement [116] are that those studies did not incorporate recent up-to-date published scientific information on Borrelia and its ability to form biofilms [117] and "persister" bacteria [118–120], which were factors addressed in our study; these were inadequate treatment trials because sample sizes were extremely small, ranging from 37 to 78 patients. Sample sizes this small lack sufficient statistical power to measure clinically relevant improvement. Furthermore, ongoing coinfections, including *Babesia* spp. and *Bartonella* spp., may have been present in the participants, and these infections are treated differently than *Borrelia burgdorferi*; overlapping causes of inflammation were not adequately addressed in the NIH studies i.e., food allergies/sensitivities, leaky gut, imbalances of the microbiome, resistant insomnia, elevated levels of environmental toxins, including heavy metals and mold, with nutritional deficiencies in magnesium, copper, zinc, and/or iodine; nor were the downstream effects of inflammation addressed. These factors include, but are not limited to, endocrine disorders (low testosterone, low adrenal function), mitochondrial dysfunction, and POTS/dysautonomia. It is important to consider all these factors on the MSIDS model, since they can result in the same symptoms seen in chronic Lyme disease/PTLDS, including resistant fatigue, headaches, dizziness, anxiety and palpitations, neuropsychiatric symptoms with depression and anxiety, cognitive difficulties/problems with executive functioning, and insomnia. If simultaneous overlapping etiologies are present, which can increase an inflammatory process and cause similar symptoms, it will be difficult to differentiate the effectiveness of anti-infective therapy alone until all underlying etiologies increasing inflammation have been properly diagnosed and treated.

4.2. Neurocognitive Deficits in PTLDS and Lyme-MSIDS

Multiple overlapping causes of inflammation may explain some of the differences in outcomes of studies comparing PTLDS patients to the larger group of patients with chronic Lyme disease. In a recent 2018 study on cognitive decline in 124 patients with PTLDS [26], 92% of patients had some level of cognitive difficulty, yet 50% had no statistically or clinically relevant cognitive decline, with only 26% showing significant cognitive decline on measures of memory and processing speed. In our study of 165 patients with "Lyme-MSIDS" who reported their symptoms before DDS and at least six months on DDS, almost 91% of patients self-reported some level of cognitive difficulty (similar numbers to the Touradji et al. study), but the group with moderate, moderately severe, or severe cognitive impairment (forgetfulness/brain fog) was three times higher at 78%. Speech and writing problems were present in more than three quarters of these patients (76.4%). These were also patients with evidence of inflammation (69.5%) and immune dysfunction (72%). Infections (including coinfections), heavy metal burdens (84.5%), nutritional deficiencies (76%), and sleep disorders (98%) as well as G.I. disorders (79.5%) can all increase inflammation and contribute in part to neurocognitive deficits. The role of infections, however, is striking. As we reported in Precision Medicine: Part 1, after six months of dapsone therapy, the group with the most significant cognitive deficits (moderate, moderately severe, and severe) statistically improved with DDS with p values < 0.001. The success of dapsone combination therapy using hydroxychloroquine, grapefruit seed extract, doxycycline, rifampin, DDS, and agents that disrupt the biofilm (stevia, oregano oil) [121] was probably due to several mechanisms of action. Clinically, this protocol has good penetration into the central nervous system (CNS), where it can exert its antibacterial effects (stopping RNA and protein production by bacteria); it works against a broad range of pathogens (i.e., *Borrelia* as well as multiple intracellular coinfections), with efficacy against different forms of *Borrelia*, including round body, stationary phase, and biofilm forms. Dapsone also has an anti-inflammatory effect, by converting myeloperoxidase (MPO) into its inactive compound II (ferryl) form [122]. Myeloperoxidase is an enzyme in neutrophils that results in the production of hypochlorous acid (HOCl), whose function is to help kill bacteria and other pathogens, although it can also cause inflammation/oxidative damage in tissues. Inflammation and inflammatory cytokine production has been linked to fatigue, pain (migratory pain was present in 92.5% of our patients, which is a hallmark symptom of active Lyme disease) [96], and neurocognitive deficits in large controlled studies [123].

4.3. The Role of Inflammation in Lyme Disease and MSIDS

How might inflammation affect patient outcomes and how might we control its effects? There are at least three major biochemical pathways that may be involved in the production of inflammatory cytokines, which include the NF-Kappa B [124] (NFK-B) and nitric oxide (NO) pathways [125,126], and biochemical reactions leading to production of advanced glycation end products (AGE's) [127]. Multiple factors on the MSIDS map, including, but not limited to, multiple infections and environmental toxins, along with a high carbohydrate diet with hyperinsulinemia [128] and imbalances in the microbiome can create inflammation through stimulating these pathways, resulting in elevated levels of chemokines as well as cytokines, including IL-1, IL-6, TNF-α, and IL-17 [48,129–133]. These inflammatory cytokines are responsible for some of the disabling symptoms seen in Lyme disease, and their production along with the creation of free radicals/oxidative stress can damage cell membranes, mitochondria, and nerve cells. A potential solution is, therefore, to not only avoid simple carbohydrates and allergic/sensitive foods while treating the full range of infections and overlapping abnormalities on the 16 point MSIDS model increasing inflammation, but also to block NFK-B and NO (antioxidants, including alpha lipoic acid and glutathione, may be helpful) [134–136], while simultaneously increasing detoxification. Low dose naltrexone (LDN) has been one medication shown to also help in this regard, by decreasing microglial activation of the brain, and subsequently lowering CNS inflammatory cytokine production. LDN can be an effective treatment for autoimmune diseases, including Crohn's disease and multiple sclerosis as well helping with fibromyalgia symptoms [137–140].

Lowering inflammation may also take place by stimulating the Nrf2 pathway in the cytoplasm of cells. Nrf2 acts as a sensor in the cytoplasm that regulates redox balance and the stress response: It is activated by oxidative stress [141]. Once activated, Nrf2 goes into the nucleus and binds to Antioxidant Response Element (ARE) genes. These are DNA binding sites that primarily activate phase II enzymes (with a minor effect on phase I) plus numerous other cytoprotective enzymes. ARE gene activation enhances detoxification, decreases inflammation, and inhibits cancer growth. This mechanism may explain many observed beneficial effects of detoxifying phytochemicals noted in the scientific literature, including a variety of substances which activate Nrf2: Sulforaphane [142](broccoli seed extract), resveratrol [143,144], green tea (epigallocatechin gallate [EGCG]), and curcumin [145]. Patients in our study were instructed to take antioxidants (NAC, alpha lipoic acid, glutathione), LDN (if not on narcotics for pain, since naltrexone blocks narcotic receptors), and Nrf2 activators during dapsone combination therapy. A more detailed statistical analysis in a larger cohort of patients will be necessary, however, to evaluate their relative efficacy of decreasing inflammation, compared to the effects of anti-infective therapy and correcting abnormalities on the 16-point MSIDS model.

4.4. Repairing Free Radical Damage: The 4 "R's": Replace, Repair, Rebalance, Re-inoculate the G.I. Microbiome

Once we addressed the multiple sources of inflammation and used drainage and detoxification support with glutathione (GSH), then repairing the damage to the body may be helpful. This can be summed up by "the 4 R's": Replace (hormones), Repair (mitochondria) [61,146], Rebalance (ANS) [82,147,148], and Re-inoculate (G.I. bacteria) [149]. Almost all (97.5%) of our patients had endocrine abnormalities; 7.5% of our patients had mitochondrial dysfunction; 41.5% had some level of POTS/dysautonomia, and 79.5% had some form of gastrointestinal dysfunction. Retrospective chart review showed hormone balancing (adrenals, sex hormones, thyroid) and addressing POTS/dysautonomia to be key factors in those with resistant fatigue and cognitive dysfunction.

Protecting and inoculating the right types of bacteria (and yeast, i.e., *Saccharomyces boulardii*) was also important. The type of bacteria in the microbiome of our gut can have different effects on inflammatory cytokine production. Some of these bacteria, such as *Prevotella* and *Clostridium* species, have recently been reported to be associated with inflammation and diverse disease manifestations, including rheumatoid arthritis [150] and multiple sclerosis (MS) [151–154]. All our patients were on probiotics to support a healthy microbiome throughout the G.I. tract (*Lactobacillus* strains are most active in the small intestine; *Bifidobacterium* strains work best in the large intestine). These strains were chosen as they have been shown in double blind studies to help with functional bowel disorders [155] (*L. acidophilus* NCFM, *bifidobacterium Bi-07*); possess anti-inflammatory and immune enhancing properties [153,156,157] (*bifidobacterium Bl-04* increases IL-10, and *B. lactis* can enhance immunity in the elderly); while helping to prevent *C. difficile*. According to the CDC, nearly half a million Americans suffered from *Clostridium difficile* infections in a single year [158] and more than 100,000 of these infections developed among residents of U.S. nursing homes [158]. Some of these may have been preventable with regular use of targeted probiotics, such as *Saccharomyces boulardii*. Double-blind studies have shown targeted probiotics to help with functional bowel disorders, and large-scale clinical studies need to be performed to evaluate their efficacy in reducing associated morbidity.

It is important to identify potential multifactorial causes of chronic diseases, since health care costs are rising, with a recent health care survey reporting that almost half of all Americans suffer from at least one of 10 chronic conditions [159]. Autoimmunity can result from antibodies produced against *Borrelia* that cross react with our own tissue antigens (molecular mimicry), while bacteria activate Toll-like receptor 2 (TLR-2), [160,161] furthering increases in the pro-inflammatory cytokines,

TNF-alpha and IL-17. Similarly, mercury (Hg), bisphenol A (BPA), asbestos, and small particle pollution have now been published in the medical literature as potential factors increasing autoimmune reactions [37,51,101,102]. Over 84% of patients had evidence of exposure to at least one heavy metal, with 68% had evidence of mercury exposure; 100%, 46.5%, and 82% of patients had evidence of exposure to *Borrelia*, *Bartonella*, and *Mycoplasma* spp., respectively; and 72.5% of our patients in this study had evidence of immune dysfunction, including production of positive antinuclear antibodies and rheumatoid factors. Although ANA's and rheumatoid factors can be seen in autoimmune diseases, including systemic lupus erythematosus (SLE) and rheumatoid arthritis, these represent non-specific markers of inflammation in our study (only three patients were positive for dsDNA and/or CCP antibodies, markers of true lupus and rheumatoid arthritis). There was also evidence of elevated inflammatory markers, including elevated sedimentation rates (ESR), C-reactive protein (CRP), and C3a/C4a, in most of our patients, although the latter can be seen with both Lyme disease [162] and toxic mold exposure [163]. Forty five percent had evidence of food allergies (not everyone was checked for evidence of leaky gut by breath test analysis), and Vitamin D deficiency was noted in 68% of patients, with several patients having elevated 1,25 dihydroxyvitamin D/25-OH vitamin D ratios (>2:1 ratio), suggestive of an active intracellular infection increasing inflammation [164]. Interestingly, the three patients identified with elevated 1,25 dihydroxyvitamin D/25 OH vitamin D ratios also had evidence of immune deficiency (decreased immunoglobulin levels, decreased antibody production to a pneumococcal challenge, and/or a genetic predisposition). In total, 139 (69.5%) participants had markers of inflammation. These biomarkers of inflammation, including the recently identified chemokine, CCL-19 [133], can be followed during the course of treatment to help confirm clinical improvement in symptoms.

Inflammation in Other Chronic Conditions: Lyme disease patients are known to have increased levels of IL-1, IL-6, and TNF-α, also found in chronic fatiguing, musculoskeletal illnesses, and other neurodegenerative disorders. These pro-inflammatory cytokines increase fatigue and pain as well as peripheral nervous system (PNS) and central nervous system (CNS) neurological symptoms [165–167]. They can be produced by not only infections [47], but environmental toxins. [125,168] In recent years "more than 100,000 new chemicals have been used in common consumer products and are released into the everyday environment" [169]. According to a 2018 report of the US population, 12.8% now report medically diagnosed multiple chemical sensitivity (MCS) and 25.9% report chemical sensitivity [170]. Treatment of chemical exposure/sensitivity, which may result in some of the same increased inflammatory cytokines seen in Lyme disease, requires a different therapeutic approach. Chemical sensitivity is best addressed by decreasing our total exposure and toxic load (i.e., reducing the body burden through far infrared saunas, chelation, and mold removal using phosphatidylcholine and glutathione) [171], while supporting the detoxification pathways (phase I and phase II liver support, methylation support, toxin binders). Our study and chart review showed that evaluating patients for associated environmental toxicity and using detoxification with glutathione (GSH) is clinically useful, especially during Herxheimer reactions. Glutathione modulates inflammation [172,173]. A 2018 PNAS report found that intracellular GSH production was increased up to 10-fold during an infection with *Borrelia burgdorferi*, and infection was a key factor in inflammation/cytokine production [174]. Glutathione is also a key factor in helping to detoxify environmental chemicals.

Environmental toxins are known to be detrimental to our health, but what is their potential role in patients with Lyme disease and how significant is our daily exposure to a broad range of pollutants? Apart from evaluating patients for exposure to heavy metals and mold toxins, which were present, respectively, in 84.5% and 71.4% of those tested, we only evaluated five individuals for pesticide exposure, some of whom had Parkinsonian symptoms. Other published scientific research suggests our exposure to a broad range of toxins, including pesticides, to be much greater. The CDC performed a 6.5-million-dollar study in 2003, evaluating 2500 patients for environmental toxins [175]. They found a total of 116 different pollutants (13 heavy metals, 14 combustion byproducts, and 10 pesticides). One of those toxins, trichloroethylene (TCE), caused a leukemia outbreak in Woburn, Massachusetts.

TCE can also cause learning disabilities and paresthesias, as can exposure to mercury and lead [38]. These are some of the same symptoms we see in neurological Lyme disease with or without coinfections. Some patients who undergo detoxification, such as using Far infra-red saunas, with or without oral (or IV) liposomal glutathione, notice clinical improvement in what was perceived to only be Lyme related symptoms. Herxheimer reactions also oftentimes improves with alkalinizing the body [176] (decreasing acidic byproducts) and using liposomal glutathione to support detoxification. How can we potentially use this information to inform future clinical studies and research and improve patient care?

4.5. Important MSIDS Variables Determining Treatment Outcomes

The key points which emerged from a detailed data mining and review of these 200 patients charts with PTLDS/chronic Lyme disease were that a combination of factors on the 16-point MSIDS map needed to be addressed to see maximum improvement in patient symptoms. This usually involved the successful treatment of:

1. **Multiple intracellular infections:** Including *Borrelia*, *Bartonella*, *Chlamydia*, and *Mycoplasma* [32], using a triple intracellular antibiotic combination therapy (doxycycline, rifampin, and dapsone) along with agents that disrupt biofilm (i.e., Stevia [177], oregano oil [178]). Although *Borrelia* has been reported to exist in the intracellular compartment [179–182], the importance of addressing *Borrelia* and associated intracellular infections in clinical studies of patients with chronic Lyme symptoms has been a subject of ongoing debate among clinicians and scientists. Although concurrent infection with more than one agent is already known to complicate management of patients [183–185], our new study on dapsone combination therapy implies a significant role of intracellular bacteria in those suffering from symptoms of chronic Lyme disease/PTLDS. Our 2016 and new study imply that there may be multiple intracellular bacterial infections present in a subset of Lyme patients with persistent symptoms, some of whom have autoimmune manifestations, and a broad screening approach is necessary, using multiple testing strategies over time.

2. **Parasitic infections:** *Babesia* oftentimes required rotations of antimalarial medication and herbal therapies, due to the ability of *Babesia microti* to persist after standard treatments with drugs, like atovaquone and azithromycin [186–188]. Patients usually reported feeling better once Babesiosis was adequately treated. *Babesia* infection is also known to interfere with the clearance of other parasites. Addressing these other parasites and co-morbid conditions oftentimes led to clinical improvement. Although dapsone combination therapy was effective in reducing symptoms of babesiosis (decreased fevers, sweats, chills, flushing) as it has an antimalarial effect, further research is needed to identify more effective treatments for babesiosis, since several patients had evidence of persistent symptoms and positive *Babesia* PCR's or RNA (FISH) testing despite standard therapies. The role of associated parasitic infections and their interactions with *Babesia* parasites and host immunity needs further study.

3. **Sleep disorders:** These needed to be addressed by treating Lyme and associated coinfections, as well as ruling out other causes of sleep related problems (such as OSA, RLS, BPH, depression, anxiety, long acting stimulant and/or caffeine use). Treatment of insomnia using various medications (i.e., trazadone, tiagabine, mirtazapine, cyclobenzaprine, and pregabalin) and herbal therapies which support sleep and the circadian rhythm (i.e., valerian root and melatonin, which also lowers IL-17) were often needed [189]. Chart review indicated that balancing hormones (phosphatidylserine can be used to lower high adrenal function at night) [190] while stimulating GABA receptors (using GABA L-theanine) also were occasionally helpful in getting the patient to sleep.

4. **Hormonal dysregulation:** Low hormones (adrenal, sex hormones, thyroid) needed to be corrected to see maximum improvement in fatigue, libido, and cognitive and weight challenges in certain patients [191,192]. Forty-one percent of patients had hormonal dysregulation, and low testosterone (low T) was occasionally seen in young men in their 20's, 30's, and 40's with low libido. One individual (39 years old) with Lyme disease had a testosterone level of 138 (normal range 250–1100 ng/dl, Quest Diagnostics), whose testosterone increased to 356 with clomiphene (Clomid) and anastrozole (Arimidex). The use of clomiphene [193] and anastrozole (an aromatase inhibitor) [194]

in men has been shown to improve testosterone/estrogen ratios without additional use of testosterone replacement therapy, which has its limitations and potential side effects.

5. **Autonomic Nervous System dysregulation:** POTS/dysautonomia needed to be adequately addressed in a subpopulation of our patients if there was resistant fatigue, dizziness with changing position, presyncopal or syncopal episodes, unexplained palpitations and anxiety, as well as resistant cognitive symptoms [82]. The most commonly used therapies resulting in clinical improvement of dysautonomia was a combination of salt, increased fluids, and/or medication, including fludrocortisone, midodrine [195], and/or droxidopa [196], for blood pressure support, and Beta blockers (metoprolol XL) for control of palpitations. Further data mining analysis will be needed to determine the most effective combination of these medications, as patients oftentimes required more than one medication to improve symptomatology. In total, 41.5% of patients had evidence of ANS dysfunction or POTS as per clinical definitions [86]. Dysautonomia has also been reported in M.E./Chronic Fatigue Syndrome [197].

6. **Immune dysfunction/immune deficiency:** This occasionally required subcutaneous or intravenous immunoglobulin therapy (IVIG), as immunoglobulins are necessary to fight infections (CVID), modulate immunity [198], heal (small fiber) neuropathy, POTS, and address autoimmune encephalopathy [199]. Improvement of CVID using embryonic stem cell therapy in Lyme disease may be an option in resistant disease [200]. More than 72% of participants had immune dysfunction. Total IgG deficiency was found in 20.6%; 19.3% had IgM deficiency (13.5% had elevated IgM antibodies, not in the range of Waldenstroms macroglobulinemia); 15.9% had IgA deficiency (which can increase the incidence of food allergies), while more than 85% had combined IgG subclass deficiencies, 1–4 (see Table 1). The most frequent subclass deficiencies seen were IgG subclasses 1 and 3, associated with phagocytosis and antibody-dependent cellular and complement-dependent cytotoxicity. Some patients with normal or low normal immunoglobulin levels were also unable to mount an adequate antibody response to a pneumococcal challenge. Immune dysfunction and immune deficiency were therefore oftentimes associated with Lyme disease in our study, but the difficulty in determining the etiology and true prevalence was that there were too many potential overlapping variables (coinfections, heavy metals, mold toxins), which can all affect immunity (all patients tested for mold had evidence of gliotoxins, which are immunosuppressive). There is also the possibility that the patients who enrolled in the dapsone trial may have been sicker and more resistant to other therapies secondary to an immune deficiency.

Another possible explanation comes from a study done by Nicole Baumgarth and researchers from the University of California at Davis. They found that infection with *Borrelia burgdorferi* in mice targets lymph nodes and production of IgG antibodies by affecting germinal centers, structures that are needed for the generation of highly functional and long-lived antibody responses. *Borrelia* subverted a B cell response in that study (B cells produce antibodies to fight infection), and instead, caused T cell independence, leading to an IgM skewed profile [201]. In our precision medicine study, we saw many more CDC IgM positive Western blots in patients with chronic persistent Lyme symptoms (N = 90, 45%), as opposed to IgG positive Western blots (N = 23, 11.5%), and 11.5% had increased IgM antibody production (N = 23). Thirty-three patients out of 171 tested (16.5%) also had low IgM antibodies. The incidence of low IgM antibodies in our study could represent the production of Lyme antibody-antigen complexes [202], and be a potential surrogate immune marker for active Lyme disease. Future studies in a larger cohort of patients will need to be performed to confirm this theory, although sequestration of antibody to *Borrelia burgdorferi* in immune complexes in the blood and spinal fluid in seronegative and neurologic Lyme disease have been reported [202,203] (one of our patients in the study who was initially negative on Lyme testing on a lumbar puncture was later found to be Lyme antibody-antigen complex positive in the spinal fluid in research assays performed at the State University of New York at Stony Brook). Over 19% of patients who failed DDS combination therapy (N = 36) had low IgG levels (14 had CVID) and 22.2% had low IgG subclass 1 (N = 8), while 36% (N = 13) had low IgG subclass 3. Immunoglobulin G and subclass deficiencies associated with Lyme and associated co-infections might therefore have contributed to DDS failures. A 2018 study [204] showed that robust B cell responses predict rapid resolution of Lyme disease. These immunological abnormalities found in our study parallel those discovered in mice exposed to *Borrelia burgdorferi* and may therefore explain, in part, persistent symptomatology in those with chronic Lyme disease/PTLDS.

7. **Food allergies/sensitivities:** Avoidance of allergic and sensitive foods, which are known to increase the same inflammatory cytokines in Lyme disease, were helpful in our cohort of patients, and 45% of participants had evidence of food allergies, with 15.9% showing evidence of an IgA deficiency. Patients were instructed to stay on a low carbohydrate, Mediterranean/Paleo style diet, eating small frequent meals to avoid blood sugar swings (reactive hypoglycemia), Candida overgrowth in the G.I. tract, and further inflammatory reactions. Hypoglycemia may cause some of the same symptoms frequently seen in Lyme disease (fatigue, headaches, palpitations, mood swings, cognitive difficulties) [205], and both Paleolithic and Mediterranean diet pattern scores have been shown to be inversely associated with biomarkers of inflammation and oxidative balance in adults [206]. Mitochondrial damage can also be a by-product of excess sugar [146], resulting in metabolic syndrome and hyperinsulinemia [207] with insulin resistance, as glycation results in advanced glycation end products (AGEs) [127]. These can bind to receptors for advanced glycation end products (RAGEs), increasing inflammation [128,192] and cytokine production, which have been associated with nerve complications (neuropathy) [208] and neurological diseases (including Alzheimer's) [209].

8. **Mitochondrial support:** In our study only 7.5% of patients reported an improvement in symptoms with the use of NT Factors, CoQ10, and acetyl-l-carnitine, and prior scientific research has shown that up to one third of patients with chronic Lyme symptoms respond to lipid replacement therapy [61,146]. Overlapping etiologies increasing inflammation that may not yet have been adequately addressed at that point in time during therapy could account for some of the discrepancies. Our definition of mitochondrial dysfunction may also have been too strict (response to mitochondrial support), since fatigue, muscle pain, nerve pain, and cognitive difficulties improved with dapsone combination therapy, and these symptoms have all been shown to be associated with mitochondrial dysfunction. Mitochondrial membranes are particularly vulnerable to free radical/oxidative stress, since they are not protected, as is DNA surrounded by histones [210]. Future studies should consider directly measuring markers of oxidative stress, such as lipid peroxides [211], Thiobarbituric acid reactive substances (TBARS), 8-OH d guanine [212], and protein carbonyls, since oxidative stress from infections and environmental chemicals has been shown to activate multiple signaling pathways, including NFK-B, leading to elevated cytokine production and inflammation [213]. One of our patients with chronic resistant symptoms and multiple infections had elevated levels of lipid peroxides (patients were not consistently measured for oxidative stress markers). Another patient with resistant neuropathy and autonomic nervous system dysfunction had a negative genetic workup to rule out inherited mitochondrial DNA (mtDNA) mutations [214]. A third patient was found to have mitochondrial dysfunction through the Cleveland Clinic with a low CoQ10 ratio, who improved with nutritional supplementation. Checking levels of amino acids, organic acids, ammonia, lactate/pyruvate ratios, creatinine phosphokinase (CPK), free/total carnitine ratios, and CoQ10 and tiglyglycine levels (a marker for mitochondrial respiratory chain disorders) can also be useful to evaluate mitochondrial function [215,216].

9. **Detoxification/Herxheimer support:** Glutathione and other detoxification support (NAC, alpha lipoic acid, methylation support, binders, drainage) were often helpful in reducing symptomatology, but due to challenges of identifying a broader range of toxins (expense, necessity of multiple blood draws and/or fat biopsies), lack of consistency in testing and treatment protocols, and because simultaneous overlapping inflammatory factors on the MSIDS model were often present, requiring different, individualized therapies, it was difficult to identify the exact role of these toxins and the effect of detoxification on environmental chemicals. Our conclusions are also limited in the absence of data on a healthy population tested under provoked conditions. More than 84% of our patients had evidence of exposure to heavy metals, including mercury, lead, and arsenic, and 71.4%

had exposure to at least one mold toxin (not every individual was tested). The need to address mineral deficiencies and support detoxification pathways becomes particularly relevant in the setting of daily exposure to multiple environmental toxins, as 76% of our patients in the study had nutritional and enzyme deficiencies.

10. **Mineral Replacement:** Seven percent of patients had evidence of copper deficiency. Copper is necessary to produce the enzyme, superoxide dismutase (SOD) [217], which helps control oxidative stress and mitigates subsequent free radical damage to cells. Sixteen percent of patients had evidence of magnesium deficiency. Magnesium is necessary in over 300 enzymes in the body, some of which are necessary for detoxification [218]. Testing for red blood cell levels of magnesium (and other minerals) was important in this context, since 13% of patients showed evidence of RBC magnesium deficiency, which would otherwise not have been found on routine serum analysis. Eighteen percent of patients were iodine deficient. Iodine helps support proper thyroid function [219]. Finally, 18% of patients were deficient in zinc, by both serum, plasma, and RBC analysis. Zinc is necessary for not only decreasing the production of inflammatory cytokines [220], but also acts as a cofactor in the enzyme, alcohol dehydrogenase [221]. Zinc deficiency may lead to aldehydes being formed from alcohol groups, and "oxidative stress, lipid peroxidation, hyperglycemia-induced glycations, and environmental exposures increase the cellular concentrations of aldehydes" [222], potentially increasing levels of chloral hydrate in the body. Chloral hydrate is an FDA-approved soporific agent used for resistant insomnia. Lyme patients with elevated levels of quinolinic acid [223], a byproduct of the L-tryptophan pathway, combined with ammonia (due to methylation defects, mitochondrial urea/organic acid disorders, and/or an imbalance of ammonia producing bacteria in the gut) along with chloral hydrate are all potential factors that might result in a worsening of neurocognitive symptoms [224], apart from exposure to Lyme and associated coinfections. These factors need to be evaluated in future clinical studies.

Several patients with cognitive dysfunction and no evidence of severe liver disease (i.e., cirrhosis) had high ammonia levels. Ammonia, a byproduct of the metabolism of nitrogen-containing compounds, is neurotoxic at elevated concentrations [225] and the liver clears most portal vein ammonia, converting it into glutamine and urea. Glutamine is metabolized in mitochondria, yielding glutamate and ammonia, and ammonia can evoke oxidative/nitrosative stress, mitochondrial abnormalities, and astrocyte swelling, which is a major component of brain edema [226]. Ammonia levels can be decreased by reducing intestinal production (lactulose, rifaximin, diet), L-ornithine, prebiotic, and probiotic supplementation [227], as well as by supplementation with zinc and L-carnosine [228]. Zinc deficiency was found in 18% of patients, which could have impacted cytokine and ammonia production, as well as the integrity of the blood-brain barrier. Zinc deficiency superimposed on oxidative stress may predispose the brain to damage mediated though blood-brain barrier disruption [229]. Future studies will need to evaluate these mineral deficiencies and their role in chronic illness.

Taking a comprehensive multifactorial approach to address all abnormalities on the MSIDS map, especially those resulting in inflammation through various pathways and leading to downstream effects on hormones and the autonomic and central nervous system, as well as sleep, was especially important in those patients with chronic resistant symptomatology despite standard therapies.

Almost three quarters (72.5%) of our patients in this study had evidence of immune dysregulation, and some of these had associated immune deficiency, including CVID (7%) and/or selective subclass deficiencies (85.5%). IgG1 and IgG3 subclasses contain proteins, which are usually mobilized against toxins (i.e., diptheria, tetanus) and viral proteins, through direct (antigen binding) or by mediating indirect effector functions, such as antibody-dependent cellular cytotoxicity (ADCC), antibody-dependent cellular phagocytosis (ADCP), and complement-dependent cytotoxicity (CDC) [230]. IgG2 antibodies are used predominantly against bacteria with capsule polysaccharides (S. pneumonia, H. influenzae), and while the role of IgG4 is still being studied, decreased levels can be associated with IgA deficiency (along with IgG2 deficiency) and a Th-1 activation in Lyme borreliosis, while elevated levels have been associated with systemic fibro-inflammatory disorders of unknown origin [231].

Prior examination of the IgG subclass distribution in Lyme borreliosis showed the predominating subclasses in both serum and CSF were IgG1 and IgG3 [232]. The T helper type 1 (Th1) IFN-gamma-predominated immune response seen in Lyme borreliosis results in the production of IgG1 and IgG3 subclasses that are complement activating and opsonizing. It has been hypothesized that increased levels of these two subclasses early in disease might contribute to recovery and counteract the development of chronicity. The IgG1 and IgG 3 subclass deficiencies noted in our patient population could therefore represent active viral (herpes viruses, i.e., EBV, CMV, HHV6) and/or intracellular bacterial infections, including *Anaplasma, Borrelia, Bartonella, Mycoplasma, Chlamydia, F. tularensis*, and *Brucella* (apart from toxin production), since these "mediated effector functions are especially important against infectious diseases where cellular and complement mediated responses are important for efficient pathogen clearance" [230,233]. These subclass deficiencies may also represent associated immune markers of active infection in Lyme and associated coinfections (along with low IgM antibodies, see Table 1), and need to be studied further in a larger cohort of well-defined patients.

The relative prevalence of CVID in the general population (1:25,000 to 1:50,000) is usually much lower than those seen in our study (N = 14 [7%], i.e., approximately 1:14), resulting in acute and chronic infections, inflammatory, and autoimmune diseases [234]. Although genetic mutations have been identified, including those causing IgA and IgM antibody deficiency with autoimmune phenomenon [235], the precise etiology is usually unknown [236]. Lyme disease has been associated with cytopathic killing of lymphocytes [237] and immunodeficiency syndromes, as long-lived humoral immunity and immunoglobulin production can be suppressed after an infection with *Borrelia burgdorferi* [238]. Coinfections, like *Mycoplasma* [34] and *Bartonella* [239,240], as well as environmental toxins have also been associated with immunological dysfunction. *Mycoplasmas* can interact with B cells [33], affecting antibody production, and mercury [50], along with other environmental toxins [51] (including gliotoxins, which have been shown to be immunosuppressive), have been linked to immune dysfunction and a worldwide increase in autoimmune disease [37,241].

Although immune deficiency is known to increase the risk of infection, is infection increasing the risk of immune deficiency? Do chronic viral infections found in our study, like HHV6, play a role in Lyme and associated coinfections? HHV-6 is ubiquitous, can establish a lifelong, latent infection in its host, and is known to be a major cause of opportunistic viral infections in immunosuppressed individuals [242]. Certain flaviviruses, like West Nile virus, found in our study (N = 13, 6.5%) have also been shown to be persistent [243]. Is the ability to clear multiple infections affected by heavy metals, like mercury, which have been associated with autoimmune phenomenon? One of the mold toxins found in our study, gliotoxins, is known to be immunosuppressive. Do mold and heavy metals, when combined with infections that are immunosuppressive, lead to more severe and resistant illness? Do these toxins increase the severity and duration of fatigue, pain, and neuropsychiatric symptoms when combined with Lyme and associated coinfections? Seventy-seven percent of patients reported depression in our study, and *Borrelia burgdorferi* and associated diseases have been associated with immune mediated and metabolic changes increasing the risk of suicide [40]. Since Lyme disease and environmental toxins both increase inflammatory cytokines, worsening mood disorders, does this increase risk? These are questions that will need to be answered in future scientific trials using a broad data mining approach.

One important characteristic of our study that limits our ability to answer the above questions is that our patient population could represent a subset of the sickest patients with PTLDS/chronic Lyme disease, and not necessarily represent the broader population with chronic "unexplained" symptoms. Although our patient population did come from broad geographical areas across the US, we propose doing a national multicenter trial with a large cohort of patients who could be assessed using the 16-point MSIDS model, evaluating patient reported symptom severity and changes in MSIDS variables before and after treatment of each abnormality on the map. As previous research has demonstrated, self-reported symptoms can be reliable predictors of health outcomes [244]. In the future, we could measure cytokine levels, chemokine levels, and other inflammatory markers pre- and post-therapy to further evaluate the efficacy of DDS CT and treating multiple abnormalities on the 16-point MSIDS model, and include a healthy cohort for a detailed comparison chart review of all 16 factors. Our study showed improvement in the primary symptoms of Lyme disease and babesiosis, using a novel "persister" drug regimen. Multiple factors on the MSIDS map were also found to interfere and contribute to ongoing resistant symptomatology. Most of our patients improved when all sources of inflammation were discovered and adequately treated, along with treating the four "R"s. This needs to be confirmed in larger clinical studies.

4.6. Healthcare Opportunities Going Forward

The Role of Biofilms and "Persisters" in Chronic Disease

Biofilms have recently been implicated as a possible factor in the pathogenesis of Alzheimer's disease [245], just as they have been in Lyme disease, and play a role in some resistant infections (including, but not limited to, chronic otitis media, rhinosinusitis, implant infections with *Staphylococcus/Streptococcus*, urinary tract infections with *Pseudomonas*, *Candida* and *pneumocystis*) [246–251]. "Persisters are a specific subpopulation of bacterial cells that have acquired temporary antibiotic-resistant phenotypes" [252] and some are produced in higher numbers in colony–biofilm culture than in the usual liquid culture. Miyaue et al. [252] reported that "persisters can be maintained in higher numbers ... even after complete withdrawal from the colony–biofilm culture. This suggests the presence of a long-retention effect, or "memory effect", in the persister cell ... " " ... Increases in persisters during colony–biofilm culture and their memory effects are common, to a greater or lesser degree, in other bacterial species" [252]. *Borrelia burgdorferi* can form both biofilms [177] and persister cells [120], and the success of DDS combination therapy with agents that disrupt biofilms (Stevia, oregano oil) may be due to its effect against these different forms.

Patients infected with *Borrelia burgdorferi* and associated coinfections are often much sicker than patients with Lyme disease alone [19,65]. They can often be resistant to standard therapies (the role of biofilms and persisters in tick-borne disease still needs to be established in well controlled studies), but many in our study also had evidence of other medical problems, which might account for their ongoing symptoms. These health issues included immune dysfunction/immune deficiency, inflammation, environmental toxin exposure with detoxification problems, gastrointestinal problems, allergies, and nutritional deficiencies, as well as sleep, hormone, and autonomic nervous system dysregulation. Therefore, as other authors have suggested, we propose that patients with "chronic Lyme disease" no longer be referred to using this nomenclature, which can be confusing [253]. We suggest that patients now be considered to have "Lyme-MSIDS", and believe that this term best describes the multiple biologic and biochemical abnormalities that can be present after an infection with *Borrelia burgdorferi* (whose etiologies go beyond tick-borne disease), causing chronic illness. Each patient is unique, and each treatment approach must be individualized (although certain guidelines for differential diagnosis and treatment remain in place based on peer reviewed literature and physician experience). The MSIDS model helps provide a framework for diagnosing and treating complex chronic Lyme disease patients that have a multiplicity of symptoms, along with a map of up to 16 potential factors that may need to be addressed. These factors can keep a patient chronically ill, but these abnormalities are not regularly accounted for in routine standards of patient care. Establishing a uniform definition of chronic Lyme disease will facilitate diagnostic and treatment decisions and allow comparison among varied cohorts of patients.

5. Conclusions

The rising numbers of individuals suffering with Lyme disease and other long-term disabling illnesses alerts us to a necessary shift in the paradigm for the diagnosis and treatment of chronic disease [39]. An integrated, interdisciplinary systems-biology approach described in this study may help us to better understand Lyme and associated diseases. Based on published scientific data, we need to examine the role of multiple infections and environmental toxicants in neurodegenerative diseases, along with other factors on the MSIDS map that increase inflammation and cause downstream effects, including immune suppression. Some of these infections, like *Anaplasma*, *Babesia*, *Bartonella*, *Rickettsia* (Rocky Mountain spotted fever), and Relapsing Fever *borrelia*, now are present in the blood supply. *Borrelia*, *Babesia*, and *Bartonella* can be transmitted from a mother to her developing fetus, resulting in potential perinatal morbidity and mortality. *Rickettsia rickettsii* (Rocky Mountain spotted fever) can cause severe illness and death in children and adults if not treated within the first few days of illness [254]. Chronic tick-borne diseases can be both emotionally and financially devastating to individuals and their families and to the productivity of our country. Obstacles to the diagnosis and treatment of Lyme disease in the U.S. have also been associated with a "detrimental impact . . . on the ability to work and fulfill caregiving roles" [255].

A precision medicine focus and paradigm shift in health care is desperately needed. In attempting to fully understand the etiology(ies) of chronic Lyme disease/PTLDS, retrospective chart review and data mining research might help us to better understand etiologies and effective treatments for a broad range of other chronic diseases. Computer assisted, data mining from large cohorts of patients from multiple medical centers using a focused, personalized, precision medical perspective, like the MSIDS model, would allow us to examine the complexities of overlapping causes of inflammation in patients with ongoing suffering from Lyme and associated tick-borne disorders.

Author Contributions: Both R.I.H. and P.R.F. contributed to the writing of this paper including Conceptualization; Research Methodology; Formal Analysis; Investigation; Data curation; Writing—Original Draft Preparation; Writing—Review & Editing; Project Administration.; R.I.H. provided care for the 200 patients in this study.

Funding: This research was funded in part by Bay Area Lyme Foundation and MSIDS Research Foundation.

Acknowledgments: We thank our Hudson Valley Healing Arts Center research team: Haley Moss Dillon, Ph.D., Sonja Siderias, AAS, LPN, Heather Orza, CPC, AAS and Renee Nelson BA for their assistance, as well as Aron G. Wiegand, MS, Egamaria Alacam, BA and Connor Duncan, BA who assisted us with data input. We acknowledge with thanks the Bay Area Lyme Foundation (BAL) and the MSIDS Research Foundation (MRF) for providing us research grants for the data mining portion of this study. The first author also would also like to express his appreciation to his colleagues and subcommittee members on the HHS Tickborne Disease Working Group for their dedication and expertise in the diagnosis and treatment of tick-borne disorders.

Disclaimer: The views expressed are those of Richard Horowitz, and do not represent the views of the Tick-Borne Disease Working Group, HHS or the United States.

References

1.   Kugeler, K.J.; Farley, G.M.; Forrester, J.D.; Mead, P.S. Geographic Distribution and Expansion of Human Lyme Disease, United States. *Emerg. Infect. Dis.* **2015**, *21*, 1455–1457. [CrossRef] [PubMed]
2.   How Many People Get Lyme Disease? | Lyme Disease | CDC. Available online: https://www.cdc.gov/lyme/stats/humancases.html (accessed on 13 February 2018).
3.   Rosenberg, R. Vital Signs: Trends in Reported Vectorborne Disease Cases—United States and Territories, 2004–2016. *MMWR Morb. Mortal. Wkly. Rep.* **2018**, *67*. [CrossRef] [PubMed]
4.   Klempner, M.S.; Hu, L.T.; Evans, J.; Schmid, C.H.; Johnson, G.M.; Trevino, R.P.; Norton, D.; Levy, L.; Wall, D.; McCall, J.; et al. Two Controlled Trials of Antibiotic Treatment in Patients with Persistent Symptoms and a History of Lyme Disease. *N. Engl. J. Med.* **2001**, *345*, 85–92. [CrossRef] [PubMed]
5.   Johnson, L.; Wilcox, S.; Mankoff, J.; Stricker, R.B. Severity of chronic Lyme disease compared to other chronic conditions: A quality of life survey. *PeerJ* **2014**, *2*, e322. [CrossRef] [PubMed]
6.   Ward, B.W. Multiple Chronic Conditions Among US Adults: A 2012 Update. *Prev. Chronic Dis.* **2014**, *11*. [CrossRef] [PubMed]

7.   Public Information Office.   Nearly 1 in 5 People Have a Disability in the U.S., Census Bureau Reports-Miscellaneous-Newsroom-U.S. Census Bureau.   Available online: https://www.census.gov/newsroom/releases/archives/miscellaneous/cb12-134.html (accessed on 20 June 2018).

8.   Lyme Disease | 2017 Case Definition. Available online: https://wwwn.cdc.gov/nndss/conditions/lyme-disease/case-definition/2017/ (accessed on 21 May 2018).

9.   Stricker, R.B.; Johnson, L. Let's tackle the testing. *BMJ* **2007**, *335*, 1008. [CrossRef] [PubMed]

10. Surveillance Case Definitions for Current and Historical Conditions | NNDSS. Available online: https://wwwn.cdc.gov/nndss/conditions/ (accessed on 8 July 2018).

11. Rudenko, N.; Golovchenko, M.; Grubhoffer, L.; Oliver, J.H. Updates on *Borrelia burgdorferi* sensu lato complex with respect to public health. *Ticks Tick-Borne Dis.* **2011**, *2*, 123–128. [CrossRef] [PubMed]

12. Girard, Y.A.; Fedorova, N.; Lane, R.S. Genetic Diversity of *Borrelia burgdorferi* and Detection of B. bissettii-Like DNA in Serum of North-Coastal California Residents. *J. Clin. Microbiol.* **2011**, *49*, 945–954. [CrossRef] [PubMed]

13. Margos, G.; Fedorova, N.; Kleinjan, J.E.; Hartberger, C.; Schwan, T.G.; Sing, A.; Fingerle, V. Borrelia lanei sp. nov. extends the diversity of *Borrelia* species in California. *Int. J. Syst. Evol. Microbiol.* **2017**, *67*, 3872–3876. [CrossRef] [PubMed]

14. Molloy, P.J.; Telford, S.R.; Chowdri, H.R.; Lepore, T.J.; Gugliotta, J.L.; Weeks, K.E.; Hewins, M.E.; Goethert, H.K.; Berardi, V.P. Borrelia miyamotoi Disease in the Northeastern United States: A Case Series. *Ann. Intern. Med.* **2015**, *163*, 91–98. [CrossRef] [PubMed]

15. Krause, P.J.; Carroll, M.; Fedorova, N.; Brancato, J.; Dumouchel, C.; Akosa, F.; Narasimhan, S.; Fikrig, E.; Lane, R.S. Human Borrelia miyamotoi infection in California: Serodiagnosis is complicated by multiple endemic Borrelia species. *PLoS ONE* **2018**, *13*, e0191725. [CrossRef] [PubMed]

16. Myalgic Encephalomyelitis/Chronic Fatigue Syndrome (ME/CFS) | Myalgic Encephalomyelitis/Chronic Fatigue Syndrome (ME/CFS) | CDC. Available online: https://www.cdc.gov/me-cfs/index.html (accessed on 21 May 2018).

17. Mozayeni, B.R.; Maggi, R.G.; Bradley, J.M.; Breitschwerdt, E.B. Rheumatological presentation of Bartonella koehlerae and Bartonella henselae bacteremias. *Medicine* **2018**, *97*. [CrossRef] [PubMed]

18. Breitschwerdt, E.B. Did Bartonella henselae contribute to the deaths of two veterinarians? *Parasit. Vectors* **2015**, *8*, 317. [CrossRef] [PubMed]

19. Maggi, R.G.; Mozayeni, B.R.; Pultorak, E.L.; Hegarty, B.C.; Bradley, J.M.; Correa, M.; Breitschwerdt, E.B. Bartonella spp. Bacteremia and Rheumatic Symptoms in Patients from Lyme Disease-endemic Region. *Emerg. Infect. Dis.* **2012**, *18*, 783–791. [CrossRef] [PubMed]

20. Miklossy, J. Historic evidence to support a causal relationship between spirochetal infections and Alzheimer's disease. *Front. Aging Neurosci.* **2015**, *7*, 46. [CrossRef] [PubMed]

21. Allen, H.B. Alzheimer's Disease: Assessing the Role of Spirochetes, Biofilms, the Immune System, and Amyloid-β with Regard to Potential Treatment and Prevention. *J. Alzheimers Dis.* **2016**, *53*, 1271–1276. [CrossRef] [PubMed]

22. Readhead, B.; Haure-Mirande, J.-V.; Funk, C.C.; Richards, M.A.; Shannon, P.; Haroutunian, V.; Sano, M.; Liang, W.S.; Beckmann, N.D.; Price, N.D.; et al. Multiscale Analysis of Independent Alzheimer's Cohorts Finds Disruption of Molecular, Genetic, and Clinical Networks by Human Herpesvirus. *Neuron* **2018**, *99*. [CrossRef] [PubMed]

23. Brookmeyer, R.; Abdalla, N.; Kawas, C.H.; Corrada, M.M. Forecasting the prevalence of preclinical and clinical Alzheimer's disease in the United States. *Alzheimers Dement. J. Alzheimers Assoc.* **2018**, *14*, 121–129. [CrossRef] [PubMed]

24. Autoimmune Disease Statistics ● American Autoimmune Related Diseases Association (AARDA) 2016. Available online: www.aarda.org/news-information/statistics/ (accessed on 21 May 2018).

25. Feder, H.M.; Johnson, B.J.B.; O'Connell, S.; Shapiro, E.D.; Steere, A.C.; Wormser, G.P.; Ad Hoc International Lyme Disease Group; Agger, W.A.; Artsob, H.; Auwaerter, P.; Dumler, J.S.; et al. A critical appraisal of "chronic Lyme disease". *N. Engl. J. Med.* **2007**, *357*, 1422–1430. [CrossRef]

26. Touradji, P.; Aucott, J.N.; Yang, T.; Rebman, A.W.; Bechtold, K.T. Cognitive Decline in Post-treatment Lyme Disease Syndrome. *Arch. Clin. Neuropsychol.*. [CrossRef] [PubMed]

27. Lerner, A.; Matthias, T. Changes in intestinal tight junction permeability associated with industrial food additives explain the rising incidence of autoimmune disease. *Autoimmun. Rev.* **2015**, *14*, 479–489. [CrossRef] [PubMed]

28. Moutailler, S.; Valiente Moro, C.; Vaumourin, E.; Michelet, L.; Tran, F.H.; Devillers, E.; Cosson, J.-F.; Gasqui, P.; Van, V.T.; Mavingui, P.; et al. Co-infection of Ticks: The Rule Rather Than the Exception. *PLoS Negl. Trop. Dis.* **2016**, *10*, e0004539. [CrossRef] [PubMed]

29. Nelder, M.P.; Russell, C.B.; Sheehan, N.J.; Sander, B.; Moore, S.; Li, Y.; Johnson, S.; Patel, S.N.; Sider, D. Human pathogens associated with the blacklegged tick Ixodes scapularis: A systematic review. *Parasit. Vectors* **2016**, *9*, 265. [CrossRef] [PubMed]

30. Breitschwerdt, E.B. Bartonellosis: One Health Perspectives for an Emerging Infectious Disease. *ILAR J.* **2014**, *55*, 46–58. [CrossRef] [PubMed]

31. Breitschwerdt, E.B. Bartonellosis, One Health and all creatures great and small. *Vet. Dermatol.* **2017**, *28*, 96-e21. [CrossRef] [PubMed]

32. Nicolson, G.; Haier, J. Role of chronic bacterial and viral infections in neurodegenerative, neurobehavioural, psychiatric, autoimmune and fatiguing illnesses: Part 2. *Br. J. Med. Pract.* **2010**, *3*, 301–310.

33. Simecka, J.W.; Ross, S.E.; Cassell, G.H.; Davis, J.K. Interactions of mycoplasmas with b cells: Antibody production and nonspecific effects. *Clin. Infect. Dis.* **1993**, *17* (Suppl. 1), 176s–182s. [CrossRef]

34. Furr, P.M.; Taylor-Robinson, D.; Webster, A.D. Mycoplasmas and ureaplasmas in patients with hypogammaglobulinaemia and their role in arthritis: microbiological observations over twenty years. *Ann. Rheum. Dis.* **1994**, *53*, 183–187. [CrossRef] [PubMed]

35. Chen, W.; Li, D.; Paulus, B.; Wilson, I.; Chadwick, V.S. High prevalence of mycoplasma pneumoniae in intestinal mucosal biopsies from patients with inflammatory bowel disease and controls. *Dig. Dis. Sci.* **2001**, *46*, 2529–2535. [CrossRef] [PubMed]

36. Maeda, Y.; Kurakawa, T.; Umemoto, E.; Motooka, D.; Ito, Y.; Gotoh, K.; Hirota, K.; Matsushita, M.; Furuta, Y.; Narazaki, M.; et al. Dysbiosis Contributes to Arthritis Development via Activation of Autoreactive T Cells in the Intestine. *Arthritis Rheumatol.* **2016**, *68*, 2646–2661. [CrossRef] [PubMed]

37. Parks, C.G.; Miller, F.W.; Pollard, K.M.; Selmi, C.; Germolec, D.; Joyce, K.; Rose, N.R.; Humble, M.C. Expert panel workshop consensus statement on the role of the environment in the development of autoimmune disease. *Int. J. Mol. Sci.* **2014**, *15*, 14269–14297. [CrossRef] [PubMed]

38. Jomova, K.; Vondrakova, D.; Lawson, M.; Valko, M. Metals, oxidative stress and neurodegenerative disorders. *Mol. Cell. Biochem.* **2010**, *345*, 91–104. [CrossRef] [PubMed]

39. Horowitz, R.I. Clinical Roundup: Selected Treatment Options for Lyme Disease. *Altern. Complement. Ther.* **2012**, *18*, 220–225. [CrossRef]

40. Bransfield, R.C. Suicide and Lyme and associated diseases. *Neuropsychiatr. Dis. Treat.* **2017**, *13*, 1575–1587. [CrossRef] [PubMed]

41. Ramesh, G.; Didier, P.J.; England, J.D.; Santana-Gould, L.; Doyle-Meyers, L.A.; Martin, D.S.; Jacobs, M.B.; Philipp, M.T. Inflammation in the Pathogenesis of Lyme Neuroborreliosis. *Am. J. Pathol.* **2015**, *185*, 1344–1360. [CrossRef] [PubMed]

42. Horowitz, R. *Why Can't I Get Better? Solving the Mystery of Lyme and Chronic Disease*, 1st ed.; St. Martin's Press: New York, NY, USA, 2013; ISBN 978-1-250-01940-0.

43. Cerar, T.; Strle, F.; Stupica, D.; Ruzic-Sabljic, E.; McHugh, G.; Steere, A.C.; Strle, K. Differences in Genotype, Clinical Features, and Inflammatory Potential of *Borrelia burgdorferi* sensu stricto Strains from Europe and the United States. *Emerg. Infect. Dis.* **2016**, *22*, 818–827. [CrossRef] [PubMed]

44. Cimmino, M.A.; Trevisan, G. Lyme arthritis presenting as adult onset Still's disease. *Clin. Exp. Rheumatol.* **1989**, *7*, 305–308. [PubMed]

45. Kologrivova, E.N.; Baraulina, A.S.; Nechaeva, S.V.; Shestakova, I.I.; Stronin, O.V.; Vlasova, N.M.; Sal'nikova, O.M. Intensity of the production of rheumatoid factor in patients with different degrees of sensitization to Borrelia garinii antigens. *Zh. Mikrobiol. Epidemiol. Immunobiol.* **2005**, 80–83.

46. Fagan, D.L.; Slaughter, C.A.; Capra, J.D.; Sullivan, T.J. Monoclonal antibodies to immunoglobulin G4 induce histamine release from human basophils in vitro. *J. Allergy Clin. Immunol.* **1982**, *70*, 399–404. [CrossRef]

47. Fallon, B.A.; Levin, E.S.; Schweitzer, P.J.; Hardesty, D. Inflammation and central nervous system Lyme disease. *Neurobiol. Dis.* **2010**, *37*, 534–541. [CrossRef] [PubMed]

48. Pachner, A.R.; Steiner, I. Lyme neuroborreliosis: Infection, immunity, and inflammation. *Lancet Neurol.* **2007**, *6*, 544–552. [CrossRef]

49. Whitmire, W.M.; Garon, C.F. Specific and nonspecific responses of murine B cells to membrane blebs of *Borrelia burgdorferi. Infect. Immun.* **1993**, *61*, 1460–1467. [PubMed]

50. Clarkson, T.W.; Magos, L. The toxicology of mercury and its chemical compounds. *Crit. Rev. Toxicol.* **2006**, *36*, 609–662. [CrossRef] [PubMed]

51. Cooper, G.S.; Parks, C.G.; Treadwell, E.L.; St Clair, E.W.; Gilkeson, G.S.; Dooley, M.A. Occupational risk factors for the development of systemic lupus erythematosus. *J. Rheumatol.* **2004**, *31*, 1928–1933. [PubMed]

52. Gallagher, C.M.; Meliker, J.R. Mercury and thyroid autoantibodies in U.S. women, NHANES 2007-2008. *Environ. Int.* **2012**, *40*, 39–43. [CrossRef] [PubMed]

53. Bransfield, R.C. The Psychoimmunology of Lyme/Tick-Borne Diseases and its Association with Neuropsychiatric Symptoms. *Open Neurol. J.* **2012**, *6*, 88–93. [CrossRef] [PubMed]

54. Pietikäinen, A.; Maksimow, M.; Kauko, T.; Hurme, S.; Salmi, M.; Hytönen, J. Cerebrospinal fluid cytokines in Lyme neuroborreliosis. *J. Neuroinflamm.* **2016**, *13*, 273. [CrossRef] [PubMed]

55. Patrick, L. Mercury toxicity and antioxidants: Part 1: Role of glutathione and alpha-lipoic acid in the treatment of mercury toxicity. *Altern. Med. Rev. J. Clin. Ther.* **2002**, *7*, 456–471.

56. Manzel, A.; Muller, D.N.; Hafler, D.A.; Erdman, S.E.; Linker, R.A.; Kleinewietfeld, M. Role of "Western diet" in inflammatory autoimmune diseases. *Curr. Allergy Asthma Rep.* **2014**, *14*, 404. [CrossRef] [PubMed]

57. Maintz, L.; Novak, N. Histamine and histamine intolerance. *Am. J. Clin. Nutr.* **2007**, *85*, 1185–1196. [CrossRef] [PubMed]

58. Akin, C. Mast cell activation syndromes presenting as anaphylaxis. *Immunol. Allergy Clin. N. Am.* **2015**, *35*, 277–285. [CrossRef] [PubMed]

59. Prasad, A.S.; Beck, F.W.J.; Bao, B.; Fitzgerald, J.T.; Snell, D.C.; Steinberg, J.D.; Cardozo, L.J. Zinc supplementation decreases incidence of infections in the elderly: Effect of zinc on generation of cytokines and oxidative stress. *Am. J. Clin. Nutr.* **2007**, *85*, 837–844. [CrossRef] [PubMed]

60. Bralley, A.; Lord, R. *Laboratory Evaluations in Molecular Medicine*; IAMM: Norcross, GA, USA, 2001.

61. Nicolson, G.; Settineri, R.; Ellithorpe, R. Lipid Replacement Therapy with a Glycophospholipid Formulation with NADH and CoQ10 Significantly Reduces Fatigue in Intractable Chronic Fatiguing Illnesses and Chronic Lyme Disease Patients. *Int. J. Clin. Med.* **2012**, *3*, 163–170. [CrossRef]

62. Neustadt, J.; Pieczenik, S.R. Medication-induced mitochondrial damage and disease. *Mol. Nutr. Food Res.* **2008**, *52*, 780–788. [CrossRef] [PubMed]

63. Nicolson, G. Lipid Replacement as an Adjunct to Therapy for Chronic Fatigue, Anti-Aging and Restoration of Mitochondrial Function. Available online: http://mytoprime.com/clinical_papers/lrt_jana_2003.html (accessed on 27 May 2018).

64. Balakrishnan, N.; Ericson, M.; Maggi, R.; Breitschwerdt, E.B. Vasculitis, cerebral infarction and persistent Bartonella henselae infection in a child. *Parasit. Vectors* **2016**, *9*, 254. [CrossRef] [PubMed]

65. Knapp, K.L.; Rice, N.A. Human Coinfection with *Borrelia burgdorferi* and Babesia microti in the United States. *J. Parasitol. Res.* **2015**, *2015*, 587131. [CrossRef] [PubMed]

66. Hájek, T.; Pasková, B.; Janovská, D.; Bahbouh, R.; Hájek, P.; Libiger, J.; Höschl, C. Higher prevalence of antibodies to *Borrelia burgdorferi* in psychiatric patients than in healthy subjects. *Am. J. Psychiatry* **2002**, *159*, 297–301. [CrossRef] [PubMed]

67. Finkel, M.J.; Halperin, J.J. Nervous System Lyme Borreliosis—Revisited. *Arch. Neurol.* **1992**, *49*, 102–107. [CrossRef] [PubMed]

68. Berczi, I. The pituitary gland, psychoneuroimmunology and infectious disease. In *Psychoneuroimmunology, Stress and Infection*; Friedman, H., Klein, T., Friedman, A., Eds.; CRC Press: Boca Raton, FL, USA, 1996; pp. 79–109.

69. Anisman, H.; Baines, M.G.; Berczi, I.; Bernstein, C.N.; Blennerhassett, M.G.; Gorczynski, R.M.; Greenberg, A.H.; Kisil, F.T.; Mathison, R.D.; Nagy, E.; et al. Neuroimmune mechanisms in health and disease: 2. Disease. *Can. Med. Assoc. J.* **1996**, *155*, 1075–1082.

70. Berczi, I.; Baragar, F.D.; Chalmers, I.M.; Keystone, E.C.; Nagy, E.; Warrington, R.J. Hormones in self tolerance and autoimmunity: A role in the pathogenesis of rheumatoid arthritis? *Autoimmunity* **1993**, *16*, 45–56. [CrossRef] [PubMed]

71. Milrad, S.F.; Hall, D.L.; Jutagir, D.R.; Lattie, E.G.; Czaja, S.J.; Perdomo, D.M.; Fletcher, M.A.; Klimas, N.; Antoni, M.H. Depression, evening salivary cortisol and inflammation in chronic fatigue syndrome: A psychoneuroendocrinological structural regression model. *Int. J. Psychophysiol.* **2017**. [CrossRef] [PubMed]

72. Haack, M.; Sanchez, E.; Mullington, J.M. Elevated Inflammatory Markers in Response to Prolonged Sleep Restriction Are Associated with Increased Pain Experience in Healthy Volunteers. *Sleep* **2007**, *30*, 1145–1152. [CrossRef] [PubMed]

73. Lorton, D.; Lubahn, C.L.; Estus, C.; Millar, B.A.; Carter, J.L.; Wood, C.A.; Bellinger, D.L. Bidirectional Communication between the Brain and the Immune System: Implications for Physiological Sleep and Disorders with Disrupted Sleep. *Neuroimmunomodulation* **2006**, *13*, 357–374. [CrossRef] [PubMed]

74. Greenberg, H.E.; Ney, G.; Scharf, S.M.; Ravdin, L.; Hilton, E. Sleep quality in Lyme disease. *Sleep* **1995**, *18*, 912–916. [PubMed]

75. Dagan, Y.; Eisenstein, M. Circadian rhythm sleep disorders: Toward a more precise definition and diagnosis. *Chronobiol. Int.* **1999**, *16*, 213–222. [CrossRef] [PubMed]

76. Mullington, J.M.; Hinze-Selch, D.; Pollmächer, T. Mediators of inflammation and their interaction with sleep: Relevance for chronic fatigue syndrome and related conditions. *Ann. N. Y. Acad. Sci.* **2001**, *933*, 201–210. [CrossRef] [PubMed]

77. Parish, J.M. Sleep-related problems in common medical conditions. *Chest* **2009**, *135*, 563–572. [CrossRef] [PubMed]

78. Vgontzas, A.N.; Papanicolaou, D.A.; Bixler, E.O.; Kales, A.; Tyson, K.; Chrousos, G.P. Elevation of Plasma Cytokines in Disorders of Excessive Daytime Sleepiness: Role of Sleep Disturbance and Obesity. *J. Clin. Endocrinol. Metab.* **1997**, *82*, 1313–1316. [CrossRef] [PubMed]

79. Garcia-Monco, J.C.; Seidman, R.J.; Benach, J.L. Experimental immunization with *Borrelia burgdorferi* induces development of antibodies to gangliosides. *Infect. Immun.* **1995**, *63*, 4130–4137. [PubMed]

80. Jacob, G.; Robertson, D.; Mosqueda-Garcia, R.; Ertl, A.C.; Robertson, R.M.; Biaggioni, I. Hypovolemia in syncope and orthostatic intolerance role of the renin-angiotensin system. *Am. J. Med.* **1997**, *103*, 128–133. [CrossRef]

81. Jordan, J.; Shannon, J.R.; Diedrich, A.; Black, B.K.; Robertson, D. Increased Sympathetic Activation in Idiopathic Orthostatic Intolerance: Role of Systemic Adrenoreceptor Sensitivity. *Hypertension* **2002**, *39*, 173–178. [CrossRef] [PubMed]

82. Karas, B.; Grubb, B.P.; Boehm, K.; Kip, K. The postural orthostatic tachycardia syndrome: A potentially treatable cause of chronic fatigue, exercise intolerance, and cognitive impairment in adolescents. *Pac. Clin. Electrophysiol. PACE* **2000**, *23*, 344–351. [CrossRef]

83. Rupprecht Tobias, A.; Elstner, M.; Weil, S.; Pfister, H.-W. Autoimmune-mediated polyneuropathy triggered by borrelial infection? *Muscle Nerve* **2008**, *37*, 781–785. [CrossRef] [PubMed]

84. Staud, R. Autonomic dysfunction in fibromyalgia syndrome: Postural orthostatic tachycardia. *Curr. Rheumatol. Rep.* **2008**, *10*, 463–466. [CrossRef] [PubMed]

85. Kanjwal, K.; Karabin, B.; Kanjwal, Y.; Grubb, B.P. Postural orthostatic tachycardia syndrome following Lyme disease. *Cardiol. J.* **2011**, *18*, 63–66. [PubMed]

86. Raj, S.R. The Postural Tachycardia Syndrome (POTS): Pathophysiology, Diagnosis & Management. *Indian Pac. Electrophysiol. J.* **2006**, *6*, 84–99.

87. Dysautonomia International: Postural Orthostatic Tachycardia Syndrome. Available online: http://www.dysautonomiainternational.org/page.php?ID=30 (accessed on 14 July 2018).

88. Rooney, P.J.; Jenkins, R.T.; Buchanan, W.W. A short review of the relationship between intestinal permeability and inflammatory joint disease. *Clin. Exp. Rheumatol.* **1990**, *8*, 75–83. [PubMed]

89. Knight, B.; Matthews, V.B.; Akhurst, B.; Croager, E.J.; Klinken, E.; Abraham, L.J.; Olynyk, J.K.; Yeoh, G. Liver inflammation and cytokine production, but not acute phase protein synthesis, accompany the adult liver progenitor (oval) cell response to chronic liver injury. *Immunol. Cell Biol.* **2005**, *83*, 364–374. [CrossRef] [PubMed]

90. Horowitz, H.W.; Dworkin, B.; Forseter, G.; Nadelman, R.B.; Connolly, C.; Luciano, B.B.; Nowakowski, J.; O'Brien, T.A.; Calmann, M.; Wormser, G.P. Liver function in early Lyme disease. *Hepatology* **1996**, *23*, 1412–1417. [CrossRef] [PubMed]

91. Zaidi, S.A.; Singer, C. Gastrointestinal and hepatic manifestations of tickborne diseases in the United States. *Clin. Infect. Dis.* **2002**, *34*, 1206–1212. [CrossRef] [PubMed]

92. Shimizu, Y. Liver in systemic disease. *World J. Gastroenterol.* **2008**, *14*, 4111–4119. [CrossRef] [PubMed]

93. Shadick, N.A.; Phillips, C.B.; Sangha, O.; Logigian, E.L.; Kaplan, R.F.; Wright, E.A.; Fossel, A.H.; Fossel, K.; Berardi, V.; Lew, R.A.; et al. Musculoskeletal and neurologic outcomes in patients with previously treated Lyme disease. *Ann. Intern. Med.* **1999**, *131*, 919–926. [CrossRef] [PubMed]

94. Shadick, N.A. The Long-Term Clinical Outcomes of Lyme Disease: A Population-Based Retrospective Cohort Study. *Ann. Intern. Med.* **1994**, *121*, 560. [CrossRef] [PubMed]

95. Clauw, D.J.; Chrousos, G.P. Chronic pain and fatigue syndromes: Overlapping clinical and neuroendocrine features and potential pathogenic mechanisms. *Neuroimmunomodulation* **1997**, *4*, 134–153. [CrossRef] [PubMed]

96. Citera, M.; Freeman, P.R.; Horowitz, R.I. Empirical validation of the Horowitz Multiple Systemic Infectious Disease Syndrome Questionnaire for suspected Lyme disease. *Int. J. Gen. Med.* **2017**, *10*, 249–273. [CrossRef] [PubMed]

97. Crane, J.D.; Ogborn, D.I.; Cupido, C.; Melov, S.; Hubbard, A.; Bourgeois, J.M.; Tarnopolsky, M.A. Massage Therapy Attenuates Inflammatory Signaling After Exercise-Induced Muscle Damage. *Sci. Transl. Med.* **2012**, *4*, 119ra13. [CrossRef] [PubMed]

98. Moser, M.M.C. Treatment for a 14-Year-Old Girl with Lyme Disease Using Therapeutic Exercise and Gait Training | Physical Therapy | Oxford Academic. Available online: https://academic.oup.com/ptj/article/91/9/1412/2735165 (accessed on 27 May 2018).

99. Nazıroğlu, M.; Akkuş, S.; Soyupek, F.; Yalman, K.; Çelik, Ö.; Eriş, S.; Uslusoy, G.A. Vitamins C and E treatment combined with exercise modulates oxidative stress markers in blood of patients with fibromyalgia: A controlled clinical pilot study. *Stress* **2010**, *13*, 498–505. [CrossRef] [PubMed]

100. Wilder, R.L.; Crofford, L.J. Do infectious agents cause rheumatoid arthritis? *Clin. Orthop.* **1991**, 36–41. [CrossRef]

101. Alves, A.G.F.; Giacomin, M.F.d.A.; Braga, A.L.F.; Sallum, A.M.E.; Pereira, L.A.A.; Farhat, L.C.; Strufaldi, F.L.; Lichtenfels, A.J.d.F.C.; Carvalho, T.d.S.; Nakagawa, N.K.; et al. Influence of air pollution on airway inflammation and disease activity in childhood-systemic lupus erythematosus. *Clin. Rheumatol.* **2018**, *37*, 683–690. [CrossRef] [PubMed]

102. Pfau, J.C.; Serve, K.M.; Noonan, C.W. Autoimmunity and Asbestos Exposure. *Autoimmune Dis.* **2014**, *2014*. [CrossRef] [PubMed]

103. Steere, A.C.; Klitz, W.; Drouin, E.E.; Falk, B.A.; Kwok, W.W.; Nepom, G.T.; Baxter-Lowe, L.A. Antibiotic-refractory Lyme arthritis is associated with HLA-DR molecules that bind a *Borrelia burgdorferi* peptide. *J. Exp. Med.* **2006**, *203*, 961–971. [CrossRef] [PubMed]

104. Zhang, Y.; Yew, W.W.; Barer, M.R. Targeting Persisters for Tuberculosis Control. *Antimicrob. Agents Chemother.* **2012**, *56*, 2223–2230. [CrossRef] [PubMed]

105. Barr, J. A Short History of Dapsone, or an Alternative Model of Drug Development. *J. Hist. Med. Allied Sci.* **2011**, *66*, 425–467. [CrossRef] [PubMed]

106. Horowitz, R.I.; Freeman, P.R. The use of dapsone as a novel "persister" drug in the treatment of chronic Lyme disease/post treatment Lyme disease syndrome. *J. Clin. Exp. Dermatol. Res.* **2016**, *7*, 345. [CrossRef]

107. WHO Model Prescribing Information: Drugs Used in Leprosy. Available online: http://apps.who.int/medicinedocs/en/d/Jh2988e/ (accessed on 27 May 2018).

108. Ma, B.; Christen, B.; Leung, D.; Vigo-Pelfrey, C. Serodiagnosis of Lyme borreliosis by western immunoblot: Reactivity of various significant antibodies against *Borrelia burgdorferi*. *J. Clin. Microbiol.* **1992**, *30*, 370–376. [PubMed]

109. Lee, B.K.; Schwartz, B.S.; Stewart, W.; Ahn, K.D. Provocative chelation with DMSA and EDTA: Evidence for differential access to lead storage sites. *Occup. Environ. Med.* **1995**, *52*, 13–19. [CrossRef] [PubMed]

110. Brewer, J.H.; Thrasher, J.D.; Straus, D.C.; Madison, R.A.; Hooper, D. Detection of mycotoxins in patients with chronic fatigue syndrome. *Toxins* **2013**, *5*, 605–617. [CrossRef] [PubMed]

111. Horowitz, R. *How Can I Get Better?: An Action Plan for Treating Resistant Lyme & Chronic Disease*, 1st ed.; St. Martin's Griffin: New York, NY, USA, 2017; ISBN 978-1-250-07054-8.

112. Jopling, W.H. Side-effects of antileprosy drugs in common use. *Lepr. Rev.* **1983**, *54*, 261–270. [CrossRef] [PubMed]

113. Krupp, L.B.; Hyman, L.G.; Grimson, R.; Coyle, P.K.; Melville, P.; Ahnn, S.; Dattwyler, R.; Chandler, B. Study and treatment of post Lyme disease (STOP-LD): A randomized double masked clinical trial. *Neurology* **2003**, *60*, 1923–1930. [CrossRef] [PubMed]

114. Fallon, B.A.; Keilp, J.G.; Corbera, K.M.; Petkova, E.; Britton, C.B.; Dwyer, E.; Slavov, I.; Cheng, J.; Dobkin, J.; Nelson, D.R.; et al. A randomized, placebo-controlled trial of repeated IV antibiotic therapy for Lyme encephalopathy. *Neurology* **2008**, *70*, 992–1003. [CrossRef] [PubMed]

115. Delong, A.K.; Blossom, B.; Maloney, E.L.; Phillips, S.E. Antibiotic retreatment of Lyme disease in patients with persistent symptoms: A biostatistical review of randomized, placebo-controlled, clinical trials. *Contemp. Clin. Trials* **2012**, *33*, 1132–1142. [CrossRef] [PubMed]

116. Cameron, D.J.; Johnson, L.B.; Maloney, E.L. Evidence assessments and guideline recommendations in Lyme disease: The clinical management of known tick bites, erythema migrans rashes and persistent disease. *Expert Rev. Anti-Infect. Ther.* **2014**, *12*, 1103–1135. [CrossRef] [PubMed]

117. Sapi, E.; Balasubramanian, K.; Poruri, A.; Maghsoudlou, J.S.; Socarras, K.M.; Timmaraju, A.V.; Filush, K.R.; Gupta, K.; Shaikh, S.; Theophilus, P.A.S.; et al. Evidence of in vivo Existence of Borrelia Biofilm in Borrelial Lymphocytomas. *Eur. J. Microbiol. Immunol.* **2016**, *6*, 9–24. [CrossRef] [PubMed]

118. Zhang, Y. Persisters, persistent infections and the Yin–Yang model. *Emerg. Microbes Infect.* **2014**, *3*, e3. [CrossRef] [PubMed]

119. Lewis, K. Persister cells, dormancy and infectious disease. *Nat. Rev. Microbiol.* **2007**, *5*, 48–56. [CrossRef] [PubMed]

120. Feng, J.; Auwaerter, P.G.; Zhang, Y. Drug Combinations against *Borrelia burgdorferi* Persisters in vitro: Eradication Achieved by Using Daptomycin, Cefoperazone and Doxycycline. *PLoS ONE* **2015**, *10*, e0117207. [CrossRef] [PubMed]

121. Feng, J.; Zhang, S.; Shi, W.; Zubcevik, N.; Miklossy, J.; Zhang, Y. Selective Essential Oils from Spice or Culinary Herbs Have High Activity against Stationary Phase and Biofilm *Borrelia burgdorferi*. *Front. Med.* **2017**, *4*. [CrossRef] [PubMed]

122. Van Zyl, J.M.; Basson, K.; Kriegler, A.; van der Walt, B.J. Mechanisms by which clofazimine and dapsone inhibit the myeloperoxidase system: A possible correlation with their anti-inflammatory properties. *Biochem. Pharmacol.* **1991**, *42*, 599–608. [CrossRef]

123. Tan, Z.S.; Beiser, A.S.; Vasan, R.S.; Roubenoff, R.; Dinarello, C.A.; Harris, T.B.; Benjamin, E.J.; Au, R.; Kiel, D.P.; Wolf, P.A.; et al. Inflammatory markers and the risk of Alzheimer disease: The Framingham Study. *Neurology* **2007**, *68*, 1902–1908. [CrossRef] [PubMed]

124. Park, M.H.; Hong, J.T. Roles of NF-κB in Cancer and Inflammatory Diseases and Their Therapeutic Approaches. *Cells* **2016**, *5*, 15. [CrossRef] [PubMed]

125. Pall, M.L. Common etiology of posttraumatic stress disorder, fibromyalgia, chronic fatigue syndrome and multiple chemical sensitivity via elevated nitric oxide/peroxynitrite. *Med. Hypotheses* **2001**, *57*, 139–145. [CrossRef] [PubMed]

126. Tripathi, P.; Tripathi, P.; Kashyap, L.; Singh, V. The role of nitric oxide in inflammatory reactions. *FEMS Immunol. Med. Microbiol.* **2007**, *51*, 443–452. [CrossRef] [PubMed]

127. Ramasamy, R.; Yan, S.F.; Schmidt, A.M. Receptor for AGE (RAGE): Signaling mechanisms in the pathogenesis of diabetes and its complications. *Ann. N. Y. Acad. Sci.* **2011**, *1243*, 88–102. [CrossRef] [PubMed]

128. Crofts, C.A.P. Hyperinsulinemia: A unifying theory of chronic disease? *Diabesity* **2015**, *1*, 34. [CrossRef]

129. Strle, K.; Drouin, E.E.; Shen, S.; El Khoury, J.; McHugh, G.; Ruzic-Sabljic, E.; Strle, F.; Steere, A.C. *Borrelia burgdorferi* stimulates macrophages to secrete higher levels of cytokines and chemokines than *Borrelia afzelii* or *Borrelia garinii*. *J. Infect. Dis.* **2009**, *200*, 1936–1943. [CrossRef] [PubMed]

130. Lochhead, R.B.; Strle, K.; Kim, N.D.; Kohler, M.J.; Arvikar, S.L.; Aversa, J.M.; Steere, A.C. MicroRNA Expression Shows Inflammatory Dysregulation and Tumor-Like Proliferative Responses in Joints of Patients With Postinfectious Lyme Arthritis. *Arthritis Rheumatol.* **2017**, *69*, 1100–1110. [CrossRef] [PubMed]

131. Dame, T.M.; Orenzoff, B.L.; Palmer, L.E.; Furie, M.B. IFN-γ Alters the Response of *Borrelia burgdorferi*-Activated Endothelium to Favor Chronic Inflammation. *J. Immunol.* **2007**, *178*, 1172–1179. [CrossRef] [PubMed]

132. Mühlradt, P.F.; Quentmeier, H.; Schmitt, E. Involvement of interleukin-1 (IL-1), IL-6, IL-2, and IL-4 in generation of cytolytic T cells from thymocytes stimulated by a Mycoplasma fermentans-derived product. *Infect. Immun.* **1991**, *59*, 3962–3968. [PubMed]

133. Soloski, M.J.; Crowder, L.A.; Lahey, L.J.; Wagner, C.A.; Robinson, W.H.; Aucott, J.N. Serum Inflammatory Mediators as Markers of Human Lyme Disease Activity. *PLoS ONE* **2014**, *9*, e93243. [CrossRef] [PubMed]

134. Stich, R.W.; Shoda, L.K.; Dreewes, M.; Adler, B.; Jungi, T.W.; Brown, W.C. Stimulation of nitric oxide production in macrophages by Babesia bovis. *Infect. Immun.* **1998**, *66*, 4130–4136. [PubMed]

135. Packer, L.; Tritschler, H.J.; Wessel, K. Neuroprotection by the metabolic antioxidant alpha-lipoic acid. *Free Radic. Biol. Med.* **1997**, *22*, 359–378. [CrossRef]

136. Patrick, L. Toxic metals and antioxidants: Part II. The role of antioxidants in arsenic and cadmium toxicity. *Altern. Med. Rev. J. Clin. Ther.* **2003**, *8*, 106–128.

137. Smith, J.P.; Stock, H.; Bingaman, S.; Mauger, D.; Rogosnitzky, M.; Zagon, I.S. Low-dose naltrexone therapy improves active Crohn's disease. *Am. J. Gastroenterol.* **2007**, *102*, 820–828. [CrossRef] [PubMed]

138. Cree, B.A.C.; Kornyeyeva, E.; Goodin, D.S. Pilot trial of low-dose naltrexone and quality of life in multiple sclerosis. *Ann. Neurol.* **2010**, *68*, 145–150. [CrossRef] [PubMed]

139. Lie, M.R.K.L.; van der Giessen, J.; Fuhler, G.M.; de Lima, A.; Peppelenbosch, M.P.; van der Ent, C.; van der Woude, C.J. Low dose Naltrexone for induction of remission in inflammatory bowel disease patients. *J. Transl. Med.* **2018**, *16*, 55. [CrossRef] [PubMed]

140. Younger, J.; Mackey, S. Fibromyalgia symptoms are reduced by low-dose naltrexone: A pilot study. *Pain Med.* **2009**, *10*, 663–672. [CrossRef] [PubMed]

141. Lewis, K.N.; Mele, J.; Hayes, J.D.; Buffenstein, R. Nrf2, a guardian of healthspan and gatekeeper of species longevity. *Integr. Comp. Biol.* **2010**, *50*, 829–843. [CrossRef] [PubMed]

142. Singh, K.; Connors, S.L.; Macklin, E.A.; Smith, K.D.; Fahey, J.W.; Talalay, P.; Zimmerman, A.W. Sulforaphane treatment of autism spectrum disorder (ASD). *Proc. Natl. Acad. Sci. USA* **2014**, *111*, 15550–15555. [CrossRef] [PubMed]

143. Valenzano, D.R.; Terzibasi, E.; Genade, T.; Cattaneo, A.; Domenici, L.; Cellerino, A. Resveratrol prolongs lifespan and retards the onset of age-related markers in a short-lived vertebrate. *Curr. Biol.* **2006**, *16*, 296–300. [CrossRef] [PubMed]

144. Wu, J.M.; Wang, Z.R.; Hsieh, T.C.; Bruder, J.L.; Zou, J.G.; Huang, Y.Z. Mechanism of cardioprotection by resveratrol, a phenolic antioxidant present in red wine (Review). *Int. J. Mol. Med.* **2001**, *8*, 3–17. [CrossRef] [PubMed]

145. Yadav, V.S.; Mishra, K.P.; Singh, D.P.; Mehrotra, S.; Singh, D.V.K. Immunomodulatory Effects of Curcumin. *Immunopharmacol. Immunotoxicol.* **2005**, *27*, 485–497. [CrossRef] [PubMed]

146. Nicolson, G.L. Metabolic syndrome and mitochondrial function: Molecular replacement and antioxidant supplements to prevent membrane peroxidation and restore mitochondrial function. *J. Cell. Biochem.* **2007**, *100*, 1352–1369. [CrossRef] [PubMed]

147. Thieben, M.J.; Sandroni, P.; Sletten, D.M.; Benrud-Larson, L.M.; Fealey, R.D.; Vernino, S.; Lennon, V.A.; Shen, W.-K.; Low, P.A. Postural orthostatic tachycardia syndrome: The Mayo clinic experience. *Mayo Clin. Proc.* **2007**, *82*, 308–313. [CrossRef]

148. Watari, M.; Nakane, S.; Mukaino, A.; Nakajima, M.; Mori, Y.; Maeda, Y.; Masuda, T.; Takamatsu, K.; Kouzaki, Y.; Higuchi, O.; et al. Autoimmune postural orthostatic tachycardia syndrome. *Ann. Clin. Transl. Neurol.* **2018**, *5*, 486–492. [CrossRef] [PubMed]

149. Fasano, A. Zonulin and its regulation of intestinal barrier function: The biological door to inflammation, autoimmunity, and cancer. *Physiol. Rev.* **2011**, *91*, 151–175. [CrossRef] [PubMed]

150. Pianta, A.; Arvikar, S.; Strle, K.; Drouin, E.E.; Wang, Q.; Costello, C.E.; Steere, A.C. Evidence of the Immune Relevance of Prevotella copri, a Gut Microbe, in Patients with Rheumatoid Arthritis. *Arthritis Rheumatol.* **2017**, *69*, 964–975. [CrossRef] [PubMed]

151. Rumah, K.R.; Linden, J.; Fischetti, V.A.; Vartanian, T. Isolation of Clostridium perfringens Type B in an Individual at First Clinical Presentation of Multiple Sclerosis Provides Clues for Environmental Triggers of the Disease. *PLoS ONE* **2013**, *8*, e76359. [CrossRef] [PubMed]

152. Weiss, G.; Christensen, H.R.; Zeuthen, L.H.; Vogensen, F.K.; Jakobsen, M.; Frøkiær, H. Lactobacilli and bifidobacteria induce differential interferon-β profiles in dendritic cells. *Cytokine* **2011**, *56*, 520–530. [CrossRef] [PubMed]

153. Foligne, B.; Nutten, S.; Grangette, C.; Dennin, V.; Goudercourt, D.; Poiret, S.; Dewulf, J.; Brassart, D.; Mercenier, A.; Pot, B. Correlation between in vitro and in vivo immunomodulatory properties of lactic acid bacteria. *World J. Gastroenterol.* **2007**, *13*, 236–243. [CrossRef] [PubMed]

154. Kumar, H.; Lund, R.; Laiho, A.; Lundelin, K.; Ley, R.E.; Isolauri, E.; Salminen, S. Gut Microbiota as an Epigenetic Regulator: Pilot Study Based on Whole-Genome Methylation Analysis. *mBio* **2014**, *5*. [CrossRef] [PubMed]

155. Ringel-Kulka, T.; Palsson, O.S.; Maier, D.; Carroll, I.; Galanko, J.A.; Leyer, G.; Ringel, Y. Probiotic bacteria Lactobacillus acidophilus NCFM and Bifidobacterium lactis Bi-07 versus placebo for the symptoms of bloating in patients with functional bowel disorders: A double-blind study. *J. Clin. Gastroenterol.* **2011**, *45*, 518–525. [CrossRef] [PubMed]

156. Gill, H.S.; Rutherfurd, K.J.; Cross, M.L.; Gopal, P.K. Enhancement of immunity in the elderly by dietary supplementation with the probiotic Bifidobacterium lactis HN019. *Am. J. Clin. Nutr.* **2001**, *74*, 833–839. [CrossRef] [PubMed]

157. Kawase, M.; He, F.; Kubota, A.; Harata, G.; Hiramatsu, M. Oral administration of lactobacilli from human intestinal tract protects mice against influenza virus infection. *Lett. Appl. Microbiol.* **2010**, *51*, 6–10. [CrossRef] [PubMed]

158. Nearly Half a Million Americans Suffered from Clostridium Difficile Infections in a Single Year. Available online: https://www.cdc.gov/media/releases/2015/p0225-clostridium-difficile.html (accessed on 6 July 2018).

159. Chronic Diseases Are Taxing Our Health Care System and Our Economy. Available online: https://www.statnews.com/2018/05/31/chronic-diseases-taxing-health-care-economy/ (accessed on 20 June 2018).

160. Allen, H.B.; Shaver, C.M.; Etzler, C.A.; Joshi, S.G. Autoimmune Diseases of the Innate and Adaptive Immune System including Atopic Dermatitis, Psoriasis, Chronic Arthritis, Lyme Disease, and Alzheimers Disease. *Immunochem. Immunopathol.* **2015**, *1*, 1–4. [CrossRef]

161. Alaedini, A.; Latov, N. Antibodies against OspA epitopes of *Borrelia burgdorferi* cross-react with neural tissue. *J. Neuroimmunol.* **2005**, *159*, 192–195. [CrossRef] [PubMed]

162. Uhde, M.; Ajamian, M.; Li, X.; Wormser, G.P.; Marques, A.; Alaedini, A. Expression of C-Reactive Protein and Serum Amyloid A in Early to Late Manifestations of Lyme Disease. *Clin. Infect. Dis.* **2016**, *63*, 1399–1404. [CrossRef] [PubMed]

163. Edmondson, D.A.; Barrios, C.S.; Brasel, T.L.; Straus, D.C.; Kurup, V.P.; Fink, J.N. Immune Response among Patients Exposed to Molds. *Int. J. Mol. Sci.* **2009**, *10*, 5471–5484. [CrossRef] [PubMed]

164. Mangin, M.; Sinha, R.; Fincher, K. Inflammation and vitamin D: The infection connection. *Inflamm. Res.* **2014**, *63*, 803–819. [CrossRef] [PubMed]

165. Sommer, C.; Kress, M. Recent findings on how proinflammatory cytokines cause pain: Peripheral mechanisms in inflammatory and neuropathic hyperalgesia. *Neurosci. Lett.* **2004**, *361*, 184–187. [CrossRef] [PubMed]

166. Loggia, M.L.; Chonde, D.B.; Akeju, O.; Arabasz, G.; Catana, C.; Edwards, R.R.; Hill, E.; Hsu, S.; Izquierdo-Garcia, D.; Ji, R.-R.; et al. Evidence for brain glial activation in chronic pain patients. *Brain J. Neurol.* **2015**, *138*, 604–615. [CrossRef] [PubMed]

167. Hutchinson, M. Glial Ties to Persistent Pain. Available online: https://www.the-scientist.com/?articles.view/articleNo/51172/title/Glial-Ties-to-Persistent-Pain/ (accessed on 28 May 2018).

168. Lichtenstein, J.H.R.; Hsu, Y.-H.; Gavin, I.M.; Donaghey, T.C.; Molina, R.M.; Thompson, K.J.; Chi, C.-L.; Gillis, B.S.; Brain, J.D. Environmental Mold and Mycotoxin Exposures Elicit Specific Cytokine and Chemokine Responses. *PLoS ONE* **2015**, *10*, e0126926. [CrossRef]

169. Yang, S.-N.; Hsieh, C.-C.; Kuo, H.-F.; Lee, M.-S.; Huang, M.-Y.; Kuo, C.-H.; Hung, C.-H. The Effects of Environmental Toxins on Allergic Inflammation. *Allergy Asthma Immunol. Res.* **2014**, *6*, 478–484. [CrossRef] [PubMed]

170. Steinemann, A. National Prevalence and Effects of Multiple Chemical Sensitivities. *J. Occup. Environ. Med.* **2018**, *60*, e152. [CrossRef] [PubMed]

171. Fitzgerald, K.N.; Brailley, J.A. *Case Studies in Integrative and Functional Medicine*; Metrametrix: Duluth, GA, USA, 2011; ISBN 978-0-9673949-5-4.

172. Wu, G.; Fang, Y.-Z.; Yang, S.; Lupton, J.R.; Turner, N.D. Glutathione Metabolism and Its Implications for Health. *J. Nutr.* **2004**, *134*, 489–492. [CrossRef] [PubMed]

173. Zhang, Z.; Zhang, X.; Fang, X.; Niimi, M.; Huang, Y.; Piao, H.; Gao, S.; Fan, J.; Yao, J. Glutathione inhibits antibody and complement-mediated immunologic cell injury via multiple mechanisms. *Redox Biol.* **2017**, *12*, 571–581. [CrossRef] [PubMed]

174. Kerstholt, M.; Vrijmoeth, H.; Lachmandas, E.; Oosting, M.; Lupse, M.; Flonta, M.; Dinarello, C.A.; Netea, M.G.; Joosten, L.A.B. Role of glutathione metabolism in host defense against *Borrelia burgdorferi* infection. *Proc. Natl. Acad. Sci. USA* **2018**, *115*, E2320–E2328. [CrossRef] [PubMed]

175. Stephenson, J. CDC Report on Environmental Toxins. *JAMA* **2003**, *289*, 1230–1233. [CrossRef] [PubMed]

176. Horowitz, R.I. Effects of Shifting the Acid-Base Balance Among Lyme Patients during Jarish Herxheimer Flares: A Small Prospective Study. In Proceedings of the 16th International Scientific Conference on Lyme Disease & Other Tick-Borne Disorders, Philadelphia, PA, USA, 15 November 2003.

177. Theophilus, P.A.S.; Victoria, M.J.; Socarras, K.M.; Filush, K.R.; Gupta, K.; Luecke, D.F.; Sapi, E. Effectiveness of Stevia Rebaudiana Whole Leaf Extract Against the Various Morphological Forms of *Borrelia Burgdorferi* in vitro. *Eur. J. Microbiol. Immunol.* **2015**, *5*, 268–280. [CrossRef] [PubMed]

178. Schillaci, D.; Napoli, E.M.; Cusimano, M.G.; Vitale, M.; Ruberto, A. Origanum vulgare subsp. hirtum essential oil prevented biofilm formation and showed antibacterial activity against planktonic and sessile bacterial cells. *J. Food Prot.* **2013**, *76*, 1747–1752. [CrossRef] [PubMed]

179. Ma, Y.; Sturrock, A.; Weis, J.J. Intracellular localization of *Borrelia burgdorferi* within human endothelial cells. *Infect. Immun.* **1991**, *59*, 671–678. [PubMed]

180. Montgomery, R.R.; Nathanson, M.H.; Malawista, S.E. The fate of *Borrelia burgdorferi*, the agent for Lyme disease, in mouse macrophages. Destruction, survival, recovery. *J. Immunol.* **1993**, *150*, 909–915. [PubMed]

181. Girschick, H.J.; Huppertz, H.I.; Rüssmann, H.; Krenn, V.; Karch, H. Intracellular persistence of *Borrelia burgdorferi* in human synovial cells. *Rheumatol. Int.* **1996**, *16*, 125–132. [CrossRef] [PubMed]

182. Livengood, J.A.; Gilmore, R.D. Invasion of human neuronal and glial cells by an infectious strain of *Borrelia burgdorferi*. *Microbes Infect.* **2006**, *8*, 2832–2840. [CrossRef] [PubMed]

183. Krause, P.J.; Telford, S.R.; Ryan, R.; Conrad, P.A.; Wilson, M.; Thomford, J.W.; Spielman, A. Diagnosis of babesiosis: Evaluation of a serologic test for the detection of Babesia microti antibody. *J. Infect. Dis.* **1994**, *169*, 923–926. [CrossRef] [PubMed]

184. Sexton, D.J.; Corey, G.R.; Carpenter, C.; Kong, L.Q.; Gandhi, T.; Breitschwerdt, E.; Hegarty, B.; Chen, S.M.; Feng, H.M.; Yu, X.J.; et al. Dual infection with Ehrlichia chaffeensis and a spotted fever group rickettsia: A case report. *Emerg. Infect. Dis.* **1998**, *4*, 311–316. [CrossRef] [PubMed]

185. Maggi, R.G.; Mascarelli, P.E.; Havenga, L.N.; Naidoo, V.; Breitschwerdt, E.B. Co-infection with Anaplasma platys, Bartonella henselae and Candidatus Mycoplasma haematoparvum in a veterinarian. *Parasit. Vectors* **2013**, *6*, 103. [CrossRef] [PubMed]

186. Lemieux, J.E.; Tran, A.D.; Freimark, L.; Schaffner, S.F.; Goethert, H.; Andersen, K.G.; Bazner, S.; Li, A.; McGrath, G.; Sloan, L.; et al. A global map of genetic diversity in Babesia microti reveals strong population structure and identifies variants associated with clinical relapse. *Nat. Microbiol.* **2016**, *1*, 16079. [CrossRef] [PubMed]

187. Wormser, G.P.; Prasad, A.; Neuhaus, E.; Joshi, S.; Nowakowski, J.; Nelson, J.; Mittleman, A.; Aguero-Rosenfeld, M.; Topal, J.; Krause, P.J. Emergence of resistance to azithromycin-atovaquone in immunocompromised patients with Babesia microti infection. *Clin. Infect. Dis.* **2010**, *50*, 381–386. [CrossRef] [PubMed]

188. Krause, P.J.; Spielman, A.; Telford, S.R.; Sikand, V.K.; McKay, K.; Christianson, D.; Pollack, R.J.; Brassard, P.; Magera, J.; Ryan, R.; et al. Persistent Parasitemia after Acute Babesiosis. *N. Engl. J. Med.* **1998**, *339*, 160–165. [CrossRef] [PubMed]

189. Kuklina, E.M.; Glebezdina, N.S.; Nekrasova, I.V. Role of Melatonin in the Regulation of Differentiation of T Cells Producing Interleukin-17 (Th17). *Bull. Exp. Biol. Med.* **2016**, *160*, 656–658. [CrossRef] [PubMed]

190. Monteleone, P.; Maj, M.; Beinat, L.; Natale, M.; Kemali, D. Blunting by chronic phosphatidylserine administration of the stress-induced activation of the hypothalamo-pituitary-adrenal axis in healthy men. *Eur. J. Clin. Pharmacol.* **1992**, *42*, 385–388. [CrossRef] [PubMed]

191. Berczi, I. Pituitary hormones and immune function. *Acta Paediatr. Suppl.* **1997**, 70–75. [CrossRef]

192. Laaksonen, D.E.; Niskanen, L.; Punnonen, K.; Nyyssönen, K.; Tuomainen, T.-P.; Salonen, R.; Rauramaa, R.; Salonen, J.T. Sex hormones, inflammation and the metabolic syndrome: A population-based study. *Eur. J. Endocrinol.* **2003**, *149*, 601–608. [CrossRef] [PubMed]

193. Shabsigh, A.; Kang, Y.; Shabsign, R.; Gonzalez, M.; Liberson, G.; Fisch, H.; Goluboff, E. Clomiphene citrate effects on testosterone/estrogen ratio in male hypogonadism. *J. Sex. Med.* **2005**, *2*, 716–721. [CrossRef] [PubMed]

194. Leder, B.Z.; Rohrer, J.L.; Rubin, S.D.; Gallo, J.; Longcope, C. Effects of Aromatase Inhibition in Elderly Men with Low or Borderline-Low Serum Testosterone Levels. *J. Clin. Endocrinol. Metab.* **2004**, *89*, 1174–1180. [CrossRef] [PubMed]

195. Abed, H.; Ball, P.A.; Wang, L.-X. Diagnosis and management of postural orthostatic tachycardia syndrome: A brief review. *J. Geriatr. Cardiol.* **2012**, *9*, 61–67. [CrossRef] [PubMed]

196. Kaufmann, H.; Norcliffe-Kaufmann, L.; Palma, J.-A. Droxidopa in neurogenic orthostatic hypotension. *Expert Rev. Cardiovasc. Ther.* **2015**, *13*, 875–891. [CrossRef] [PubMed]

197. Freeman, R.; Komaroff, A.L. Does the Chronic Fatigue Syndrome Involve the Autonomic Nervous System? *Am. J. Med.* **1997**, *102*, 357–364. [CrossRef]

198. Kisand, K.E.; Prükk, T.; Kisand, K.V.; Lüüs, S.-M.; Kalbe, I.; Uibo, R. Propensity to excessive proinflammatory response in chronic Lyme borreliosis. *APMIS* **2007**, *115*, 134–141. [CrossRef] [PubMed]

199. Younger, D.S.; Orsher, S. Lyme Neuroborreliosis: Preliminary Results from an Urban Referral Center Employing Strict CDC Criteria for Case Selection. Available online: https://www.hindawi.com/journals/nri/2010/525206/ (accessed on 28 May 2018).

200. Horowitz, R.I.; Freeman, P.R. Improvement of common variable immunodeficiency using embryonic stem cell therapy in a patient with lyme disease: A clinical case report. *Clin. Case Rep.* **2018**, *6*, 1166–1171. [CrossRef] [PubMed]

201. Tunev, S.S.; Hastey, C.J.; Hodzic, E.; Feng, S.; Barthold, S.W.; Baumgarth, N. Lymphoadenopathy during Lyme Borreliosis Is Caused by Spirochete Migration-Induced Specific B Cell Activation. *PLoS Pathog.* **2011**, *7*, e1002066. [CrossRef] [PubMed]

202. Schutzer, S.E.; Coyle, P.K.; Belman, A.L.; Golightly, M.G.; Drulle, J. Sequestration of antibody to *Borrelia burgdorferi* in immune complexes in seronegative Lyme disease. *Lancet* **1990**, *335*, 312–315. [CrossRef]

203. Coyle, P.K.; Schutzer, S.E.; Deng, Z.; Krupp, L.B.; Belman, A.L.; Benach, J.L.; Luft, B.J. Detection of *Borrelia burgdorferi*-specific antigen in antibody-negative cerebrospinal fluid in neurologic Lyme disease. *Neurology* **1995**, *45*, 2010–2015. [CrossRef] [PubMed]

204. Blum, L.K.; Adamska, J.Z.; Martin, D.S.; Rebman, A.W.; Elliott, S.E.; Cao, R.R.L.; Embers, M.E.; Aucott, J.N.; Soloski, M.J.; Robinson, W.H. Robust B Cell Responses Predict Rapid Resolution of Lyme Disease. *Front. Immunol.* **2018**, *9*. [CrossRef] [PubMed]

205. Hypoglycemia-Symptoms and Causes-Mayo Clinic. Available online: https://www.mayoclinic.org/diseases-conditions/hypoglycemia/symptoms-causes/syc-20373685 (accessed on 11 July 2018).

206. Whalen, K.A.; McCullough, M.L.; Flanders, W.D.; Hartman, T.J.; Judd, S.; Bostick, R.M. Paleolithic and Mediterranean Diet Pattern Scores Are Inversely Associated with Biomarkers of Inflammation and Oxidative Balance in Adults. *J. Nutr.* **2016**, *146*, 1217–1226. [CrossRef] [PubMed]

207. Xu, H.; Barnes, G.T.; Yang, Q.; Tan, G.; Yang, D.; Chou, C.J.; Sole, J.; Nichols, A.; Ross, J.S.; Tartaglia, L.A.; et al. Chronic inflammation in fat plays a crucial role in the development of obesity-related insulin resistance. *J. Clin. Investig.* **2003**, *112*, 1821–1830. [CrossRef] [PubMed]

208. Peppa, M.; Vlassara, H. Advanced glycation end products and diabetic complications: A general overview. *Horm. Athens Greece* **2005**, *4*, 28–37. [CrossRef]

209. Sullivan, P.G.; Brown, M.R. Mitochondrial aging and dysfunction in Alzheimer's disease. *Prog. Neuropsychopharmacol. Biol. Psychiatry* **2005**, *29*, 407–410. [CrossRef] [PubMed]

210. Ljungman, M.; Hanawalt, P.C. Efficient protection against oxidative DNA damage in chromatin. *Mol. Carcinog.* **1992**, *5*, 264–269. [CrossRef] [PubMed]

211. Niki, E. Lipid peroxidation products as oxidative stress biomarkers. *BioFactors* **2008**, *34*, 171–180. [CrossRef]

212. Fenga, C.; Gangemi, S.; Teodoro, M.; Rapisarda, V.; Golokhvast, K.; Docea, A.O.; Tsatsakis, A.M.; Costa, C. 8-Hydroxydeoxyguanosine as a biomarker of oxidative DNA damage in workers exposed to low-dose benzene. *Toxicol. Rep.* **2017**, *4*, 291–295. [CrossRef] [PubMed]

213. Martindale, J.L.; Holbrook, N.J. Cellular response to oxidative stress: Signaling for suicide and survival. *J. Cell. Physiol.* **2002**, *192*, 1–15. [CrossRef] [PubMed]

214. Cohen, B.H.; Gold, D.R. Mitochondrial cytopathy in adults: What we know so far. *Cleve. Clin. J. Med.* **2001**, *68*, 625–626, 629–642. [CrossRef] [PubMed]

215. Bennett, M.J.; Powell, S.; Swartling, D.J.; Gibson, K.M. Tiglylglycine excreted in urine in disorders of isoleucine metabolism and the respiratory chain measured by stable isotope dilution GC-MS. *Clin. Chem.* **1994**, *40*, 1879–1883. [PubMed]

216. Naviaux, R.K. Mitochondrial DNA disorders. *Eur. J. Pediatr.* **2000**, *159* (Suppl. 3), S219–S226. [CrossRef]

217. Fetherolf, M.M.; Boyd, S.D.; Taylor, A.B.; Kim, H.J.; Wohlschlegel, J.A.; Blackburn, N.J.; Hart, P.J.; Winge, D.R.; Winkler, D.D. Copper-zinc superoxide dismutase is activated through a sulfenic acid intermediate at a copper ion entry site. *J. Biol. Chem.* **2017**, *292*, 12025–12040. [CrossRef] [PubMed]

218. Jahnen-Dechent, W.; Ketteler, M. Magnesium basics. *Clin. Kidney J.* **2012**, *5*, i3–i14. [CrossRef] [PubMed]

219. Chung, H.R. Iodine and thyroid function. *Ann. Pediatr. Endocrinol. Metab.* **2014**, *19*, 8–12. [CrossRef] [PubMed]

220. Foster, M.; Samman, S. Zinc and Regulation of Inflammatory Cytokines: Implications for Cardiometabolic Disease. *Nutrients* **2012**, *4*, 676–694. [CrossRef] [PubMed]

221. Auld, D.S.; Bergman, T. Medium- and short-chain dehydrogenase/reductase gene and protein families: The role of zinc for alcohol dehydrogenase structure and function. *Cell. Mol. Life Sci.* **2008**, *65*, 3961–3970. [CrossRef] [PubMed]

222. Hao, Q.; Maret, W. Aldehydes release zinc from proteins. A pathway from oxidative stress/lipid peroxidation to cellular functions of zinc. *FEBS J.* **2006**, *273*, 4300–4310. [CrossRef] [PubMed]

223. Halperin, J.J.; Heyes, M.P. Neuroactive kynurenines in Lyme borreliosis. *Neurology* **1992**, *42*, 43–50. [CrossRef] [PubMed]

224. Albrecht, J.; Zielińska, M.; Norenberg, M.D. Glutamine as a mediator of ammonia neurotoxicity: A critical appraisal. *Biochem. Pharmacol.* **2010**, *80*, 1303–1308. [CrossRef] [PubMed]

225. Ytrebø, L.M.; Sen, S.; Rose, C.; Ten Have, G.A.M.; Davies, N.A.; Hodges, S.; Nedredal, G.I.; Romero-Gomez, M.; Williams, R.; Revhaug, A.; et al. Interorgan ammonia, glutamate, and glutamine trafficking in pigs with acute liver failure. *Am. J. Physiol.-Gastrointest. Liver Physiol.* **2006**, *291*, G373–G381. [CrossRef] [PubMed]

226. Albrecht, J.; Norenberg, M.D. Glutamine: A Trojan horse in ammonia neurotoxicity. *Hepatology* **2006**, *44*, 788–794. [CrossRef] [PubMed]

227. Mittal, V.V.; Sharma, B.C.; Sharma, P.; Sarin, S.K. A randomized controlled trial comparing lactulose, probiotics, and L-ornithine L-aspartate in treatment of minimal hepatic encephalopathy. *Eur. J. Gastroenterol. Hepatol.* **2011**, *23*, 725–732. [CrossRef] [PubMed]

228. Takuma, Y.; Nouso, K.; Makino, Y.; Hayashi, M.; Takahashi, H. Clinical trial: Oral zinc in hepatic encephalopathy: Clinical trial: Oral zinc in hepatic encephalopathy. *Aliment. Pharmacol. Ther.* **2010**, *32*, 1080–1090. [CrossRef] [PubMed]

229. Noseworthy, M.D.; Bray, T.M. Zinc deficiency exacerbates loss in blood-brain barrier integrity induced by hyperoxia measured by dynamic MRI. *Proc. Soc. Exp. Biol. Med. Soc. Exp. Biol. Med. N. Y. N* **2000**, *223*, 175–182. [CrossRef]

230. Irani, V.; Guy, A.J.; Andrew, D.; Beeson, J.G.; Ramsland, P.A.; Richards, J.S. Molecular properties of human IgG subclasses and their implications for designing therapeutic monoclonal antibodies against infectious diseases. *Mol. Immunol.* **2015**, *67*, 171–182. [CrossRef] [PubMed]

231. Pieringer, H.; Parzer, I.; Wöhrer, A.; Reis, P.; Oppl, B.; Zwerina, J. IgG4- related disease: An orphan disease with many faces. *Orphanet J. Rare Dis.* **2014**, *9*, 110. [CrossRef] [PubMed]

232. Widhe, M.; Ekerfelt, C.; Forsberg, P.; Bergström, S.; Ernerudh, J. IgG subclasses in Lyme borreliosis: A study of specific IgG subclass distribution in an interferon-gamma-predominated disease. *Scand. J. Immunol.* **1998**, *47*, 575–581. [PubMed]

233. Pausa, M.; Pellis, V.; Cinco, M.; Giulianini, P.G.; Presani, G.; Perticarari, S.; Murgia, R.; Tedesco, F. Serum-resistant strains of *Borrelia burgdorferi* evade complement-mediated killing by expressing a CD59-like complement inhibitory molecule. *J. Immunol.* **2003**, *170*, 3214–3222. [CrossRef]

234. Cunningham-Rundles, C. The many faces of common variable immunodeficiency. *Hematol. Educ. Program Am. Soc. Hematol. Am. Soc. Hematol. Educ. Program* **2012**, *2012*, 301–305. [CrossRef]

235. Ombrello, M.J.; Remmers, E.F.; Sun, G.; Freeman, A.F.; Datta, S.; Torabi-Parizi, P.; Subramanian, N.; Bunney, T.D.; Baxendale, R.W.; Martins, M.S.; et al. Cold urticaria, immunodeficiency, and autoimmunity related to PLCG2 deletions. *N. Engl. J. Med.* **2012**, *366*, 330–338. [CrossRef] [PubMed]

236. Hausmann, O.; Warnatz, K. Immunodeficiency in adults a practical guide for the allergist. *Allergo J. Int.* **2014**, *23*, 261–268. [CrossRef] [PubMed]

237. Dorward, D.W.; Fischer, E.R.; Brooks, D.M. Invasion and cytopathic killing of human lymphocytes by spirochetes causing Lyme disease. *Clin. Infect. Dis.* **1997**, *25* (Suppl. 1), 2S–8S. [CrossRef]

238. Elsner, R.A.; Hastey, C.J.; Olsen, K.J.; Baumgarth, N. Suppression of Long-Lived Humoral Immunity Following *Borrelia burgdorferi* Infection. *PLoS Pathog.* **2015**, *11*, e1004976. [CrossRef] [PubMed]

239. Kaufman, D.L.; Kogelnik, A.M.; Mozayeni, R.B.; Cherry, N.A.; Breitschwerdt, E.B. Neurological and immunological dysfunction in two patients with Bartonella henselae bacteremia. *Clin. Case Rep.* **2017**, *5*, 931–935. [CrossRef] [PubMed]

240. Breitschwerdt, E.; Sontakke, S.; Hopkins, S. Neurological manifestations of Bartonellosis in immunocompetent patients: A composite of reports from 2005–2012. *J. Neuroparasitol.* **2012**, *3*, 1–15. [CrossRef]

241. Bossou, Y.M.; Serssar, Y.; Allou, A.; Vitry, S.; Momas, I.; Seta, N.; Menotti, J.; Achard, S. Impact of Mycotoxins Secreted by Aspergillus Molds on the Inflammatory Response of Human Corneal Epithelial Cells. *Toxins* **2017**, *9*, 197. [CrossRef] [PubMed]

242. Strausbaugh, L.J.; Caserta, M.T.; Mock, D.J.; Dewhurst, S. Human Herpesvirus 6. *Clin. Infect. Dis.* **2001**, *33*, 829–833. [CrossRef]

243. Office of HIV/AIDS and Infectious Disease Policy, A.S. for H. (ASH) Report of Other TBDS and Co-Infections Subcommittee. Available online: https://www.hhs.gov/ash/advisory-committees/tickbornedisease/reports/other-tbds-2018-5-9/index.html (accessed on 21 May 2018).

244. Christian, L.M.; Glaser, R.; Porter, K.; Malarkey, W.B.; Beversdorf, D.; Kiecolt-Glaser, J.K. Poorer self-rated health is associated with elevated inflammatory markers among older adults. *Psychoneuroendocrinology* **2011**, *36*, 1495–1504. [CrossRef] [PubMed]

245. Allen, H.B.; Morales, D.; Jones, K.; Joshi, S. Alzheimers Disease: A Novel Hypothesis Integrating Spirochetes, Biofilm, and the Immune System. *J. Neuroinfectious Dis.* **2016**, *7*. [CrossRef]

246. Costerton, J.W.; Stewart, P.S.; Greenberg, E.P. Bacterial biofilms: A common cause of persistent infections. *Science* **1999**, *284*, 1318–1322. [CrossRef] [PubMed]

247. Parsek, M.R.; Singh, P.K. Bacterial Biofilms: An Emerging Link to Disease Pathogenesis. *Annu. Rev. Microbiol.* **2003**, *57*, 677–701. [CrossRef] [PubMed]

248. Hoa, M.; Syamal, M.; Schaeffer, M.A.; Sachdeva, L.; Berk, R.; Coticchia, J. Biofilms and chronic otitis media: An initial exploration into the role of biofilms in the pathogenesis of chronic otitis media. *Am. J. Otolaryngol.* **2010**, *31*, 241–245. [CrossRef] [PubMed]

249. Al-Mutairi, D.; Kilty, S.J. Bacterial biofilms and the pathophysiology of chronic rhinosinusitis. *Curr. Opin. Allergy Clin. Immunol.* **2011**, *11*, 18–23. [CrossRef] [PubMed]

250. Costerton, J.W.; Montanaro, L.; Arciola, C.R. Biofilm in implant infections: Its production and regulation. *Int. J. Artif. Organs* **2005**, *28*, 1062–1068. [CrossRef] [PubMed]

251. Cushion, M.T.; Collins, M.S.; Linke, M.J. Biofilm formation by Pneumocystis spp. *Eukaryot. Cell* **2009**, *8*, 197–206. [CrossRef] [PubMed]

252. Miyaue, S.; Suzuki, E.; Komiyama, Y.; Kondo, Y.; Morikawa, M.; Maeda, S. Bacterial Memory of Persisters: Bacterial Persister Cells Can Retain Their Phenotype for Days or Weeks After Withdrawal From Colony–Biofilm Culture. *Front. Microbiol.* **2018**, *9*. [CrossRef] [PubMed]

253. Wormser, G.P. Should Patients Infected with *Borrelia Burgdorferi* No Longer Be Referred to as Having Lyme Disease? *Am. J. Med.* **2018**. [CrossRef] [PubMed]

254. Abrahamian, F.M. Consequences of delayed diagnosis of Rocky Mountain spotted fever in children—West Virginia, Michigan, Tennessee, and Oklahoma, May–July 2000. *Ann. Emerg. Med.* **2001**, *37*, 537–540. [CrossRef] [PubMed]

255. Hirsch, A.G.; Herman, R.J.; Rebman, A.; Moon, K.A.; Aucott, J.; Heaney, C.; Schwartz, B.S. Obstacles to diagnosis and treatment of Lyme disease in the USA: A qualitative study. *BMJ Open* **2018**, *8*, e021367. [CrossRef] [PubMed]

18

Sclerostin Modulation Holds Promise for Dental Indications

Mohamed G. Hassan [1,2,3], **Abbas R. Zaher** [2], **Juan Martin Palomo** [4] **and Leena Palomo** [5,*]

[1]   Division of Craniofacial Anomalies, Department of Orofacial Sciences, University of California San Francisco, San Francisco, CA 94143, USA; mgamal@dent.svu.edu.eg

[2]   Department of Orthodontics, Faculty of Dentistry, Alexandria University, Alexandria 21526, Egypt; azaher@drabbaszaher.com

[3]   Department of Orthodontics, Faculty of Oral and Dental Medicine, South Valley University, Qena 83523, Egypt

[4]   Department of Orthodontics, School of Dental Medicine, Case Western Reserve University, Cleveland, OH 44106-4905, USA; palomo@case.edu

[5]   Department of Periodontics, School of Dental Medicine, Case Western Reserve University, Cleveland, OH 44106-4905, USA

*   Correspondence: leena.palomo@case.edu

Abstract: Sclerostin modulation is a novel therapeutic bone regulation strategy. The anti-sclerostin drugs, proposed in medicine for skeletal bone loss may be developed for jaw bone indications in dentistry. Alveolar bone responsible for housing dentition share common bone remodeling mechanisms with skeletal bone. Manipulating alveolar bone turnover can be used as a strategy to treat diseases such as periodontitis, where large bone defects from disease are a surgical treatment challenge and to control tooth position in orthodontic treatment, where moving teeth through bone in the treatment goal. Developing such therapeutics for dentistry is a future line for research and therapy. Furthermore, it underscores the interprofessional relationship that is the future of healthcare.

Keywords: sclerostin; anti-sclerostin; bone remodeling; alveolar bone; orthodontic; tooth movement; periodontitis; bone loss

1. Introduction

The idea of pharmacologic alveolar bone modulation as a strategy to treat oral conditions is not new, nor is it a new concept to apply existing drugs for new indications Alveolar bone and skeletal bone remodeling share similar mechanisms. Both involve osteoblast and osteoclast balance regulated through signaling systems involving common hormones, cytokines and pathways. There are also important differences between alveolar bone and skeletal bone remodeling. Although these have not been well elucidated through well controlled studies, it is acceptable to say that Bisphosphonate drugs have been used this way [1]. Historically, bisphosphonates were in wide use for prevention and treatment of osteoporosis, Paget's disease, metastatic bone conditions and conditions where cytokine over activity leads to upregulation in osteoclasts [2–4]. Bisphosphonates reduce net bone loss related to high bone turnover rates by interfering with osteoclasts [2,5]. Strategically targeting the osteoclastic resorption process is the pharmacologic niche for Alendronate and Risedronate to slow osteoporotic bone resorption in otherwise healthy postmenopausal women and people on long term corticosteroids. Other bisphosphonates, given in much higher doses through IV, such as Pamidronate were mainly used in cancer indications to limit bone pain secondary to metastasis [6,7].

However, even as bisphosphonates were heralded for their anti-skeletal fracture outcomes in the case reports emerged linked them to a negative side effect called bisphosphonate related osteonecrosis of the jaws (BRONJ) [8,9]. Although it was rare, BRONJ is very severe, disfiguring and has high rates of morbidity and mortality [10]. While BRONJ, its infancy as a condition, was being studied and defined it was noted that daily compliance related to oral dosing for prevention and treatment of postmenopausal osteoporosis became a limitation, Zolendronate evolved from the cancer related indication for this purpose in a twice yearly bolus [11,12]. Related to BRONJ, well controlled multi-worldwide randomized placebo trials found Zolendronate to safe even when given through IV administration twice yearly [13]. The bisphosphonate strategy in dental applications in the alveolar bone met its limit due to the severe nature of BRONJ [14], however the concept of host modulation of alveolar bone in dental applications continued to grow [15,16].

Although the bisphosphonates for dental applications were limited due to the severity of BRONJ, other drugs with similar capacity to regulate bone turnover, such as those from the sclerostin family, may be useful for dental applications. Dental applications in orthodontics and periodontics can conceptually benefit from modulating bone turnover. The aim of this article is to report on potential dental indications for sclerostins.

Sclerostin modulating drugs are known for their most common indication, osteoporosis. They are also used to treat lesser known diseases such as sclerosteosis, loss of function of the gene encoding for sclerostin and Van Buchem's disease, deletion of a downstream promoter of the sclerostin gene. Sclerostins are being heavily researched for many reasons. Since bone turnover modulation shares similar pathways and signaling systems not just in alveolar and skeletal bone, these drugs hold potential indications for several diseases/conditions including rheumatoid arthritis, bone health complications in diabetes and osteogenesis imperfecta. Intravenous administration is the most common route of administration but phase III and IV studies on other routes continue.

Sclerostin is a negative osteoblast regulator. Sclerostins open the door modulating bone turnover through signaling agents which regulate bone homeostasis. The regulation of osteocyte-specific genes plays a major role in the process of bone remodeling common to both skeletal and alveolar bone [17,18]. Using their processes, osteocytes can communicate with cells on the bone surface and in the bone marrow [19,20]. Sclerostin, one of the proteins by which osteocytes regulate the function and number of the cells responsible for remodeling, is the product of the SOST gene [21,22]. Investigations of sclerostin deprived systems show enhanced bone formation. Altered sclerostin expression and restored bone formation after treatment with anti-sclerostin antibody in postmenopausal women and animal models suggest that sclerostin inhibition may be a viable approach for developing novel anabolic agents for diseases characterized by bone loss [23–27]. Sclerostin antibody (Scl-Ab) is receiving increasing attention as a bone-forming agent, as supported by studies in animals in which significant increases in bone volume and whole bone mechanical strength have been noted and in clinical trials showing increases in systemic bone formation markers and bone mineral density (BMD) [27–30]. The use of Scl-Ab leads to an increase in both osteoblast activity and osteoblast number, resulting in enhanced bone formation [31,32]. Studies with Scl-Ab treatment have demonstrated that osteoid synthesis and deposition appear to be upregulated globally as assessed by serum markers including P1NP (serum type 1 pro-collagen C-terminal/N-terminal) and osteocalcin [33]. Sclerostin secreted exclusively by osteocytes, is a glycoprotein that binds low-density lipoprotein receptor-related protein 5 and blocks the Wnt signaling pathway [34]. It suppresses osteoblastogenesis and reduces the viability of osteoblasts and osteocytes, leading to unbalanced bone turnover in favor of bone resorption not only by antagonizing Wnt but also by blocking bone morphogenetic protein signaling, both are essential for the maintenance of osteoblastogenesis [35–37]. Accordingly, it was shown that mechanical stimulation in vivo reduced the osteocytic sclerostin expression [38]. Also, it is possible that osteocyte death is a signal for bone formation because the level of sclerostin would decrease. Sclerostin levels are increased in mechanical unloading, aging and menopause, whereas they are decreased in hyperparathyroidism [39,40].

Adverse reactions at drug injection site have been noted. But the greater concern is to explain and understand the safety concerns that come with manipulation of the WNT pathway, because of its involvement in multiple cell functions. There is a potential for excess bone formation which includes potential to develop entrapment palsies, increased intracranial pressure and osteosarcoma. Furthermore, growing evidence suggests that WNT signaling inhibitors may contribute to chronic kidney disease-associated bone mineral disorder [41,42].

2. Orthodontic Tooth Movement

Orthodontic tooth movement (OTM) is considered as organized sterile inflammatory process, associated with the bone remodeling cascade [43]. Bone remodeling is necessary for OTM to occur. This unique cascade includes the osteoclast activation in areas where orthodontic pressure is applied. Here, localized bone resorption must necessarily occur in order for tooth movement. In this case, resorption is not a bad thing. On the tension areas of the tooth, counter to the force application, the opposite process occurs, as osteoblast action outweighs osteoclast action. There is bone formation [44–47].

Bone change associated with both pressure and tension areas in OTM involve a complicated communication between three main tissues: alveolar bone, periodontal ligament, cementum (Figure 1) [48]. The signaling pathways, chemical mediators and signaling cytokines useful in alveolar bone remodeling needed for OTM are the same as those in skeletal bone remodeling. The expression of PDL cytokines and chemical mediators has been reported to be significantly altered during OTM. The levels of IL-1α, IL-1β, IL-6, IL-10, IL-17, IL-33 and TNFα are significantly increased shortly after force application, except IL-6 that remains high after 12 days then it starts to decrease to its normal levels after 3 weeks of force application [49–58].

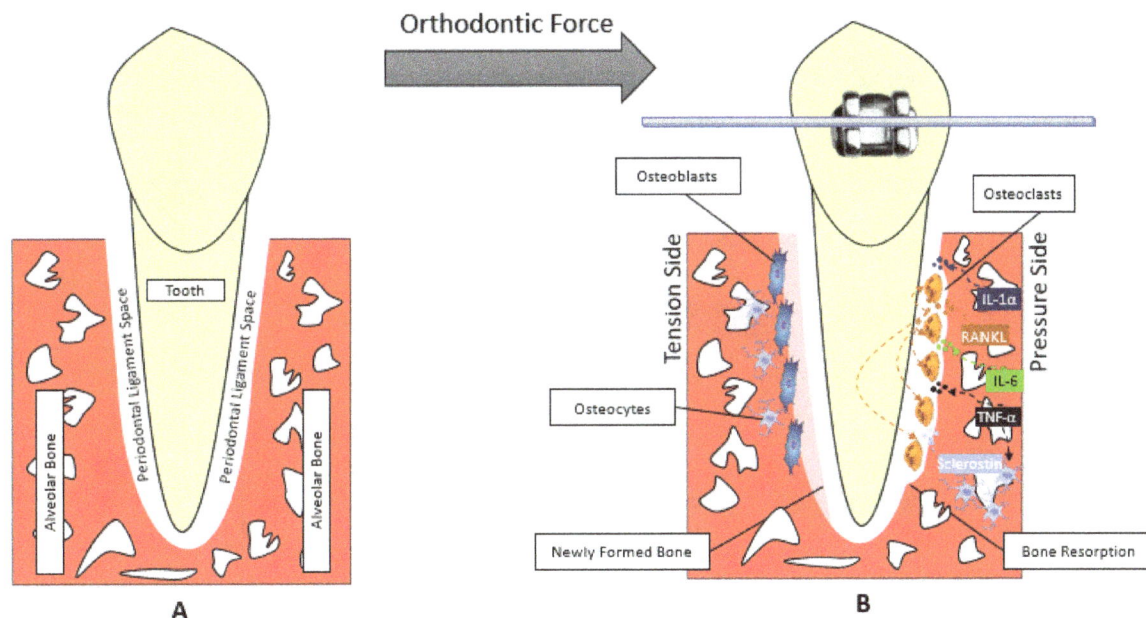

Figure 1. Model of the orthodontic tooth movement. (**A**) Before applying orthodontic force. (**B**) Applying orthodontic force to the tooth compresses the PDL. The compressed side of periodontal ligament is called the pressure side and the side where PDL is pulled is called the tension side. At the pressure side, Bone resorption is carried out mainly by osteoclasts and the help of other chemical mediators like sclerostin.

The alteration of the PDL microenvironment (cytokines and chemical mediators) regulates the formation and function of osteoclasts [59]. In alveolar bone remodeling, just as in skeletal bone, there are two factors are controlling the osteoclastogenesis; the first is the RANKL and the second is macrophage colony-stimulating factor (M-CSF). RANKL is a downstream regulator of osteoclast formation and activation, through which cytokines produce their osteoresorptive effect.

RANKL levels shortly increase after force application. Later, the increased RANKL expression is accompanied by upregulation of RANK expression, this RANK upregulation remains for 3 days following OTM. This binding leads to rapid differentiation of hematopoietic osteoclast precursors to mature osteoclasts [60,61].

Recently, the role of osteocytes during OTM has been well documented. The osteocytes in bone are thought to orchestrate "mechanotransduction" by reacting to various forms of mechanical stimulations through biologic cascades; this could be done by altering their sclerostin releases. In this way OTM manipulates bone loss in a useful way, such that tooth movement can occur. Bone loss in the OTM context is a good outcome such that tooth movement can occur into the site of bone resorption. (Figure 2). The response of the osteocytes to strain in vitro is controlled by the production of various chemical mediators like nitric oxide, prostaglandins, TNF-α and sclerostin. This mechanism is responsible for the activation of the PDL cells and the differentiation of precursors into osteoblasts or osteoclasts. Osteocyte response to mechanical loading during OTM using osteocyte knocked-out mice has been demonstrated, the changes in the level and the distribution of sclerostin in the PDL during OTM and linked it to the associated bone remodeling [62–64]. Given all the understanding of sclerostin and sclerostin-antibody pathways, we need to imply this knowledge in solving some of frequent problems occur during and/or after orthodontic treatment [65]. For example, is it possible to manage root wounds associated with orthodontic therapy using sclerostin-antibody treatment? Can we use the post-operative administration of anti-sclerostin to minimize teeth relapse and enhance retention? Is it possible and safe to use sclerostin or anti-sclerostin to accelerate or decelerate OTM? Well controlled studies are needed to answer these questions in an effort to introduce, efficacious, risk-free orthodontic therapy.

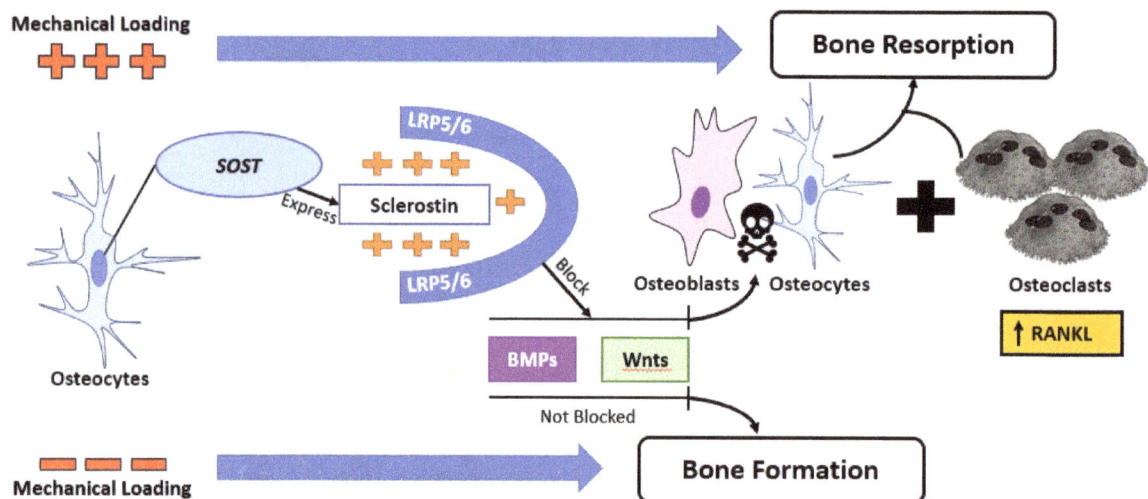

Figure 2. Relationship between mechanical loading and sclerostin expression. Mechanical loading upregulates sclerostin expression, leading to an inhibition of canonical Wnt signaling and exaggerate bone loss by upregulating osteoclastogenesis through the RANKL pathway.

3. Periodontal Therapy

Destruction in periodontal disease occurs in the supporting structures of the teeth, namely: gingiva, periodontal ligament, cementum and alveolar bone, through a complex pathogenic process starting with the interaction between bacterial plaque biofilm and the host immune response. Gingivitis, the initial phase, is a reversible inflammatory response to biofilms. Gingivitis is limited to soft tissues adjacent to teeth. If unchecked gingivitis inflammation progresses first to the periodontal ligament then to the supporting alveolar bone. With progressive bone destruction, tooth mobility ensues and finally the tooth is lost. Reconstructing these bone defects is the periodontists treatment challenge, often dealt with using surgical procedures such as grafting and tissue regenerative strategies.

Periodontitis and osteoporosis are both highly prevalent diseases associated with bone destruction [66]. Additionally, the two diseases have been considered as having overlapping pathogenesis and osteoporosis is a risk factor for the progression of periodontal destruction and potentially tooth loss [67]. The difference between osteoporosis and periodontitis is that periodontitis etiology involves host inflammation triggered by the build-up of bacterial plaque biofilm. This inflammation leads to subsequent loss of periodontal ligament, cementum and alveolar bone, the attachment apparatus of the tooth. Tissue destruction takes place in the perivascular extracellular gingival matrix. Here inflammation breaks down the collagen (Type I and III) and gingival proteoglycans. As inflammation spreads apically down the dental root surface, alveolar bone turnover shifts in favor of breakdown. In health, supporting alveolar bone is 1.5–2 mm apical to the cemento-enamel junction. In disease the distance is increased, the tooth is less supported and as a result more susceptible to abscess, trauma and ultimately tooth loss.

In the alveolar bone component, osteoclasts, triggered by mast cells, neutrophils, macrophages, lymphocytes and plasma cells, through inflammatory cytokine mediators such as IL-1, -6, -8, -10 and TNF-alpha are responsible for alveolar bone resorption. These same cytokines are implicated in mediating bone loss in both postmenopausal osteoporosis and periodontitis [68]. One important difference between alveolar bone loss through this mechanism versus skeletal bone loss through this mechanism is that in alveolar bone loss due to periodontitis, local inflammatory response to bacteria on dental surfaces, upregulates the cytokine mediators.

Osteocytic sclerostin expression has been linked to alveolar bone resorption during suppressed bone formation in rats with ligature-induced periodontitis. Kim et al. divided the rats into control and periodontitis groups. At 1, 3, 10 and 20 days after ligature, histologic an analysis of alveolar bone was performed and the numbers sclerostin-positive osteocytes were estimated, respectively. They noticed that sclerostin expression is increased when osteoid formation is suppressed. This may reinforce the hypothesis of the role of osteocytes as source of sclerostin during periodontitis-induced alveolar bone loss [69]. Clinical studies verified the results obtained from the animal studies regarding the involvement of sclerostin in alveolar bone loss associated with periodontitis. Sclerostin and sclerostin-RANKL ratio was found to be significantly lower in gingival crevicular fluid samples of healthy individuals than with patients with periodontitis [70].

The involvement of sclerostin in the inflammatory process associated with periodontitis and resulting in alveolar bone loss made many researchers to investigate the effect of the sclerostin antibody (Scl-Ab) on bone healing and the management of alveolar bone loss associating periodontitis. Animal trials showed that removal of SOST or blocking the expression of sclerostin reduces significantly bone loss associated with periodontitis in mouse models [71].

Due in part to these similarities between conditions, the concept of using same or similar pharmacotherapeutic intervention for both conditions is not new. The bisphosphonate family of medications, have been proposed as modulators of host bone loss resulting in pathologic amounts of bone loss. Farther upstream, at the macrophage level in the osteoclast activation cascade, parathyroid hormone is being explored to alter macrophage plasticity in tissues other than bone should be explored to treat bone loss in a locally delivered surgical periodontal treatment [72]. Similarly, NSAIDS and doxyclycline in sub anti-microbial doses, has been shown to modulate the host inflammatory response to down regulate collagen destruction [73,74].

The sclerostins fit this conceptual treatment model. Agents which inhibit sclerostins, such as anti-sclerostin antibodies show therapeutic outcomes such as increased bone formation, bone mass and density. Sclerostin inhibition using such neutralizing monoclonal antibodies have been proposed for postmenopausal osteoporosis and considered in preclinical models of osteogenesis imperfecta, rheumatoid arthritis and bone repair [75]. In the very same way, current findings show promise of sclerostins modulating oral bone related scenarios. Early animal studies show rats with a genetic sclerostin deficiency show increased jawbone growth. Additionally, in an experimental animal model sclerostin antibody administration reverses alveolar bone loss [76]. Furthermore, sclerostin immunolocalization has been demonstrated in periodontal tissues other than bone. Both cementocytes and periodontal ligament cultures show increasing sclerostin protein when adjacent tissues were exposed to cells genetically capable of producing sclerostins. As such both periodontal ligament cells and cementocytes show the potential participate in bone turnover when modulating osteocytes through sclerostin binding [77]. The critical question remains in what delivery system and in what dosages. More focused investigation into these approaches is to be expected.

4. Conclusions

Modulation of the alveolar bone has been discussed as the way of the future in dentistry. In periodontitis, alveolar bone loss can be countered using a pharmacotherapeutic if sclerostin therapy proves efficacious. This could be adjunctive to the conventional mechanical therapy involving the removal of pathologic biofilms accumulated on dental surfaces. In orthodontics, it can be used to influence tooth movement, either adjunctive to current treatment regimens using braces or aligners or plastic or metal retainers.

Regulating alveolar bone turnover is important in several dental disciplines. In periodontics, reducing this turnover is a strategic means to prevent and treat disease. In orthodontics, modulating turnover can increase tooth movement or decrease relapse. Pharmacologic intervention in modulating host response in dentistry fits within the conceptual framework in which other drugs such as bisphosphonates have been attempted but side effects limited the utilization. Skeletal bone and alveolar bone share some common bone turnover mechanisms. Sclerostin is a central intracellular signaling protein with the ultimate effect of inhibiting osteoblastic bone formation. Regulating sclerostin is a novel way to modulate alveolar bone. This is one more example of interprofessional collaboration. Dentistry can borrow from medicine to the benefit of its patients.

Author Contributions: Conceptualization, L.P.; Supervision, L.P.; Writing—Original draft, M.G.H.; Writing—Review & editing, A.R.Z. and J.M.P.

Funding: This research received no external funding.

References

1. Reddy, M.S.; Geurs, N.C.; Gunsolley, J.C. Periodontal host modulation with antiproteinase, anti-inflammatory, and bone-sparing agents: A systematic review. *Ann. Periodontol.* **2003**, *8*, 12–37. [CrossRef] [PubMed]
2. Goldhaber, P. Collagen and bone. *J. Am. Dent. Assoc.* **1964**, *68*, 825–832. [CrossRef] [PubMed]
3. Reinhardt, R.A.; Masada, M.P.; Payne, J.B.; Allison, A.C.; DuBois, L.M. Gingival fluid IL-1 beta and IL-6 levels in menopause. *J. Clin. Periodontol.* **1994**, *21*, 22–25. [CrossRef] [PubMed]
4. Bethesda. *National Institutes of Arthritis and Musculoskeletal Skin Diseases: Osteoporosis Research, Education, and Health Promotion*; US Department of Health and Human Services, NIH Publication: Washington, DC, USA, 1991; p. 37126.
5. Pacifici, R. Estrogen, cytokines, and pathogenesis of postmenopausal osteoporosis. *J. Bone Miner. Res.* **1996**, *11*, 1043–1051. [CrossRef] [PubMed]
6. Lipton, A. Bisphosphonate therapy in the oncology setting. *Expert Opin. Emerg. Drugs* **2003**, *8*, 469–488. [CrossRef] [PubMed]
7. Body, J.-J. Bisphosphonates for malignancy-related bone disease: Current status, future developments. Support. *Care Cancer* **2006**, *14*, 408–418. [CrossRef] [PubMed]
8. Ruggiero, S.L.; Mehrotra, B.; Rosenberg, T.J.; Engroff, S.L. Osteonecrosis of the jaws associated with the use of bisphosphonates: A review of 63 cases. *J. Oral. Maxillofac. Surg.* **2004**, *62*, 527–534. [CrossRef] [PubMed]
9. Bone, H.G.; Hosking, D.; Devogelaer, J.-P.; Tucci, J.R.; Emkey, R.D.; Tonino, R.P.; Rodriguez-Portales, J.A.; Downs, R.W.; Gupta, J.; Santora, A.C.; et al. Alendronate Phase III Osteoporosis Treatment Study Group. Ten years' experience with alendronate for osteoporosis in postmenopausal women. *N. Engl. J. Med.* **2004**, *350*, 1189–1199. [CrossRef] [PubMed]

10. Marx, R.E. Pamidronate (Aredia) and zoledronate (Zometa) induced avascular necrosis of the jaws: A growing epidemic. *J. Oral Maxillofac. Surg.* **2003**, *61*, 1115–1117. [CrossRef]

11. Black, D.M.; Schwartz, A.V.; Ensrud, K.E.; Cauley, J.A.; Levis, S.; Quandt, S.A.; Satterfield, S.; Wallace, R.B.; Bauer, D.C.; Palermo, L.; et al. FLEX Research Group. Effects of continuing or stopping alendronate after 5 years of treatment: The Fracture Intervention Trial Long-term Extension (FLEX): A randomized trial. *JAMA* **2006**, *296*, 2927–2938. [CrossRef] [PubMed]

12. Black, D.M.; Reid, I.R.; Boonen, S.; Bucci-Rechtweg, C.; Cauley, J.A.; Cosman, F.; Cummings, S.R.; Hue, T.F.; Lippuner, K.; Lakatos, P.; et al. The effect of 3 versus 6 years of zoledronic acid treatment of osteoporosis: A randomized extension to the HORIZON-Pivotal Fracture Trial (PFT). *J. Bone Miner. Res.* **2012**, *27*, 243–254. [CrossRef] [PubMed]

13. Adler, R.A.; El-Hajj Fuleihan, G.; Bauer, D.C.; Camacho, P.M.; Clarke, B.L.; Clines, G.A.; Compston, J.E.; Drake, M.T.; Edwards, B.J.; Favus, M.J.; et al. Managing osteoporosis in patients on long-term bisphosphonate treatment: Report of a task force of the American society for bone and mineral research. *J. Bone Miner. Res.* **2016**, *31*, 1910. [CrossRef] [PubMed]

14. Soileau, K.M. Oral post-surgical complications following the administration of bisphosphonates given for osteopenia related to malignancy. *J. Periodontol.* **2006**, *77*, 738–743. [CrossRef] [PubMed]

15. La, V.D.; Tanabe, S.; Bergeron, C.; Gafner, S.; Grenier, D. Modulation of matrix metalloproteinase and cytokine production by licorice isolates licoricidin and licorisoflavan A: Potential therapeutic approach for periodontitis. *J. Periodontol.* **2011**, *82*, 122–128. [CrossRef] [PubMed]

16. Jin, Q.; Cirelli, J.A.; Park, C.H.; Sugai, J.V.; Taba, M.; Kostenuik, P.J.; Giannobile, W.V. RANKL inhibition through osteoprotegerin blocks bone loss in experimental periodontitis. *J. Periodontol.* **2007**, *78*, 1300–1308. [CrossRef] [PubMed]

17. Bonewald, L.F. The amazing osteocyte. *J. Bone Miner. Res.* **2011**, *26*, 229–238. [CrossRef] [PubMed]

18. Bellido, T. Osteocyte-driven bone remodeling. *Calcif. Tissue Int.* **2014**, *94*, 25–34. [CrossRef] [PubMed]

19. Taylor, A.F.; Saunders, M.M.; Shingle, D.L.; Cimbala, J.M.; Zhou, Z.; Donahue, H.J. Mechanically stimulated osteocytes regulate osteoblastic activity via gap junctions. *Am. J. Physiol. Cell Physiol.* **2007**, *292*, C545–C552. [CrossRef] [PubMed]

20. Bonewald, L.F.; Johnson, M.L. Osteocytes, mechanosensing and Wnt signaling. *Bone* **2008**, *42*, 606–615. [CrossRef] [PubMed]

21. Van Bezooijen, R.L.; ten Dijke, P.; Papapoulos, S.E.; Löwik, C.W. SOST/sclerostin, an osteocyte-derived negative regulator of bone formation. *Cytokine Growth Factor Rev.* **2005**, *16*, 319–327. [CrossRef] [PubMed]

22. Van Bezooijen, R.L.; Svensson, J.P.; Eefting, D.; Visser, A.; van der Horst, G.; Karperien, M.; Quax, P.H.A.; Vrieling, H.; Papapoulos, S.E.; ten Dijke, P.; et al. Wnt but not BMP signaling is involved in the inhibitory action of sclerostin on BMP-stimulated bone formation. *J. Bone Miner. Res.* **2007**, *22*, 19–28. [CrossRef] [PubMed]

23. Honasoge, M.; Rao, A.D.; Rao, S.D. Sclerostin: Recent advances and clinical implications. *Curr. Opin. Endocrinol. Diabetes Obes.* **2014**, *21*, 437–446. [CrossRef] [PubMed]

24. Ten Dijke, P.; Krause, C.; de Gorter, D.J.J.; Löwik, C.W.; van Bezooijen, R.L. Osteocyte-derived sclerostin inhibits bone formation: Its role in bone morphogenetic protein and Wnt signaling. *J. Bone Joint Surg. Am.* **2008**, *90* (Suppl. 1), 31–35. [CrossRef] [PubMed]

25. Silverman, S.L. Sclerostin. *J. Osteoporos.* **2010**, *2010*, 941419. [CrossRef] [PubMed]

26. Mirza, F.S.; Padhi, I.D.; Raisz, L.G.; Lorenzo, J.A. Serum sclerostin levels negatively correlate with parathyroid hormone levels and free estrogen index in postmenopausal women. *J. Clin. Endocrinol. Metab.* **2010**, *95*, 1991–1997. [CrossRef] [PubMed]

27. Padhi, D.; Jang, G.; Stouch, B.; Fang, L.; Posvar, E. Single-dose, placebo-controlled, randomized study of AMG 785, a sclerostin monoclonal antibody. *J. Bone Miner. Res.* **2011**, *26*, 19–26. [CrossRef] [PubMed]

28. Ominsky, M.S.; Vlasseros, F.; Jolette, J.; Smith, S.Y.; Stouch, B.; Doellgast, G.; Gong, J.; Gao, Y.; Cao, J.; Graham, K.; et al. Two doses of sclerostin antibody in cynomolgus monkeys increases bone formation, bone mineral density, and bone strength. *J. Bone Miner. Res.* **2010**, *25*, 948–959. [CrossRef] [PubMed]

29. Tian, X.; Setterberg, R.B.; Li, X.; Paszty, C.; Ke, H.Z.; Jee, W.S.S. Treatment with a sclerostin antibody increases cancellous bone formation and bone mass regardless of marrow composition in adult female rats. *Bone* **2010**, *47*, 529–533. [CrossRef] [PubMed]

30. Ross, R.D.; Edwards, L.H.; Acerbo, A.S.; Ominsky, M.S.; Virdi, A.S.; Sena, K.; Miller, L.M.; Sumner, D.R. Bone matrix quality after sclerostin antibody treatment. *J. Bone Miner. Res.* **2014**, *29*, 1597–1607. [CrossRef] [PubMed]

31. Van Bezooijen, R.L.; Bronckers, A.L.; Gortzak, R.A.; Hogendoorn, P.C.W.; van der Wee-Pals, L.; Balemans, W.; Oostenbroek, H.J.; Van Hul, W.; Hamersma, H.; Dikkers, F.G.; et al. Sclerostin in mineralized matrices and van Buchem disease. *J. Dent. Res.* **2009**, *88*, 569–574. [CrossRef] [PubMed]

32. Galli, C.; Passeri, G.; Macaluso, G.M. Osteocytes and WNT: The mechanical control of bone formation. *J. Dent. Res.* **2010**, *89*, 331–343. [CrossRef] [PubMed]

33. Ominsky, M.S.; Li, C.; Li, X.; Tan, H.L.; Lee, E.; Barrero, M.; Asuncion, F.J.; Dwyer, D.; Han, C.-Y.; Vlasseros, F.; et al. Inhibition of sclerostin by monoclonal antibody enhances bone healing and improves bone density and strength of nonfractured bones. *J. Bone Miner. Res.* **2011**, *26*, 1012–1021. [CrossRef] [PubMed]

34. Baron, R.; Rawadi, G. Targeting the Wnt/beta-catenin pathway to regulate bone formation in the adult skeleton. *Endocrinology* **2007**, *148*, 2635–2643. [CrossRef] [PubMed]

35. Winkler, D.G.; Sutherland, M.K.; Geoghegan, J.C.; Yu, C.; Hayes, T.; Skonier, J.E.; Shpektor, D.; Jonas, M.; Kovacevich, B.R.; Staehling-Hampton, K.; et al. Osteocyte control of bone formation via sclerostin, a novel BMP antagonist. *EMBO J.* **2003**, *22*, 6267–6276. [CrossRef] [PubMed]

36. Devarajan-Ketha, H.; Craig, T.A.; Madden, B.J.; Robert Bergen, H.; Kumar, R. The sclerostin-bone protein interactome. *Biochem. Biophys. Res. Commun.* **2012**, *417*, 830–835. [CrossRef] [PubMed]

37. Poole, K.E.S.; van Bezooijen, R.L.; Loveridge, N.; Hamersma, H.; Papapoulos, S.E.; Löwik, C.W.; Reeve, J. Sclerostin is a delayed secreted product of osteocytes that inhibits bone formation. *FASEB J.* **2005**, *19*, 1842–1844. [CrossRef] [PubMed]

38. Robling, A.G.; Bellido, T.; Turner, C.H. Mechanical stimulation in vivo reduces osteocyte expression of sclerostin. *J. Musculoskelet. Neuronal Interact.* **2006**, *6*, 354. [PubMed]

39. Amrein, K.; Amrein, S.; Drexler, C.; Dimai, H.P.; Dobnig, H.; Pfeifer, K.; Tomaschitz, A.; Pieber, T.R.; Fahrleitner-Pammer, A. Sclerostin and its association with physical activity, age, gender, body composition, and bone mineral content in healthy adults. *J. Clin. Endocrinol. Metab.* **2012**, *97*, 148–154. [CrossRef] [PubMed]

40. Lin, C.; Jiang, X.; Dai, Z.; Guo, X.; Weng, T.; Wang, J.; Li, Y.; Feng, G.; Gao, X.; He, L. Sclerostin mediates bone response to mechanical unloading through antagonizing Wnt/beta-catenin signaling. *J. Bone Miner. Res.* **2009**, *24*, 1651–1661. [CrossRef] [PubMed]

41. Pelletier, S.; Dubourg, L.; Carlier, M.C.; Hadj-Aissa, A.; Fouque, D. The relation between renal function and serum sclerostin in adult patients with CKD. *Clin. J. Am. Soc. Nephrol.* **2013**, *8*, 819–823. [CrossRef] [PubMed]

42. Kanbay, M.; Siriopol, D.; Saglam, M.; Kurt, Y.G.; Gok, M.; Cetinkaya, H.; Karaman, M.; Unal, H.U.; Oguz, Y.; Sari, S.; et al. Serum sclerostin and adverse outcomes in nondialyzed chronic kidney disease patients. *J. Clin. Endocrinol. Metab.* **2014**, *99*, E1854–E1861. [CrossRef] [PubMed]

43. Huang, H.; Williams, R.C.; Kyrkanides, S. Accelerated orthodontic tooth movement: Molecular mechanisms. *Am. J. Orthod. Dentofac. Orthop.* **2014**, *146*, 620–632. [CrossRef] [PubMed]

44. Beersen, W. Remodelling of collagen fibers in the periodontal ligament and the supra-alveolar region. *Angle Orthod.* **1979**, *49*, 218–224.

45. Melsen, B. Tissue reaction to orthodontic tooth movement—A new paradigm. *Eur. J. Orthod.* **2001**, *23*, 671–681. [CrossRef] [PubMed]

46. Graber, L.W.; Vanarsdall, R.L.; Vig, K.W.L. *Orthodontics: Current Principles and Techniques*, 5th ed.; Elsevier/Mosby: Philadelphia, PA, USA, 2012.

47. Melsen, B. Biological reaction of alveolar bone to orthodontic tooth movement. *Angle Orthod.* **1999**, *69*, 151–158. [PubMed]

48. Nogueira, A.V.B.; de Molon, R.S.; Nokhbehsaim, M.; Deschner, J.; Cirelli, J.A. Contribution of biomechanical forces to inflammation-induced bone resorption. *J. Clin. Periodontol.* **2017**, *44*, 31–41. [CrossRef] [PubMed]

49. De Taddei, S.R.A.; Moura, A.P.; Andrade, I.; Garlet, G.P.; Garlet, T.P.; Teixeira, M.M.; da Silva, T.A. Experimental model of tooth movement in mice: A standardized protocol for studying bone remodeling under compression and tensile strains. *J. Biomech.* **2012**, *45*, 2729–2735. [CrossRef] [PubMed]

50. Smuthkochorn, S.; Palomo, J.M.; Hans, M.G.; Jones, C.S.; Palomo, L. Gingival crevicular fluid bone turnover biomarkers: How postmenopausal women respond to orthodontic activation. *Am. J. Orthod. Dentofac. Orthop.* **2017**, *152*, 33–37. [CrossRef] [PubMed]

51. Teixeira, C.C.; Khoo, E.; Tran, J.; Chartres, I.; Liu, Y.; Thant, L.M.; Khabensky, I.; Gart, L.P.; Cisneros, G.; Alikhani, M. Cytokine expression and accelerated tooth movement. *J. Dent. Res.* **2010**, *89*, 1135–1141. [CrossRef] [PubMed]

52. Kapoor, P.; Kharbanda, O.P.; Monga, N.; Miglani, R.; Kapila, S. Effect of orthodontic forces on cytokine and receptor levels in gingival crevicular fluid: A systematic review. *Prog. Orthod.* **2014**, *15*, 65. [CrossRef] [PubMed]

53. Alikhani, M.; Alyami, B.; Lee, I.S.; Almoammar, S.; Vongthongleur, T.; Alikhani, M.; Alansari, S.; Sangsuwon, C.; Chou, M.Y.; Khoo, E.; et al. Saturation of the biological response to orthodontic forces and its effect on the rate of tooth movement. *Orthod. Craniofac. Res.* **2015**, *18* (Suppl. 1), 8–17. [CrossRef] [PubMed]

54. Hazan-Molina, H.; Reznick, A.Z.; Kaufman, H.; Aizenbud, D. Periodontal cytokines profile under orthodontic force and extracorporeal shock wave stimuli in a rat model. *J. Periodont. Res.* **2015**, *50*, 389–396. [CrossRef] [PubMed]

55. Madureira, D.F.; de Taddei, S.A.; Abreu, M.H.; Pretti, H.; Lages, E.M.B.; da Silva, T.A. Kinetics of interleukin-6 and chemokine ligands 2 and 3 expression of periodontal tissues during orthodontic tooth movement. *Am. J. Orthod. Dentofac. Orthop.* **2012**, *142*, 494–500. [CrossRef] [PubMed]

56. Fox, S.W.; Fuller, K.; Bayley, K.E.; Lean, J.M.; Chambers, T.J. TGF-beta 1 and IFN-gamma direct macrophage activation by TNF-alpha to osteoclastic or cytocidal phenotype. *J. Immunol.* **2000**, *165*, 4957–4963. [CrossRef] [PubMed]

57. Kotake, S.; Udagawa, N.; Takahashi, N.; Matsuzaki, K.; Itoh, K.; Ishiyama, S.; Saito, S.; Inoue, K.; Kamatani, N.; Gillespie, M.T.; et al. IL-17 in synovial fluids from patients with rheumatoid arthritis is a potent stimulator of osteoclastogenesis. *J. Clin. Investig.* **1999**, *103*, 1345–1352. [CrossRef] [PubMed]

58. Gao, Y.; Morita, I.; Maruo, N.; Kubota, T.; Murota, S.; Aso, T. Expression of IL-6 receptor and GP130 in mouse bone marrow cells during osteoclast differentiation. *Bone* **1998**, *22*, 487–493. [CrossRef]

59. Alhashimi, N.; Frithiof, L.; Brudvik, P.; Bakhiet, M. Chemokines are upregulated during orthodontic tooth movement. *J. Interf. Cytokine Res.* **1999**, *19*, 1047–1052. [CrossRef] [PubMed]

60. Grant, M.; Wilson, J.; Rock, P.; Chapple, I. Induction of cytokines, MMP9, TIMPs, RANKL and OPG during orthodontic tooth movement. *Eur. J. Orthod.* **2013**, *35*, 644–651. [CrossRef] [PubMed]

61. Kitaura, H.; Kimura, K.; Ishida, M.; Sugisawa, H.; Kohara, H.; Yoshimatsu, M.; Takano-Yamamoto, T. Effect of cytokines on osteoclast formation and bone resorption during mechanical force loading of the periodontal membrane. *Sci. World J.* **2014**, *2014*, 617032. [CrossRef] [PubMed]

62. Yamaguchi, M. RANK/RANKL/OPG during orthodontic tooth movement. *Orthod. Craniofac. Res.* **2009**, *12*, 113–119. [CrossRef] [PubMed]

63. Henneman, S.; Von den Hoff, J.W.; Maltha, J.C. Mechanobiology of tooth movement. *Eur. J. Orthod.* **2008**, *30*, 299–306. [CrossRef] [PubMed]

64. Matsumoto, T.; Iimura, T.; Ogura, K.; Moriyama, K.; Yamaguchi, A. The role of osteocytes in bone resorption during orthodontic tooth movement. *J. Dent. Res.* **2013**, *92*, 340–345. [CrossRef] [PubMed]

65. Nishiyama, Y.; Matsumoto, T.; Lee, J.-W.; Saitou, T.; Imamura, T.; Moriyama, K.; Yamaguchi, A.; Iimura, T. Changes in the spatial distribution of sclerostin in the osteocytic lacuno-canalicular system in alveolar bone due to orthodontic forces, as detected on multimodal confocal fluorescence imaging analyses. *Arch. Oral Biol.* **2015**, *60*, 45–54. [CrossRef] [PubMed]

66. Eke, P.I.; Dye, B.A.; Wei, L.; Slade, G.D.; Thornton-Evans, G.O.; Borgnakke, W.S.; Taylor, G.W.; Page, R.C.; Beck, J.D.; Genco, R.J. Update on prevalence of periodontitis in adults in the United States: NHANES 2009 to 2012. *J. Periodontol.* **2015**, *86*, 611–622. [CrossRef] [PubMed]

67. Jeffcoat, M. The association between osteoporosis and oral bone loss. *J. Periodontol.* **2005**, *76*, 2125–2132. [CrossRef] [PubMed]

68. Kinney, J.S.; Ramseier, C.A.; Giannobile, W.V. Oral fluid-based biomarkers of alveolar bone loss in periodontitis. *Ann. N. Y. Acad. Sci.* **2007**, *1098*, 230–251. [CrossRef] [PubMed]

69. Kim, J.-H.; Lee, D.-E.; Cha, J.-H.; Bak, E.-J.; Yoo, Y.-J. Receptor activator of nuclear factor-κB ligand and sclerostin expression in osteocytes of alveolar bone in rats with ligature-induced periodontitis. *J. Periodontol.* **2014**, *85*, e370–e378. [CrossRef] [PubMed]

70. Balli, U.; Aydogdu, A.; Dede, F.O.; Turer, C.C.; Guven, B. Gingival crevicular fluid levels of sclerostin, osteoprotegerin, and receptor activator of nuclear factor-κB ligand in periodontitis. *J. Periodontol.* **2015**, *86*, 1396–1404. [CrossRef] [PubMed]

71. Ren, Y.; Han, X.; Ho, S.P.; Harris, S.E.; Cao, Z.; Economides, A.N.; Qin, C.; Ke, H.; Liu, M.; Feng, J.Q. Removal of SOST or blocking its product sclerostin rescues defects in the periodontitis mouse model. *FASEB J.* **2015**, *29*, 2702–2711. [CrossRef] [PubMed]

72. Bashutski, J.D.; Eber, R.M.; Kinney, J.S.; Benavides, E.; Maitra, S.; Braun, T.M.; Giannobile, W.V.; McCauley, L.K. Teriparatide and osseous regeneration in the oral cavity. *N. Engl. J. Med.* **2010**, *363*, 2396–2405. [CrossRef] [PubMed]

73. Preshaw, P.M. Host modulation therapy with anti-inflammatory agents. *Periodontology* **2018**, *76*, 131–149. [CrossRef] [PubMed]

74. Golub, L.M.; Elburki, M.S.; Walker, C.; Ryan, M.; Sorsa, T.; Tenenbaum, H.; Goldberg, M.; Wolff, M.; Gu, Y. Non-antibacterial tetracycline formulations: Host-modulators in the treatment of periodontitis and relevant systemic diseases. *Int. Dent. J.* **2016**, *66*, 127–135. [CrossRef] [PubMed]

75. Li, X.; Ominsky, M.S.; Warmington, K.S.; Morony, S.; Gong, J.; Cao, J.; Gao, Y.; Shalhoub, V.; Tipton, B.; Haldankar, R.; et al. Sclerostin antibody treatment increases bone formation, bone mass, and bone strength in a rat model of postmenopausal osteoporosis. *J. Bone Miner. Res.* **2009**, *24*, 578–588. [CrossRef] [PubMed]

76. Taut, A.D.; Jin, Q.; Chung, J.-H.; Galindo-Moreno, P.; Yi, E.S.; Sugai, J.V.; Ke, H.Z.; Liu, M.; Giannobile, W.V. Sclerostin antibody stimulates bone regeneration after experimental periodontitis. *J. Bone Miner. Res.* **2013**, *28*, 2347–2356. [CrossRef] [PubMed]

77. Jäger, A.; Götz, W.; Lossdörfer, S.; Rath-Deschner, B. Localization of SOST/sclerostin in cementocytes in vivo and in mineralizing periodontal ligament cells in vitro. *J. Periodont. Res.* **2010**, *45*, 246–254. [CrossRef] [PubMed]

Permissions

The contributors of this book come from diverse backgrounds, making this book a truly international effort. This book will bring forth new frontiers with its revolutionizing research information and detailed analysis of the nascent developments around the world.

We would like to thank all the contributing authors for lending their expertise to make the book truly unique.

They have played a crucial role in the development of this book. Without their invaluable contributions this book wouldn't have been possible. They have made vital efforts to compile up to date information on the varied aspects of this subject to make this book a valuable addition to the collection of many professionals and students.

This book was conceptualized with the vision of imparting up-to-date information and advanced data in this field. To ensure the same, a matchless editorial board was set up. Every individual on the board went through rigorous rounds of assessment to prove their worth. After which they invested a large part of their time researching and compiling the most relevant data for our readers.

The editorial board has been involved in producing this book since its inception. They have spent rigorous hours researching and exploring the diverse topics which have resulted in the successful publishing of this book. They have passed on their knowledge of decades through this book. To expedite this challenging task, the publisher supported the team at every step. A small team of assistant editors was also appointed to further simplify the editing procedure and attain best results for the readers.

Apart from the editorial board, the designing team has also invested a significant amount of their time in understanding the subject and creating the most relevant covers. They scrutinized every image to scout for the most suitable representation of the subject and create an appropriate cover for the book.

The publishing team has been an ardent support to the editorial, designing and production team. Their endless efforts to recruit the best for this project, has resulted in the accomplishment of this book. They are a veteran in the field of academics and their pool of knowledge is as vast as their experience in printing. Their expertise and guidance has proved useful at every step. Their uncompromising quality standards have made this book an exceptional effort. Their encouragement from time to time has been an inspiration for everyone.

The publisher and the editorial board hope that this book will prove to be a valuable piece of knowledge for researchers, students, practitioners and scholars across the globe.

List of Contributors

Marianne J. Middelveen
Atkins Veterinary Services, Calgary, AB T3B 4C9, Canada

Eva Sapi and Katherine R. Filush
Department of Biology and Environmental Science, University of New Haven, West Haven, CT 06516, USA

Jennie Burke
Australian Biologics, Sydney, NSW 2000, Australia

Agustin Franco
School of Health Sciences, Universidad Catolica Santiago de Guayaquil, Guayaquil 090615, Ecuador

Melissa C. Fesler and Raphael B. Stricker
Union Square Medical Associates, 450 Sutter Street, Suite 1504, San Francisco, CA 94108, USA

Tony Klouda
Freelance Consultant, 71A Lady Margaret Road, London NW5 2NN, UK

Cathy Green
Freelance Consultant, 28/4 Royal William Yard, Plymouth, Devon PL1 3GD, UK

Miniratu Soyoola and Paula Quigley
DAI Global Health, Waterside Centre, North Street, Lewes, East Sussex BN7 2PE, UK

Tendayi Kureya
Development Data, Lunzua Road, Off Addis Ababa, Rhodespark, Lusaka, Zambia

Caroline Barber
Transaid, 137 Euston Rd, Kings Cross, London NW1 2AA, UK

Kenneth Mubuyaeta
Disacare, Off Chilimbulu Road, behind Libala High School, Lusaka, Zambia

Janet L. Williams and Marc S. Williams
Genomic Medicine Institute, Geisinger, Danville, PA 17822, USA

Wendy K. Chung
Departments of Pediatrics and Medicine, Columbia University, New York, NY 10025, USA

Alex Fedotov
Irving Institute for Clinical and Translational Research, Columbia University, New York, NY 10025, USA

Krzysztof Kiryluk
Department of Medicine, Division of Nephrology, Columbia University, New York, NY 10025, USA

ChunhuaWeng
Department of Biomedical Informatics, Columbia University, New York, NY 10025, USA

John J. Connolly and Margaret Harr
Children's Hospital of Philadelphia, Philadelphia, PA 19104, USA

Hakon Hakonarson
Children's Hospital of Philadelphia, Philadelphia, PA 19104, USA
Perelman School of Medicine, University of Pennsylvania, Philadelphia, PA 19104, USA

Kathleen A. Leppig
Genetic Services, Kaiser Permanente of Washington, Seattle, WA 98101, USA

Eric B. Larson
Kaiser Permanente Washington Health Research Institute, Seattle, WA 98101, USA

Gail P. Jarvik
Departments of Medicine (Medical Genetics) and Genome Sciences, University of Washington, Seattle, WA 98195, USA

David L. Veenstra
Department Pharmacy, University of Washington, Seattle, WA 98195, USA

Christin Hoell and Maureen E. Smith
Center for Genetic Medicine, Northwestern University, Chicago, IL 60611, USA

Ingrid A. Holm
Division of Genetics and Genomics, Boston Children's Hospital, and Department of Pediatrics, Harvard Medical School, Boston, MA 02115, USA

Josh F. Peterson
Departments of Biomedical Informatics and Medicine, School of Medicine, Vanderbilt University, Nashville, TN 37232, USA

Robert M. Burkes, Takudzwa Mkorombindo, Udit Chaddha and Alok Bhatt
Department of Internal Medicine, University of Louisville, 550 S. Jackson Street, ACB 3rd Floor, Louisville, KY 40202, USA

Karim El-Kersh and Rodrigo Cavallazzi
Division of Pulmonary, Critical Care, and Sleep Medicine Disorders, Department of Internal Medicine, University of Louisville, 550 S. Jackson Street, Pulmonary, Critical Care and Sleep Disorders Medicine Offices, ACB 3rd Floor, Louisville, KY 40202, USA

Nancy Kubiak
Department of General Internal Medicine, University of Louisville, Palliative Care, and Medical Education, 550 S. Jackson Street, General Internal Medicine and Palliative Care Offices, ACB 3rd Floor, Louisville, KY 40202, USA

Sara Kintzle, Nicholas Barr, Gisele Corletto and Carl A. Castro
USC Suzanne Dworak-Peck School of Social Work, University of Southern California, 1150 S. Olive Street Suite 1406, Los Angeles, CA 90015, USA

Åsa Alftberg
Department of Social Work, Faculty of Health and Society, Malmö University, SE-205 06 Malmö, Sweden

Gerd Ahlström and Lina Behm
Department of Health Sciences, Faculty of Medicine, Lund University, SE-221 00 Lund, Sweden

Per Nilsen
Department of Medical and Health Sciences, Division of Community Medicine, Linköping University, SE-581 83 Linköping, Sweden

Anna Sandgren, Eva Benzein and Birgitta Wallerstedt
Center for Collaborative Palliative Care, Department of Health and Caring Sciences, Faculty of Health and Life Sciences, Linnaeus University, SE-351 95 Växjö, Sweden

Birgit H. Rasmussen
Department of Health Sciences, Faculty of Medicine, SE-221 00 Lund, Sweden
The Institute for Palliative Care, Region Skane and Lund University, Lund, Sweden

Cynthia Yeung and Adrian Baranchuk
Department of Medicine, Queen's University, Kingston, ON K7L 3N6, Canada

Lawrence V. Fulton and Matthew S. Brooks
Department of Health Administration, Texas State University, HPB 250, 601 University Drive, San Marcos, TX 78666, USA

Samira Behboudi-Gandevani and Saeideh Ziaei
Department of Midwifery and Reproductive Health, Medical Sciences Faculty, Tarbiat Modares University, 14115-111 Tehran, Iran

Anoshirvan Kazemnejad
Department of Biostatistics, Medical Sciences Faculty, Tarbiat Modares University, 14115-111 Tehran, Iran

Farideh Khalajabadi Farahani
National Population Studies and Comprehensive Management Institute, 1531635711 Tehran, Iran

Mojtaba Vaismoradi
Faculty of Nursing and Health Sciences, Nord University, 8049 Bodø, Norway

Amanda Roome
Department of Anthropology, Binghamton University, Binghamton, NY 13902, USA

Rita Spathis
School of Pharmacy and Pharmaceutical Sciences, Binghamton University, Binghamton, NY 13902, USA

Leah Hill
Quality Control, Regeneron Pharmaceuticals, Albany, NY 12144, USA

John M. Darcy
US Clinical Development and Medical Affairs in the Division of Immunology, Hepatology and Dermatology, Novartis, East Hanover, NJ 07936, USA

Ralph M. Garruto
Department of Anthropology, Binghamton University, Binghamton, NY 13902, USA
Department of Biological Sciences, Binghamton University, Binghamton, NY 13902, USA

Pia Andersen
Department of Research and Development, Region Kronoberg, 351 88 Växjö, Sweden
Division of Community Medicine, Department of Medical and Health Sciences, Linköping University, 581 83 Linköping, Sweden

Sara Holmberg
Department of Research and Development, Region Kronoberg, 351 88 Växjö, Sweden
Division of Occupational and Environmental Medicine, Institute of Laboratory Medicine, Lund University, 221 00 Lund, Sweden

Lena Lendahls
Department of Research and Development, Region Kronoberg, 351 88 Växjö, Sweden
Department of Health and Caring Sciences, Faculty of Health and Life Sciences, Linnaeus University, 391 82 Kalmar, Sweden

Per Nilsen and Margareta Kristenson
Division of Community Medicine, Department of Medical and Health Sciences, Linköping University, 581 83 Linköping, Sweden

Modhi Alshammari, Kelly A. Reynolds, Marc Verhougstraete and Mary Kay O'Rourke
Mel and Enid Zuckerman College of Public Health, Department of Community, Environment and Policy, University of Arizona, Tucson, AZ 85719, USA

Surender Rajasekaran and Anthony Olivero
Department of Pediatric Critical Care Medicine, Helen DeVos Children's Hospital, 100 Michigan Street NE, Grand Rapids, MI 49503, USA
Department of Pediatrics, Michigan State University College of Human Medicine, 15 Michigan Street NE, Grand Rapids, MI 49503, USA

Mark Pressler
Department of Pediatrics, Michigan State University College of Human Medicine, 15 Michigan Street NE, Grand Rapids, MI 49503, USA

Jessica L. Parker and Nicholas J. Andersen
Office of Research Administration, Spectrum Health, 100 Michigan Street NE, Grand Rapids, MI 49503, USA

Alex Scales
Department of Emergency Medicine, Helen DeVos Children's Hospital, 100 Michigan Street NE, Grand Rapids, MI 49503, USA

John R. Ballard
Design Solutions, Inc., 1266 Park Road, Chanhassen, MN 55317, USA

Robert McGough
Department of Electrical and Computer and Engineering, Michigan State University, 2120 Engineering Building, East Lansing, MI 48824, USA

Dorthe Varning Poulsen and Ulrika K. Stigsdotter
Department of Geosciences and Natural Resource Management, University of Copenhagen, Rolighedsvej 23, n1958 Frederiksberg C, Denmark

Annette Sofie Davidsen
The Research Unit for General Practice, University of Copenhagen, Øster Farimagsgade 5, 1014 København K, Denmark

Göran Holst
The Swedish Red Cross University College, SE-141 21 Stockholm, Sweden

Maria Johansson and Gerd Ahlström
Department of Health Sciences, Faculty of Medicine, Lund University, SE-221 00 Lund, Sweden

Preethi Balan, Mun Loke Wong and Chaminda Jayampath Seneviratne
Discipline of Oral Sciences, Faculty of Dentistry, National University of Singapore, Singapore 119083, Singapore

Hong-Gu He, Fengchunzhi Cao and Violeta Lopez
Alice Lee Centre for Nursing Studies, Yong Loo Lin School of Medicine, National University of Singapore, Singapore 117597, Singapore

Yap-Seng Chong
Singapore Institute for Clinical Sciences, Agency for Science, Technology and Research, Singapore 117549, Singapore
Department of Obstetrics and Gynaecology, Yong Loo Lin School of Medicine, National University of Singapore, Singapore 119074, Singapore

Shu-E. Soh
Singapore Institute for Clinical Sciences, Agency for Science, Technology and Research, Singapore 117549, Singapore
Department of Paediatrics, Yong Loo Lin School of Medicine, National University of Singapore, Singapore 119228, Singapore

Mohamed G. Hassan
Division of Craniofacial Anomalies, Department of Orofacial Sciences, University of California San Francisco, San Francisco, CA 94143, USA
Department of Orthodontics, Faculty of Dentistry, Alexandria University, Alexandria 21526, Egypt
Department of Orthodontics, Faculty of Oral and Dental Medicine, South Valley University, Qena 83523, Egypt

Abbas R. Zaher
Department of Orthodontics, Faculty of Dentistry, Alexandria University, Alexandria 21526, Egypt

Juan Martin Palomo
Department of Orthodontics, School of Dental Medicine, Case Western Reserve University, Cleveland, OH 44106-4905, USA

Leena Palomo
Department of Periodontics, School of Dental Medicine, Case Western Reserve University, Cleveland, OH 44106-4905, USA

Index

www.ingramcontent.com/pod-product-compliance
Lightning Source LLC
Chambersburg PA
CBHW080510200326
41458CB00012B/4153